Advances in Salivary Diagnostics

Charles F. Streckfus

Editor

Advances in Salivary Diagnostics

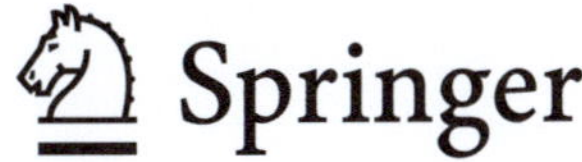 Springer

Editor
Charles F. Streckfus, DDS, MA, FAAOM, FAGD
Department of Diagnostic
and Biomedical
University of Texas School
of Dentistry at Houston
Houston, Texas
USA

ISBN 978-3-662-51335-4   ISBN 978-3-662-45399-5   (eBook)
DOI 10.1007/978-3-662-45399-5
Springer Heidelberg New York Dordrecht London

Preface

Too often we still think of saliva as being "just spit"; however, as outlined in the ensuing paragraphs below, saliva is a diverse medium with numerous applications to both medicine and dentistry. Interest in saliva as a diagnostic medium has advanced exponentially in the last three decades. The need for further research in the field of salivary diagnostics has been emphasized by agency-wide action plans emanating from the Office of the Surgeon General [1] and the National Institutes for Craniofacial and Dental Research [2].

The literature is replete with articles concerning human saliva. A PubMed.gov search using "human saliva" as the keywords revealed more than 35,710 articles since 1905, with 232 manuscripts focused on salivary diagnostics starting in the year 1971. As stated previously, the bulk of these publications have emerged in the last three decades. We are now using saliva to examine the state of the whole body, and this, in turn, opens doors to new frontiers that we cannot afford to miss.

In this book, we have compiled a knowledge base of the current state-of-the-art technology concerning salivary diagnostics. The book begins with an extensive description of the anatomy, histology, and physiology of the salivary glands and the basic constituents of their secretions. The following chapter describes the rich history of the evolution of salivary diagnostics from the ancient Egyptians to the present. The third chapter reflects the varied techniques and devices employed for the collection of saliva. Collectively, these three chapters provide the background necessary for the understanding of the technical chapters that ensue.

The next three chapters describe the encompassing field of "omics." These chapters describe advances in genomics, proteomics, and nanotechnology for assessing traumatic injuries. The final three chapters deal with salivary diagnostics for oral diseases, salivary gland tissue engineering, and future diagnostics, and finally a chapter illustrating how the salivary proteome may be used to study serious disease progression.

In summary, technology has moved beyond measuring just oral health and is now used to measure the overall health of the individual. Saliva, as stated by Dr. Irwin Mandel, may indeed be the "mirror" for the body as further specific and sensitive molecularly based assays are developed [3]. It is the collective dream of the authors of this book that it may be possible that the next dental visit could be the time that one gets a good overview of their oral health, but also their general health by using saliva as a diagnostic fluid.

Houston, TX   Charles F. Streckfus, DDS, MA, FAAOM, FAGD

References

1. US Department of Health and Human Services. Oral Health in America. A report of the surgeon general. Rockville: US Department of Health and Human Services, National Institute of Dental and Craniofacial Research, National Institutes of Health; 2000. p. 279–80.
2. National Institute of Dental and Craniofacial Research, National Institutes of Health. Workshop on development of new technologies for saliva and other oral fluid-based diagnostics. Virginia: Airlie House Conference Center; 1999. p. 12–4.
3. Mandel ID. A contemporary view of salivary research. Crit Rev Oral Biol Med. 1993;4:599.

Contents

Contributors

Francisco Manuel Lemos Amado, PhD Department of Chemistry, University of Aveiro, Aveiro, Portugal

Juliana A. Barros, DDS, MS Department of Restorative Dentistry and Prosthodontics, The University of Texas School of Dentistry at Houston, Houston, TX, USA

Lenora Bigler, PhD Department of Diagnostic and Biomedical Sciences, University of Texas School of Dentistry at Houston, Houston, TX, USA

Steven A. Bigler, MD Department of Pathology, Mississippi Baptist Medical Center, Jackson, MS, USA

Tiziana Cabras, PhD Dipartimento di Scienza della Vita e dell'Ambiente, Università degli Studi di Cagliari, Cagliari, Italy

Massimo Castagnola, PhD Istituto di Biochimica e di Biochimica Clinica, Università Cattolica, Roma, Italy

Shane V. Caswell, PhD, ATC Sports Medicine Assessment, Research and Testing Laboratory, George Mason University, Manassas, VA, USA

Nelson Cortes, PhD Sports Medicine Assessment, Research and Testing Laboratory, George Mason University, Manassas, VA, USA

Marta Alexandra Mendonça Nóbrega Cova, MSc Department of Chemistry, University of Aveiro, Aveiro, Portugal

Courtney Edwards, MD Department of Surgery, Lehigh Valley Health Network, Allentown, PA, USA

Mary C. Farach-Carson, PhD Department of Biochemistry, Cell Biology and Bioengineering, Rice University, Houston, TX, USA

Rita Maria Pinho Ferreira, PhD Department of Chemistry, University of Aveiro, Aveiro, Portugal

Cynthia Guajardo-Streckfus, BS Department of Pediatric Anesthesiology, Baylor College of Medicine, Texas Children's Hospital, Houston, TX, USA

Daniel A. Harrington, PhD Department of Biochemistry and Cell Biology, Rice University, Houston, TX, USA

Rafid Shahriyar Karim, BSc/MBBS – Year 5 Saliva Translational Research Group, The University of Queensland Diamantina Institute, The University of Queensland, Woolloongabba, QLD, Australia

Jennifer E. Kerr, PhD Department of Biology – Oral Microbiology, Notre Dame of Maryland University, Baltimore, MD, USA

Arutha Kulasinghe, BSC (Hons) Medical Microbiology Saliva Translational Research Group, The University of Queensland Diamantina Institute, The University of Queensland, Woolloongabba, QLD, Australia

Lance Liotta, MD, PhD Center for Applied Proteomics and Molecular Medicine, George Mason University, Manassas, VA, USA

Mariane Martinez, PhD candidate Department of Biochemistry and Cell Biology, Rice University, Houston, TX, USA

Irene Messana, PhD Department of Life and Environmental Sciences, University of Cagliari, Monserrato, Italy

Kelsey Mitchell, BS Sports Medicine Assessment, Research and Testing Laboratory, George Mason University, Manassas, VA, USA

Center for Applied Proteomics and Molecular Medicine, George Mason University, Manassas, VA, USA

Ezinne I. Ogbureke, BDS, DMD Department of General Dentistry and Dental Public Health, The University of Texas School of Dentistry at Houston, Houston, TX, USA

Kalu U. E. Ogbureke, BDS, MSc, DMSc, JD, FDSRCS, FDSRCPS, FDSRCSEd, FRCPath, FACD Department of Diagnostic and Biomedical Sciences, The University of Texas School of Dentistry at Houston, Houston, TX, USA

Shalizeh A. Patel, DDS Department of Restorative Dentistry and Prosthodontics, The University of Texas School of Dentistry at Houston, Houston, TX, USA

Emanuel F. Petricoin, PhD Center for Applied Proteomics and Molecular Medicine, George Mason University, Manassas, VA, USA

School of Systems Biology, George Mason University, Manassas, VA, USA

Swati Pradhan-Bhatt, PhD Department of Biological Sciences, University of Delaware, Newark, DE, USA

Center for Translational Cancer Research (CTCR), Helen F. Graham Cancer Center and Research Institute, Christiana Care Health Systems, Newark, DE, USA

Chamindie Punyadeera, PhD Saliva Translational Research Group, The University of Queensland Diamantina Institute, Woolloongabba, QLD, Australia

Paul Desmond Slowey, BSc (Hons), PhD Department of Corporate Management, Oasis Diagnostics® Corporation, Vancouver, WA, USA

Charles F. Streckfus, DDS, MA, FAAOM, FAGD Department of Diagnostic and Biomedical Sciences, University of Texas School of Dentistry at Houston, Houston, TX, USA

Department of Diagnostic and Biomedical Sciences, Baylor College of Medicine, UT School of Nursing, Houston, TX, USA

Gena D. Tribble, PhD Department of Periodontics, University of Texas Health Science Center, School of Dentistry, Houston, TX, USA

Rui Miguel Pinheiro Vitorino, PhD QOPNA, Mass Spectrometry Center, Department of Chemistry, University of Aveiro, Aveiro, Portugal

Danielle Wu, PhD Department of Biochemistry and Cell Biology, Rice University, Houston, TX, USA

Xi Zhang, BPharm, MBiotech Saliva Translational Research Group, The University of Queensland Diamantina Institute, The University of Queensland, Woolloongabba, QLD, Australia

Introduction

Shalizeh A. Patel and Juliana A. Barros

Abstract

Saliva, crucial to the function and protection of the oral cavity, has recently become also a "diagnostic fluid." Protein composition and function of saliva are altered during disease, allowing it to become a medium in detection of many systemic illnesses. Furthermore, its safe and noninvasive collection makes saliva an ideal specimen over blood. To appreciate the role of salivary proteomics in predicting disease, saliva's production, composition, and excretion in health must be understood. A summary of salivary gland anatomy, histology, saliva formation, and secretion is reviewed in this chapter.

General

Salivary glands are exocrine organs that are responsible for the production of saliva. This complex fluid has several important functions: (1) it lubricates the oral mucosa and the ingested food; (2) it protects and maintains the health of both soft and hard tissues in the oral cavity [1]. Salivary glands are classified by size, location, and histology. There are three major paired glands: parotid, submandibular, and sublingual, all responsible for approximately 90 % of the whole saliva production in the mouth (Fig. 1.1) [2]. Moreover, smaller glands, spread throughout the labial, lingual, palatal, buccal, glossopalatine, and retromolar surfaces of the mouth, secrete the other 10 % [3].

Whole saliva is mostly made of water (99.5 %) and other functional components such proteins, enzymes, electrolytes, and smaller organic molecules as described in Table 1.1 [4]. At least 40 proteins have been identified in salivary secretions, and most of these are identified in helping maintain the integrity of teeth against a constant barrage of physical, chemical, and microbial trauma. In addition to these proteins and lipids, salivary electrolytes and organic molecules like urea and glucose are also important elements of the oral defense system. The interaction among these components is essential in maintaining a balanced and healthy oral environment [5].

The protein-rich secretions of the salivary glands contain a milieu of antibacterial enzymes, immunoglobulins, lubricants, inorganic elements,

S.A. Patel, DDS (⊠) • J.A. Barros, DDS, MS
Department of Restorative Dentistry and Prosthodontics, The University of Texas School of Dentistry at Houston, Houston, TX, USA
e-mail: shalizeh.patel@uth.tmc.edu

C.F. Streckfus (ed.), *Advances in Salivary Diagnostics*,
DOI 10.1007/978-3-662-45399-5_1, © Springer-Verlag Berlin Heidelberg 2015

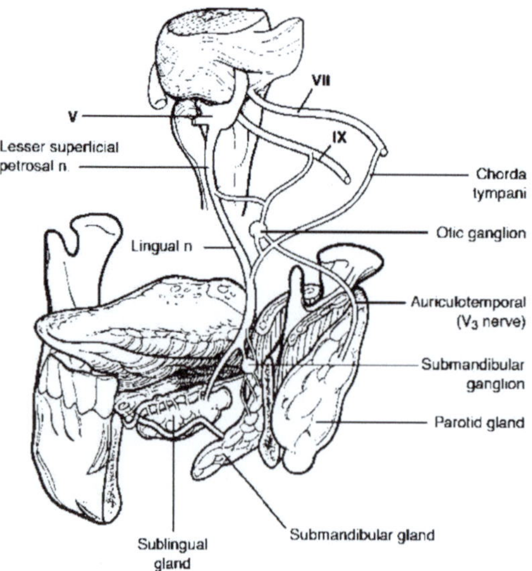

Fig. 1.1 The three major salivary glands (**a**) parotid gland, (**b**) submandibular gland, and (**c**) sublingual gland with their nerve innervation are highlighted (Reprinted with permission from Holsinger and Bui [2])

Table 1.1 The composition of saliva

Composition of saliva	

Proteins:
  Enzymes
  Glycoprotein
  Peptides
	Albumin; amylase; β(beta)-glucuronidase, carbohydrates; cystatins; epidermal growth factor; esterases; fibronectin; gustin; histatins; immunoglobulin A, G, and M; kallikrein; lactate dehydrogenase; lactoferrin; lipase; lysozyme; mucins; nerve growth factor; parotid aggregins; peptidases; phosphatases, proline-rich proteins; ribonucleases; salivary peroxidases; secretory component; secretory IgA; serum proteins; tyrosine-rich proteins; vitamin-binding proteins

Small organic molecules	Creatinine, glucose, lipids, nitrogen, sialic acid, urea, uric acid
Electrolytes	Ammonia, bicarbonate, calcium, chloride, fluoride, iodide, magnesium, phosphates, potassium, nonspecific buffers, sodium, sulfates, thiocyanate

Adapted from Fox et al. [4]

Table 1.2 The salivary components involved in the "protective" function of saliva

Function: protective	Salivary components involved
Lubrication	Water, mucins, proline-rich glycoproteins coat surfaces of oral mucosa, throat, and food
Antibacterial, antifungal, antiviral	Salivary proteins (e.g., lysozyme, lactoferrin, lactoperoxidase, mucins): histatins, cystatins, secretory IgA, proline-rich glycoproteins
Mucosal integrity	Mucins, electrolytes, water
Lavage, cleansing	Water
Buffering capacity	Bicarbonate and phosphate, proteins
Remineralization	Calcium, phosphate, proline-rich glycoproteins

Adapted from Fox et al. [4]

divided mainly into three major areas: (1) protective, (2) food related, and (3) communication/speech. The salivary components involved in the "protective" function of saliva are described in Table 1.2 [4].

Protective

Saliva protects and lubricates oral cavity. Mucins, produced mainly by the submandibular and sublingual secretory cells, are the lubricant component of saliva [6, 7]. Mucins control the permeability of mucosal surfaces, by creating a salivary film that is able to limit the penetration of various potential irritants and toxins in foods and beverages, as well as hazardous agents such as tobacco smoke. Furthermore, mucins, in combination with electrolytes and water, act as a natural "water proofing" agent that helps maintain the oral tissues in a hydrated state thus preserving its mucosal integrity. Saliva also contains antifungal and antiviral systems, such as secreting antibodies (secretory IgA), directly involved in neutralizing viruses [8]. Consequently, water, IgA, and proline provide a constant oral "cleansing" or "lavage" function. This physical flow of saliva continuously removes potentially harmful bacteria. Next, bicarbonate and phosphate ions

and incredibly high numbers of bacteria (10^8–10^9 bacteria per ml of saliva). That being said, saliva continues to be the tooth's first defense against cariogenic pathogens [5]. Salivary function can be

Table 1.3 The salivary components involved in the "food-related and communication" functions of saliva

	Salivary components involved
Function: food related	
Preparation for digestion	Water, mucins, proline-rich glycoproteins
Digestion	Amylase, ribonuclease, lipase
Mucosal integrity	Mucins, electrolytes, water
Taste	Water, gustin (zinc-binding salivary protein)
Function: communication	
Speech	Water, mucins

Adapted from Fox et al. [4]

and proteins assist in the achievement of oral homeostasis and the maintenance of a specific pH by buffering extreme oral acids and bases. Teeth are remineralized through the deposition of calcium, phosphorus, and statherin (a calcium-binding protein) [9].

Food-Related and Communication

Another important function of saliva is its contribution to the initial phase of digestion (Table 1.3) [4]. The salivary glands provide lubricatory molecules that coat food and the soft and hard tissues of the oral cavity. Lubrication allows food to travel easily through the digestive system and provides smooth tissue surfaces with minimal friction. Without lubrication, food becomes impacted around teeth, making eating difficult and unpleasant, and it also contributes to plaque formation. Saliva enhances taste and swallowing as well. The presence of saliva is critical in stimulating chemical sensations on taste buds [10]. During mastication, the salivary flow intensifies, which in turn stimulates taste receptors and augments the diffusion and chemical interaction between food particles and the associated taste buds. Saliva, as a result, is a fundamental factor in maintaining optimal nutritional status. Moreover, the lubrication from water and mucins assists in the ability to speak and makes verbal communicate possible [11].

Gross Anatomy of the Salivary Glands

The Parotid Gland

The parotid gland, the largest of the salivary glands, weighs approximately 15–30 g and is 6×4 cm in dimensions. The parotid gland is located bilaterally on each side of the face in front of the ears and extends to the lower borders of the mandible. Each gland is covered by fibrous connective tissue capsule that secretes serous fluid, a watery and protein-rich solution. The parotid gland is shaped like an inverted pyramid. It is positioned inferior to the zygomatic arch, anteroinferior to the external acoustic meatus, anterior to the mastoid process, and posterior to the ramus of the mandible (Fig. 1.2). The gland is divided into a base, an apex, and lateral, anterior, and posterior surfaces. Its laterosurface is situated right below the skin and superficial fascia of the head. The anterior surface of the gland is grooved by the ramus of the mandible and masseter muscle (from this depression the maxillary artery leaves the gland). The posterior surface is grooved by the mastoid process, the sternocleidomastoid muscle, and styloid process. From this site, the external carotid and the facial nerve enter the gland. The apex of the gland is located between the angle of the mandible and the sternocleidomastoid muscle. From this area, the retromandibular vein and the facial nerve leave the gland [12] (Fig. 1.2).

The parotid gland has a large duct (Stensen's duct) that crosses the masseter muscle and opens near the upper second molar in the oral cavity (Fig. 1.3). Blood supply is provided by the terminal branches of external carotid artery (ECA). The facial nerve and its branches form an important landmark, dividing the parotid into superficial and deep lobes. The main sensory nerve within this gland is the auriculotemporal nerve (Fig. 1.2). Secretomotor supply to the parotid is derived from the glossopharyngeal nerve (IX), via the tympanic branch, tympanic plexus, lesser petrosal nerve, and the pterygopalatine ganglion. The parotid contains superficial lymph nodes in its superior lobe. These nodes drain deeply to the

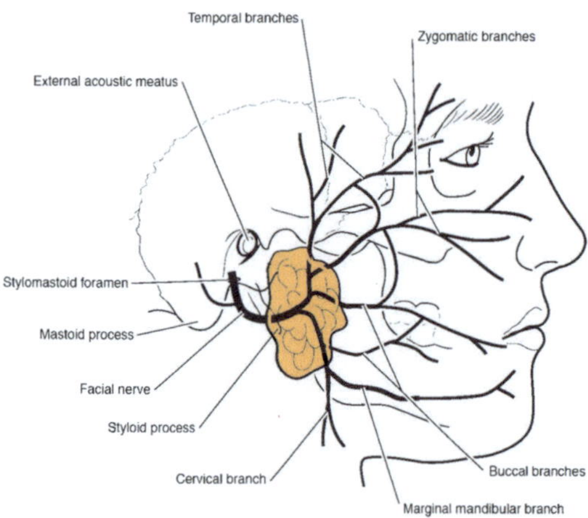

Fig. 1.2 Lateral view of the parotid gland and its nerve supply (Adapted with permission from Holsinger and Bui [2])

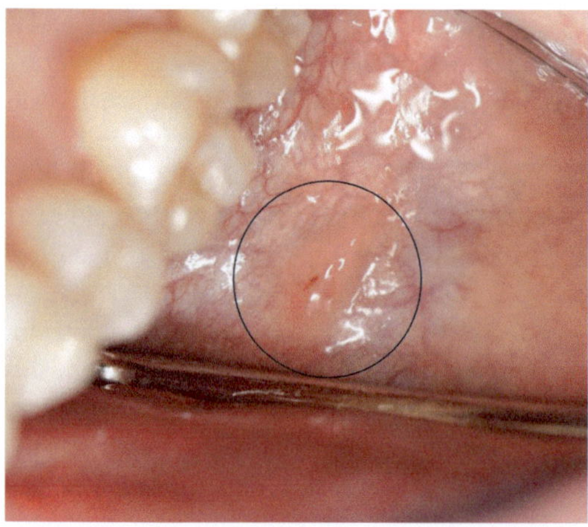

Fig. 1.3 The orifice of the Stensen's duct of the parotid gland located near the second maxillary molar

deep cervical nodes or superficially to the superficial cervical nodes [6].

The Submandibular Gland

The submandibular gland is approximately half of the weight (7–10 g) and size (4–5 cm) of the parotid gland. This gland is also encapsulated, but there is no fibrous connective tissue. The submandibular gland is located in the submandibular triangle formed by the anterior and posterior bellies of the digastric muscle and the inferior margin of the mandible

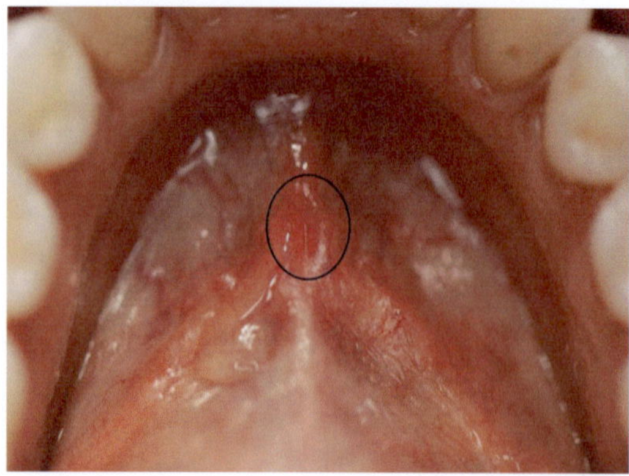

Fig. 1.4 The orifices of the Wharton's ducts are located on anterior part of the floor of the mouth

(Fig. 1.1b). The gland present three surfaces: lateral (connected to medial surface of the mandible), medial (connected to the mylohyoid, hyoglossus, and digastric muscles), and inferior (shielded by the skin and platysma muscle). The gland is divided into superficial and deep lobes, the latter being the majority part of the gland. The deep lobe projects from the mylohyoid and hyoglossus muscles. The submandibular duct, also referred to as Wharton's duct, exits from the deep part of the gland adjacent to the mandibular second molar and ascends anteriorly to the floor of the mouth (Fig. 1.4). As the duct exits the gland, it lies inferior to the lingual nerve. The blood supply originates from the facial and lingual artery and submental and facial veins. The innervation of this gland relies on submandibular ganglion and lingual nerve located superiorly to the deep process of the gland (Fig. 1.1) [2, 6, 12].

The Sublingual Gland

The sublingual gland is the smallest of the major salivary glands. It is almond shaped and is located underneath the mucous membrane of the floor of the mouth between the mandible and genioglossus muscle (Fig. 1.1c). The sublingual gland is not covered by a fascial capsule. This gland has approximately 8–20 small ducts (the ducts of

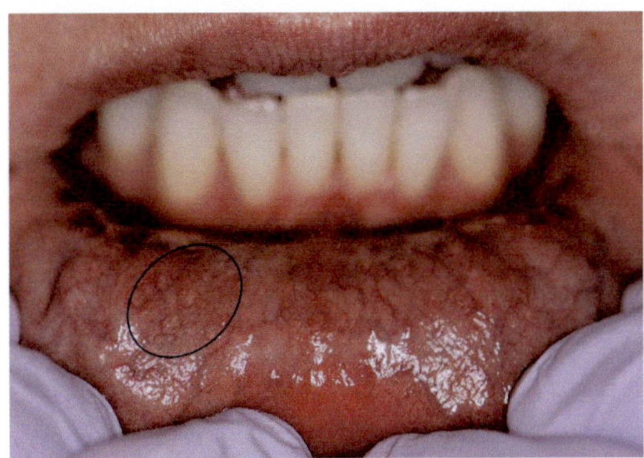

Fig. 1.5 The minor salivary glands within the *circle*

Rivinus), which exit the superior aspect of the gland and open along the sublingual fold on the floor of the mouth. Occasionally, several of these ducts may join to form a common duct (the duct of Bartholin), which typically empties into the Wharton's duct. The secretions from sublingual and submandibular glands flow through this duct and excrete into the floor of the mouth below the tongue. The sublingual and submental arteries are the main source of circulation in this salivary gland. The lingual, the chorda tympani, and the sympathetic nerves are responsible for its innervation (Fig. 1.1) [2, 6, 12].

Minor Salivary Glands

The minor salivary glands are widely distributed throughout the oral mucosa, palate, uvula, floor of the mouth, posterior tongue, retromolar and peritonsillar area, pharynx, larynx, and paranasal sinuses. There are hundreds (600–1,000) of these small glands ranging in size from 1 to 5 mm (Fig. 1.5). Unlike the major glands, the minor glands present a single duct that secretes directly into the oral cavity. These glands can secrete serous, mucous, or mixed saliva. Additionally, minor salivary glands may be found at the superior pole of the tonsils (Weber's glands) and at the base of the tongue (von Ebner's glands). Parasympathetic innervation is derived from the lingual nerve, except for the minor glands of the palate, which receive their parasympathetic fibers from the palatine nerves, fed by the sphenopalatine ganglion.

Histology of the Salivary Glands

The major salivary glands consist of a main excretory duct, which drains into the oral cavity on one side, and on the reverse side it branches into series of smaller ducts (progressively lesser in diameter) referred to as striated, intercalated, and finally into even tinier ones termed intercellular canaliculi [2, 6, 13]. These highly divided branches terminate into globular secretory end pieces known as acini (Fig. 1.6).

The end pieces may contain the two leading types of secretory cells: serous and mucous. Serous cells produce water and protein-rich content, whereas mucous cells produce mucin. This subcomponent of mucus is viscous; thus, it coats and protects mucosal surfaces. Salivary glands are supported by connective tissue, which house the nerve, vascular, and lymphatic supplies (Fig. 1.7). Parotid glands are mostly composed of serous cells, while the submandibular and sublingual glands are mixed glands of both serous and mucous cells (Figs. 1.7 and 1.8) [2, 6, 13].

Salivary Secretory End Pieces

In parotid glands, secretory end pieces present themselves as an encapsulated spherical structure with 8–12 of only serous cells (Fig. 1.9). Each of these cells is pyramidal in shape: the broad base is adjacent to the connective tissue called stroma, while its narrow apex faces the central lumen (Fig. 1.9). The submandibular gland has similar secretory end pieces; however, it contains both mucous- and serous-secreting cells (Fig. 1.10). Mucous cells form the main lining of these submandibular gland secretory acini, while a group of serous-secreting cells lie on the periphery and are referred to as serous demilune (Fig. 1.11) [5, 6].

Another group of cells, present in both parotid and submandibular secretory end pieces, are called myoepithelial cells (Fig. 1.12) [14]. These flat and stellate-shaped structures, with their copious branching extensions, are situated between the basal lamina and secretory cells and are linked to such cells via desmosomes (Fig. 1.13n). Myoepithelial cells are epithelial in

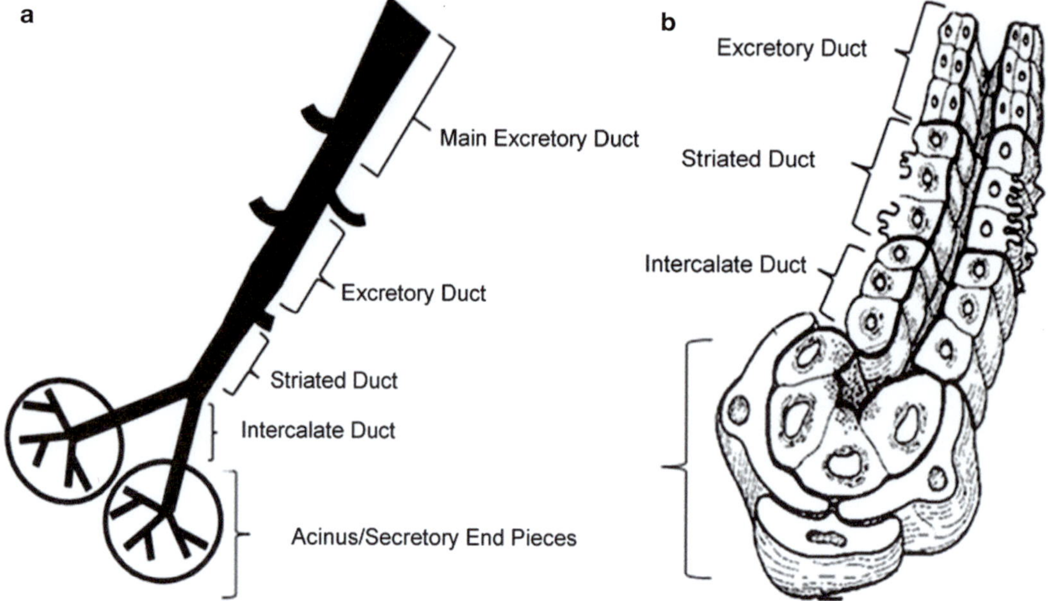

Fig. 1.6 (**a**) Ductal system of the salivary gland, (**b**) A cross-sectional view of different cells which make up the ductal system. The rough caricature illustrates the emergence of smaller ducts to larger ones and eventually to the main excretory duct which opens into the oral cavity (Adapted with permission from Holsinger and Bui [2])

Fig. 1.7 Parotid gland contains serous producing cells (*a*). Connective tissue septum separates each lobule (*b*). Intralobular ducts (*c*) transport primary saliva from secretory end pieces to the main excretory ducts and eventually to the oral cavity

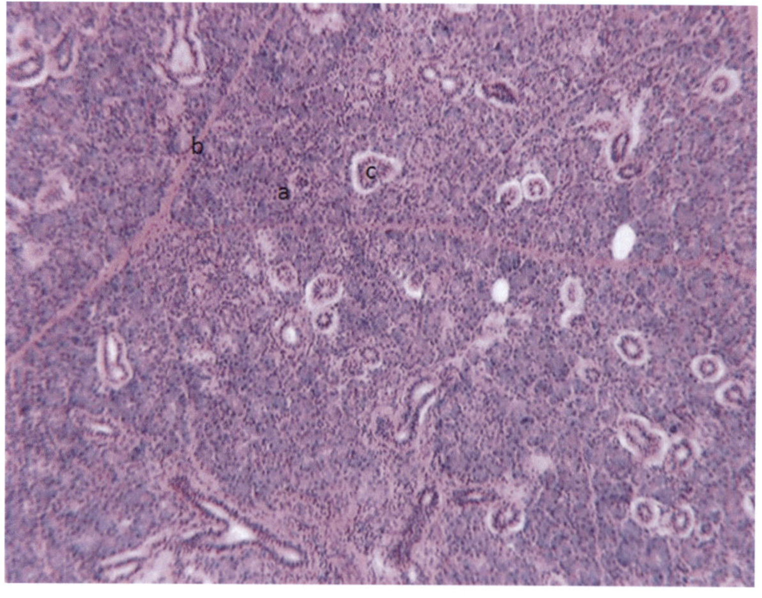

origin but have contractile functions. Their numerous extensions, filled with filaments of actin, outspread from the cell body to embrace secretory end pieces. In the presence of an appropriate stimulus, they contract and exert pressure on secretory cells, forcing them to push their content (primary saliva) from the lumen into the ductal system and eventually into the oral cavity. In addition to their role in secretory secretion, these cells help maintain cell polarity and structural

Fig. 1.8 Submandibular gland contains both serous- (*a*) and mucous (*b*)-secreting cells

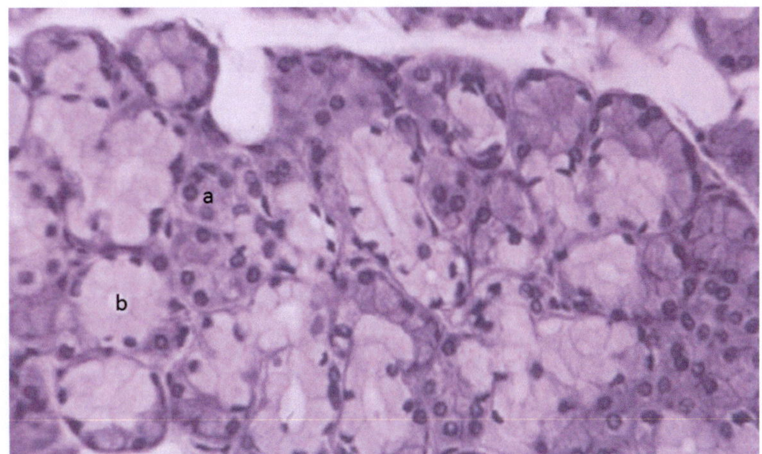

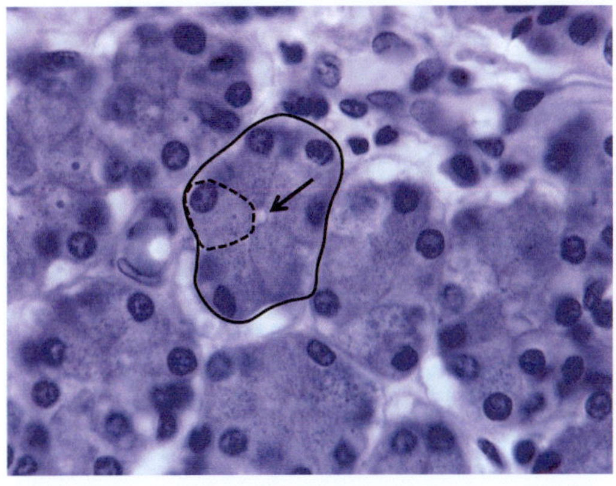

Fig. 1.9 Parotid secretory end pieces (*solid circle*) are globular structures with 8–12 serous cells and an associated lumen (*arrow*). The *dashed lines* highlight one serous cell

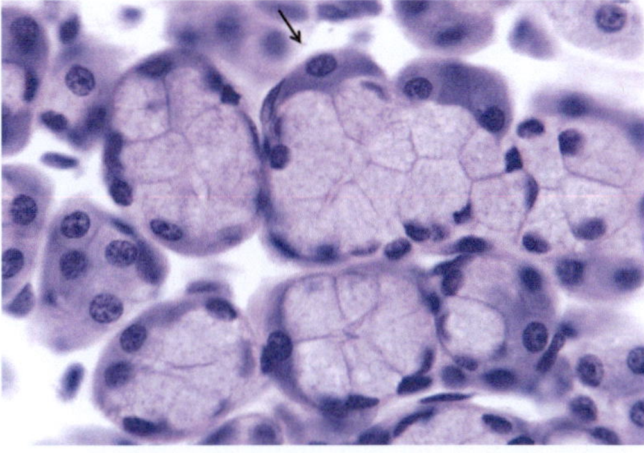

Fig. 1.11 Submandibular gland has both serous and mucous producing cells. The serous cells are located on the periphery of each acinus in a shape of a half-moon (*arrow*), referred to as serous semilune

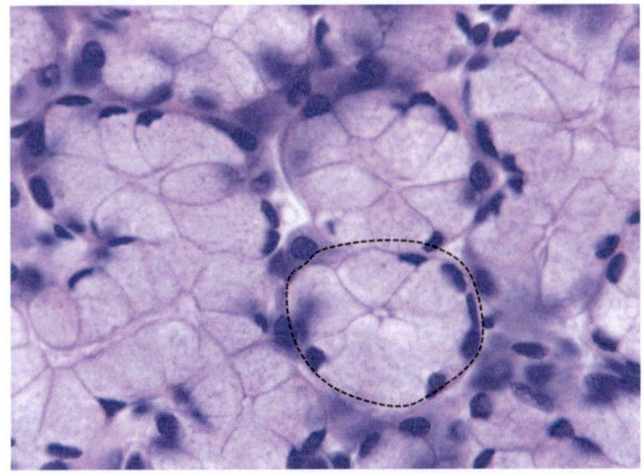

Fig. 1.10 Submandibular and sublingual glands' secretory end pieces are made of few mucous cells arranged in a spherical unit, called acinus (*dotted line*)

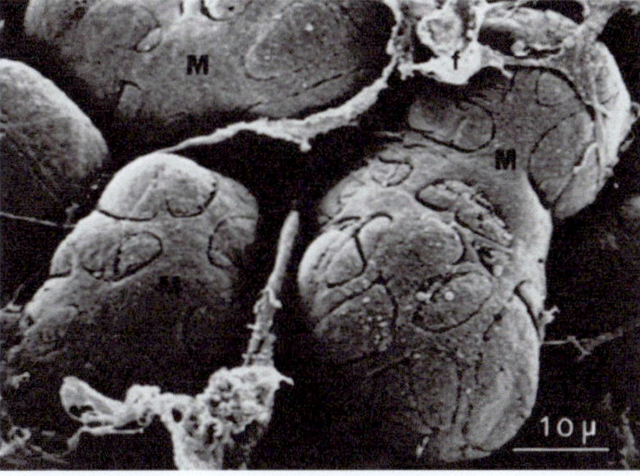

Fig. 1.12 The secretory end pieces of the sublingual gland. The myoepithelial cells (*M*) are characterized by their flattened cell body and their extensive cellular extensions (Reprinted with permission from Nagato et al. [14])

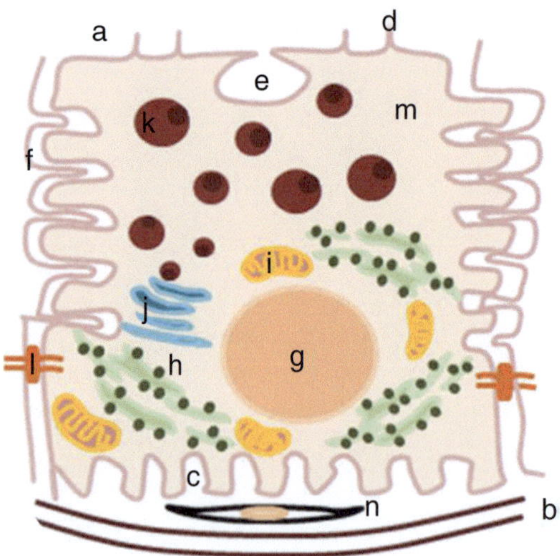

Fig. 1.13 A single serous cell illustration: (*a*) lumen, (*b*) basal lamina, (*c–f*) special infoldings, (*g–k*) essential organelles, (*l*) desmosomes, (*m*) cellular cytoplasm, (*n*) related myoepithelial cell (Adapted with permission from Nanci [6])

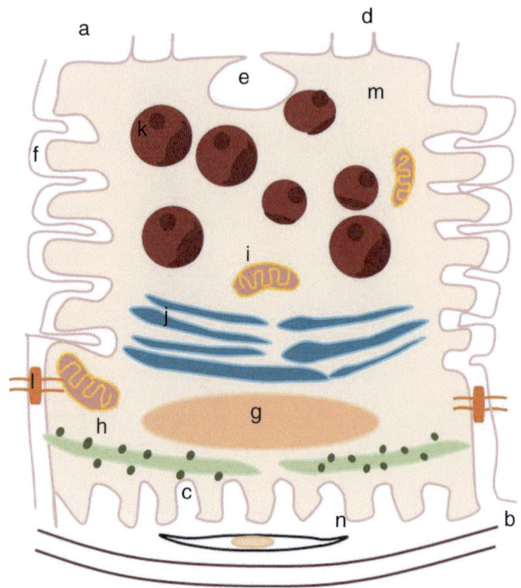

Fig. 1.14 A single mucous cell illustration: (*a*) lumen, (*b*) basal lamina, (*c–f*) special infoldings, (*g–k*) essential organelles, (*l*) desmosomes, (*m*) cellular cytoplasm, (*n*) related myoepithelial cell. Note that the large granules (*k*) push the major organelles toward the basal lamina (*b*) giving the illusion of the pressed nucleus around the edges of each cell (Adapted with permission from Nanci [6])

organization of the secretory end pieces by providing signaling pathways [6].

Serous Secretory Cells

Serous cells in both parotid and submandibular glands have a nucleus, numerous rough endoplasmic reticuli, a few mitochondria, and a large Golgi complex (Fig. 1.13g–j). A number of secretory granules (mature and immature), where the salivary macromolecular components are kept, can be seen in the apical cytoplasm (Fig. 1.13k). These granules in the parotid glands have a dense sphere embedded in a less dense matrix; on the other hand, these granules in the submandibular glands are multilayered with a matrix, a sphere, and a crescent piece (Fig. 1.14k). However, these spherical structures in both glands contain secretory products. The cell membrane at the base of the serous cell contains infoldings, apical membrane is comprised of intercellular canaliculi and a few rounded microvilli, and the lateral membranes have interdigitated folds. These all are membrane specialization traits involved in increasing cell's surface area (Fig. 1.13c–f). Serous cells are linked to their neighboring cells within an acinus by an array of structures grouped as intercellular junctions,

specifically termed as tight, adhering and gap junctions, and desmosomes (Fig. 1.13l). A tight junction controls the passage of water and certain ions in and from the lumen to the intercellular spaces. Adhering junctions and desmosomes mostly function to hold adjoining cells together. Gap junctions, joining the cytoplasm of adjacent cells, allow the passage of small molecules, such as ion metabolites and cyclic adenosine monophosphate between cells. Such cellular interchange regulates the activity of all the cells within an acinus, allowing this spherical complex to function as one unit [5, 6, 13].

Mucous Secretory Cells

Secretory end pieces that are composed of mucous cells are more tubular in shape. A large number of secretory vesicles, mainly containing mucus, are located in the apical cytoplasm and thus push the nucleus, Golgi complex (relatively large in size), and the endoplasmic reticuli to the basal portion of the cell (Figs. 1.10 and 1.14). Like serous cell, intercellular junctions join

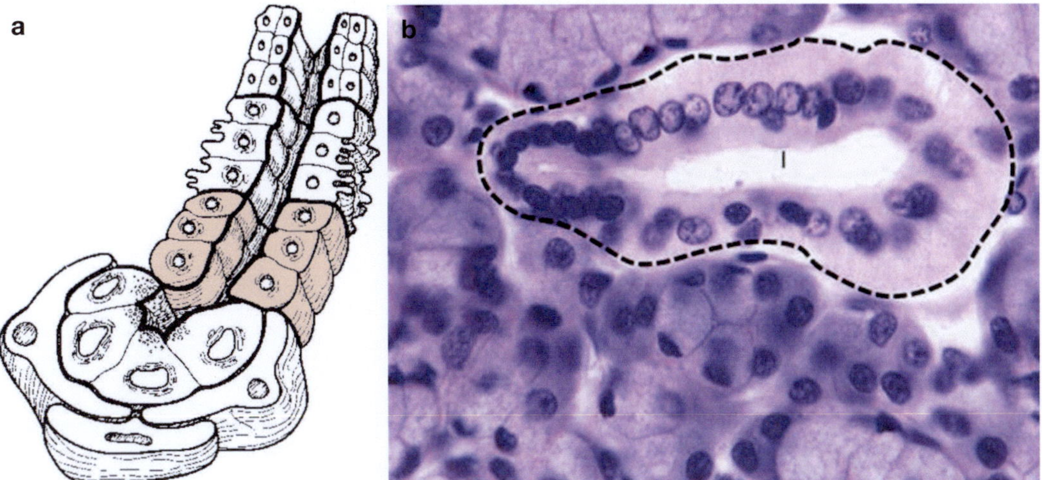

Fig. 1.15 (**a**) A drawing of salivary ductal system highlighting the intercalated duct cells (Reprinted with permission from: Holsinger and Bui [2]); (**b**) Cross-sectional histology of an intercalated duct (*dotted lines*), with its cuboidal epithelial cells and lumen (*l*) where the modification of primary saliva is initiated

adjacent mucous cells and allow communication between neighboring cells [5, 6, 13].

Salivary Ductal System

Intercalated Ducts

Saliva from the lumen of the secretory end pieces are transferred into intercalated ducts (Fig. 1.15). The first cells of these ducts are directly adjacent to the secretory cells of the end pieces, and their lumens are continuous. These ducts are usually longer in the parotid than in the submandibular glands and contribute greatly to the formation of organic content of human saliva. They are made of simple cuboidal epithelium accompanied with myoepithelial cells on their basal membrane. These duct cells have few cellular organelles such as a nucleus, some rough endoplasmic reticulum, a small Golgi complex, and some secretory granules. Few microvilli on the apical surface do project into the lumen, while junctional complexes such as desmosomes, gap junctions, and folded processes are involved in connecting these duct cells together. The intercalated ducts add macromolecular components, such as lysozyme and lactoferrin, into saliva. Undifferentiated salivary gland stem cells are also thought to exist in these ducts, which can proliferate and differentiate to replace damaged or dying cells in both the secretory end pieces and striated ducts [6].

Striated Ducts

More in the submandibular than the parotid glands, these intercalated duct cells merge to form striated ducts thus constituting the largest portion of the ductal system (Fig. 1.16). Striated ducts are mainly located within the lobules of the gland, consequently referred to as intralobular ducts. This striation appearance at the base of these duct cells is formed by rows of mitochondria alternating with highly folded plasma membranes. This complex ductal anatomy enables these cells to participate in modifying the primary saliva by reabsorbing electrolytes, largely sodium, to formulate its hypotonic nature. Desmosomes and hemidesmosomes are used to join these cells to the basal lamina, and the lateral borders are pleated to allow them to fit together with adjacent cells like a jigsaw puzzle [5, 6, 13].

Excretory Ducts

Striated ducts line to form excretory ducts—also referred to as interlobular ducts simply due to their location (between the lobules of the gland). These ducts are comprised of stratified and pseudostratified columnar epithelium with numerous mitochondria (Fig. 1.17). These cells are connected to

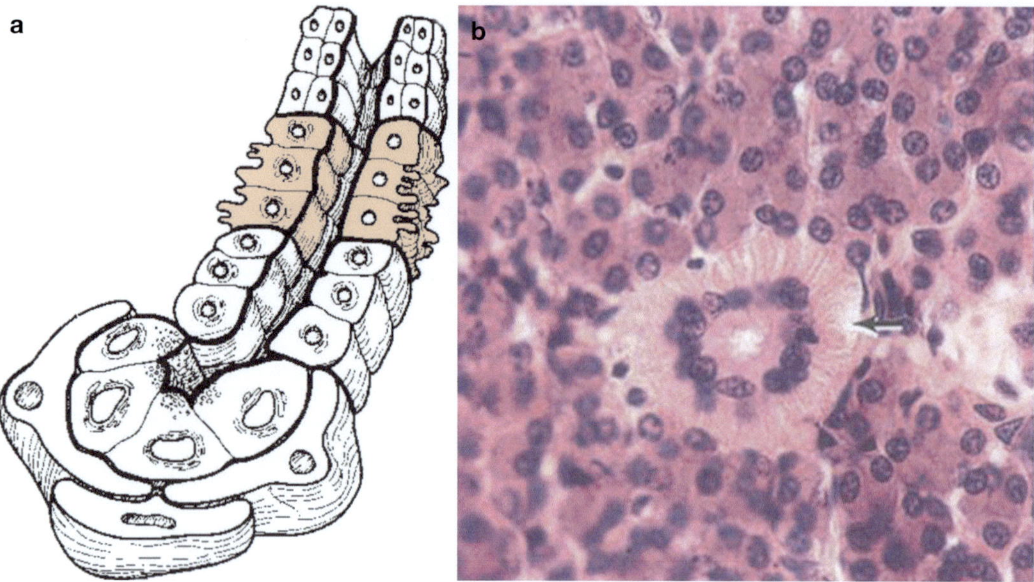

Fig. 1.16 (**a**) A drawing of salivary ductal system highlighting the striated duct cells (Reprinted with permission from Holsinger and Bui [2]); (**b**) Cross-sectional histology of striated ducts of the salivary gland ductal system. *Arrow* points to the striation characteristics of these cells mainly formed by rows of mitochondria and highly folded plasma membrane

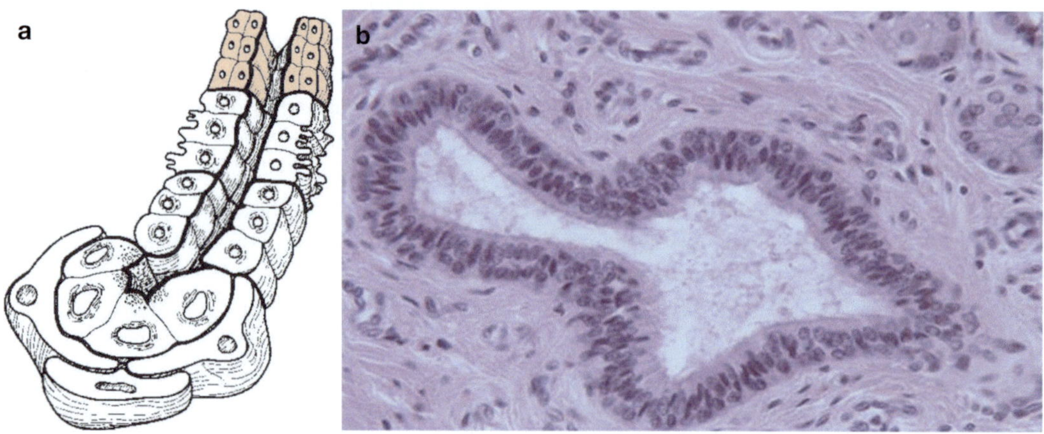

Fig. 1.17 (**a**) A drawing of salivary ductal system highlighting the excretory duct cells (Reprinted with permission from Holsinger and Bui [2]); (**b**) Cross-sectional histology of excretory ducts of the salivary gland ductal system

the associated basal lamina by hemidesmosomes. Goblet cells—columnar epithelial cells that secrete mucin—may be found in the excretory ducts of parotid glands, but not in the submandibular ones. These ducts take part in the resorption of electrolytes from the saliva.

Main Excretory Ducts

Excretory ducts merge to form the main excretory duct, which exits the gland and drains saliva into the mouth. This duct is called the Stensen's duct in the parotid and the Wharton's duct in the submandibular gland (Figs. 1.3 and 1.4). The

Stensen's duct opens into the mouth opposite the upper second molar, whereas the Wharton's duct opens at the apex of the sublingual papilla lateral to the lingual frenulum. Stensen's duct is lined by pseudostratified epithelium and occasional goblet cells with a layer of underlying smooth muscular cells. Wharton's duct has also pseudostratified epithelium, but unlike the Stensen's, it includes a number of mitochondria, lysosomes, smooth endoplasmic reticuli, and small vesicles [5, 6, 13].

Nerve Supply

Postganglionic nerve fibers of both parasympathetic and sympathetic divisions of the autonomic nervous system innervate the salivary glands and increase both protein secretion and volume flow (Fig. 1.1). Preganglionic parasympathetic fibers originate in the superior or inferior salivary nuclei in the brainstem and travel via the facial nerve (VII) to innervate sublingual and submandibular glands and by glossopharyngeal nerve (IX) to innervate parotid glands. Direct sympathetic innervation takes place via preganglionic nerves in the thoracic segments (T1–T3), which synapse in the superior cervical ganglion with the postganglionic neurons. Indirectly, the sympathetic nervous system innervates the blood vessels that supply the glands. The main parasympathetic neurotransmitter is acetylcholine where norepinephrine is the key sympathetic transmitter.

Blood Supply

External carotid artery enters the salivary glands and branches into smaller arteries and arterioles that tend to follow the path of the excretory ducts. These arterioles fragment into capillaries and surround the secretory end pieces and eventually connect with a venous portal system, which follows the arterial supply. The endothelium of these capillaries (both arterial and venous) is fenestrated, and its pressure increases during salivary secretion (Fig. 1.18).

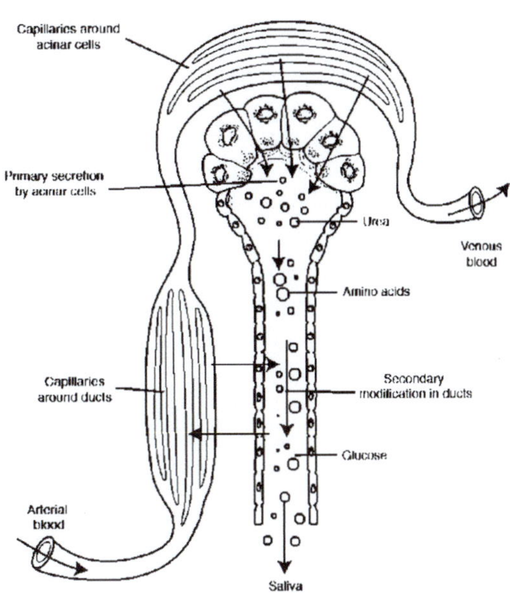

Fig. 1.18 Blood supply system involved in the salivary gland system (Reprinted with permission from Holsinger and Bui [2])

Salivary Secretion

Whole saliva is a mixed fluid of 99 % water and 1 % electrolytes and protein in the mouth. A healthy adult produces a range of 1.0–1.5 l of whole saliva per day: 20 % from parotid, 60 % from submandibular, and 7–8 % from sublingual glands. However, smaller glands in the labial, palatine, buccal, lingual, and sublingual submucosa can contribute to the remaining 10 % of the overall salivary output. When stimulated, the parotid gland drastically increases its contribution to 50 % of the total salivary secretion [3].

In the presence of an appropriate stimulus, such as mastication or gustation, mechanoreceptors in the periodontal ligament or chemoreceptors in the taste buds (afferent sensory) transmit signals via trigeminal nerve to the salivary nuclei in the brainstem. This activates the parasympathetic and sympathetic postganglionic efferent autonomic nervous system leading to glandular stimulation and thus a change in salivary production. In general, parasympathetic stimulation increases flow rate, whereas sympathetic pathway increases salivary proteins yet decreases its flow level. In addition to afferent stimuli, salivary nuclei can receive impulses from higher centers in the brain. Consequently, a surge of neurotransmitters either inhibit or stimulate preganglionic efferent signals, influencing salivary yield. Upon stimulation, neurotransmitters or neuropeptides bind to specific receptors and ultimately trigger a number of ion transport pathways in the cell membrane of salivary ductal tissues. As a result, acinar serous and mucous cells produce primary saliva, while the ductal system modifies it before its secretion into the mouth. This salivary production and modification system is referred to as the two-step model in salivary biology [5].

Two-Step Salivary Secretion Model

Part 1: Acinar Cell Secretion

At unstimulated state (rest), acinar cells have a high concentration (above electrochemical equilibrium) of potassium (K^+) and chloride (Cl^-). This is due to the coordinated ion exchange activities of both Na^+/ K^+ adenosine triphosphatase (ATPase) and Na^+/K^+/$2Cl^-$ contransporter complex, accordingly (Fig. 1.19).

Upon stimulation, neurotransmitters such as acetylcholine bind to receptor-specific sites on the acinar cell membrane activating a cascade of reactions. Ion channels, such as Ca^{2+}-activated K^+ and apical Cl^- channels, play an important role in K^+ and Cl^- passage from the acinar cytoplasm to the interstitium and lumen, respectively. Simultaneously, Cl^- uptake is also regulated by a second mechanism through Cl^-/HCO_3^- (bicarbonate) and Na^+/H^+ exchangers. The increase of the luminal concentration of Cl^- triggers the transport of sodium (Na^+) through the tight junctions to establish cellular neutrality. Subsequently, osmotic pressure moves water into the lumen through specific water channels, aquaporin 5 (Aqp5), located in the apical membrane of acinar cell, forming an isotonic solution, with similar electrolyte composition as the plasma, also known as the primary saliva (Fig. 1.20) [15, 16].

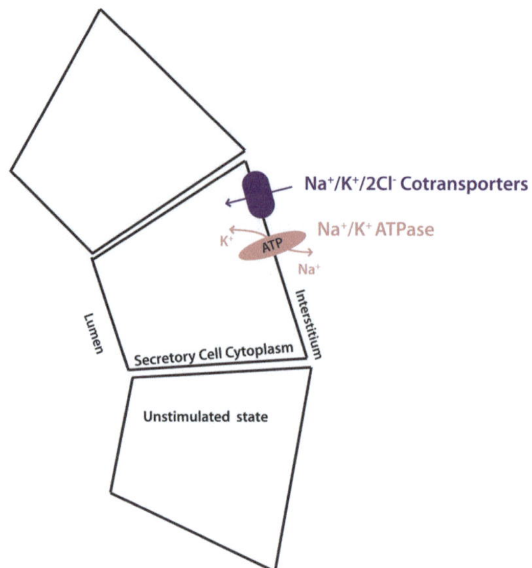

Fig. 1.19 Acinar cell secretion at a rested state with high cytoplasmic concentration of potassium

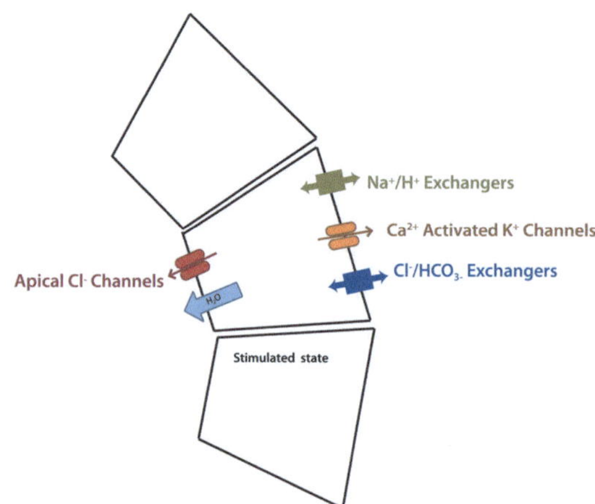

Fig. 1.20 Acinar cell secretion at a stimulated state leading to primary saliva formation

Part 2: Ductal Cell Secretion

As primary saliva travels through the ductal system, more neural impulses stimulate specific receptors on the ductal cell surfaces triggering Na^+, K^+ ATPase mechanism. This signaling cascade initiates reabsorption of Na^+ and Cl^- in the ductal cell membranes followed by K^+ and HCO_3^- discharge. Epithelial Na^+ channels, expressed in the apical membrane of salivary ducts, play an essential part

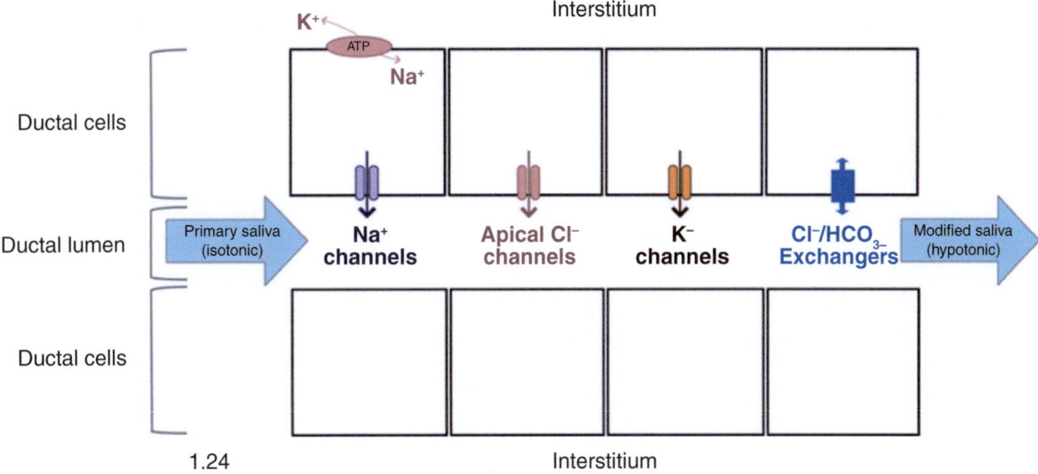

Fig. 1.21 Ductal cell secretion at a stimulated state where primary saliva is modified

in the ductal Na$^+$ resorption [17]. Apical Cl$^-$ channels and Cl$^-$/ HCO$_3^-$ exchangers are also hypothesized to be involved in the active resorption of Cl$^-$ in salivary gland ducts [18]. On the other hand, K$^+$ is added to the saliva in transit via K$^+$ channels. This exchange of ions modifies the primary isotonic saliva to a more hypotonic fluid when unstimulated. The concentration of these salivary electrolytes is subjected to the flow rate: when stimulated, the Na$^+$ and Cl$^-$ uptake decrease due to limited absorption time, thus making the saliva less hypotonic. Furthermore, HCO$_3^-$ concentration will increase creating a more alkaline and buffered saliva during stimulation (Fig. 1.21) [15, 16].

Saliva Proteins

In addition to regulating the ion and water contents of saliva, acinar cells play an important role in producing and secreting salivary proteins. Secretory proteins are synthesized by ribosomes, a dense structure attached on the endoplasmic reticulum in the acinar cell. Saliva is transferred to the lumen of the endoplasmic reticulum, where it is modified depending on function (disulfide bonds and N- and O-linked glycosylation are formed) and is next translocated into Golgi complex. They are further

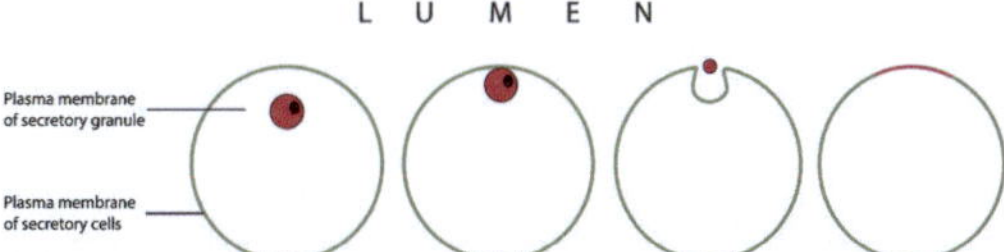

Fig. 1.22 The process of releasing the content of secretory granules into the lumen is called exocytosis

altered, condensed, and packed into secretory granules. These granules are stored in apical cytoplasm of secretory cells waiting to be released. This process of releasing the content of these granules is termed exocytosis (Fig. 1.22). This involves the fusion of the granule membrane with lumen plasma membrane of the secretory cells followed by the rupture of the fused membranes. Exocytosis is mainly controlled by the autonomic nervous system: sympathetic stimulation triggers protein release from parotid and submandibular gland secretory cells, whereas parasympathetic stimulation causes such release from parotid and sublingual glands acini [16].

Parotid and Submandibular Glands Secretion

Different glands may produce different proteins as each protein may have a specific function (Table 1.4). Serous acinar cells in parotid and

Table 1.4 Salivary proteins and their functions as they relate to saliva

Composition and properties of saliva			
Component	Glands	Cell type	Function
Serous glycoproteins	Parotid and submandibular	Acinar cell	Prevent plaque formation
Proline-rich protein (PRP)			Ca^{2+} binding
			Antimicrobial
			Lubrication
Mucous glycoproteins	Submandibular and sublingual	Acinar cell	Antimicrobial
Mucins (MUC5B, MUC7)			Lubrication
			Protease protective
Digestive enzymes	Parotid and submandibular	Acinar cell	Starch breakdown
α(alpha)-amylase			
Calcium-binding protein	Parotid and submandibular	Acinar cell	Maintain tooth integrity
Statherin			Inhibit Ca^{2+} and P precipitation
Proline-rich protein (PRP)			Modulate bacterial binding
Antimicrobial proteins and peptides	Parotid and submandibular		
Lysozyme		Duct cell	Antimicrobial
Lactoferrin		Acinar cell	Antimicrobial and anti-inflammatory
Salivary peroxidase (SP) and myeloperoxidase (MP)			Antimicrobial, decomposition of H_2O_2
Cystatins		Acinar cell	Antiviral, protease inhibitors
Histatins		Acinar cell	Antifungal, antibacterial
Agglutinins	Parotid		Aggregate bacteria
Glycoprotein gp340			

Adapted from Pfaffe et al. [26]

submandibular glands are involved in producing proline-rich proteins (PRP), digestive enzymes, calcium-binding proteins, and antimicrobial proteins and peptides. PRPs contain less than 50 % carbohydrates; thus, they are referred to as glycoproteins. They have an important role in lubricating and protecting the oral cavity. In addition, these proteins have antimicrobial effects (may cause bacterial apoptosis by inhibiting metabolic functions and cell adherence) along with the ability to bind to Ca^{2+} to prevent plaque and calculus formation. Most of the digestive enzymes produced by these glands, such as α(alpha)-amylase, are responsible in breaking starch into simpler carbohydrates, glucose, and essentially act as the body's first line of protective system in processing the incoming food. The calcium-binding proteins (statherin and PRPs) are the other subgroups of proteins secreted by salivary parotid and submandibular glands. Statherin and PRPs can modulate bacterial binding to the tooth surfaces by inhibiting or postponing calcium phosphate salts precipitation, consequently reducing the cariogenic activity of microorganisms of the oral flora [19]. Antimicrobial proteins can either be secreted by glandular or ductal cells as described in Table 1.4. Lysozymes, a ductal-secreting protein, can compromise the integrity of bacterial cell walls, thus leading to its breakdown in the presence of hypotonic saliva [20]. Lactoferrin can directly or indirectly play a role in bactericidal activities in the mouth [21]. As an iron-binding protein, it removes iron, an essential element required for bacterial survival and growth. Secondly, it agglutinates bacterial cells and prevents their adherence to the host cells. Moreover, it potentially can synergize the effects of lysozymes and immunoglobulins in killing bacteria [22]. Cystatin, another multifunctional antimicrobial protein found in saliva, targets not only bacteria (by inhibiting bacterial proteases), but it also has antiviral capabilities [23]. Histatin, a peptide present in whole saliva, regulates oral inflammation by inhibiting the release of histamine secreted by surrounding mast cells. More importantly, these peptides have antifungal properties, another testament in saliva's ability to defend and protect the host [24].

Parotid Gland Secretion

Agglutinin is a glycoprotein secreted only by the parotid gland that reduces bacterial adherence in the oral cavity by agglomerating them into a mass and facilitating their removal [25].

Submandibular and Sublingual Glands Secretion

Submandibular and sublingual glands are involved in generating mucous glycoproteins referred to as mucin. This carbohydrate-rich protein (more than 64 %) is hydrophilic and assists in lubricating the oral cavity. In addition, its viscous composition allows bacterial aggregation and its removal leading to a more balance and infection-free environment [23].

Conclusion

With its complex anatomy, histology and function, it is no surprise that saliva, this basic yet rich fluid, is our bodies' first defense against external and internal harmful microorganisms and daily routine. Its presence allows one to enjoy unassuming functions such as tasting, digesting, and swallowing food. Its constant cleansing and buffering capabilities decrease cariogenic activities of oral bacteria and maintain the health of dentition. In a diseased state, where the output of saliva is affected (xerostomia or dry mouth), the oral cavity is put at a greater risk for infection. Furthermore, activities such as speaking, eating, tasting, and swallowing become challenging and sometimes unbearable. Thus to understand xerostomia, its side effect and potential cure, one must fully grasp how this intricate gland is structured and functions at health [25].

Acknowledgments The authors would like to thank the following colleagues:

Dr. Streckfus for his continuous mentorship

Dr. Barry Rittman for his gracious support of this chapter by providing all the histology pictures

Dedication

Shalizeh A. Patel

To my parents: *for all the sacrifices they've made for me*

To my husband: *for loving me unconditionally*

To my daughters: *for making life so beautiful*

Juliana A. Barros

To my Dad for encouraging and supporting my dreams

To my husband and kids for making life meaningful

References

1. Etzel K. Role of salivary glands in nutrition. In: Dobrosielski-Vergona K, editor. Biology of the salivary glands. Boca Raton: CRC Press, Inc; 1993. p. 129–52.
2. Holsinger CF, Bui DT. Anatomy, function, and evaluation of the salivary glands. In: Myers EN, Ferris RL, editors. Salivary gland disorders. Berlin/Heidelberg: Springer; 2007. p. 1–16.
3. Edgar WM. Saliva and dental health: clinical implications of saliva: report of a consensus meeting. Br Dent J. 1990;169(3–4):96–8.
4. Fox PC, van der Ven PF, Sonies BC, Weiffenbach JM, Baum BJ. Xerostomia: evaluation of a symptom with increasing significance. JADA. 1985;110:519–25.
5. Bardow A, Lagerlof F, Nauntofte B, Tenovuo J. The role of saliva. In: Fejerskov O, Kidd E, editors. Dental caries: the disease and its clinical management. 2nd ed. Singapore: Wiley; 2008. p. 190–207.
6. Nanci A. Salivary glands. In: Ten Cate's oral histology. 8th ed. Nanci A, Development, structure, and function. St. Louis: Elsevier; 2013. p. 253–77.
7. Roth G, Calmes R. Salivary glands and saliva. In: Oral biology. Eds. Roth G and Calmes R, St Louis: CV Mosby; 1981. p. 196–236.
8. McNabb PC, Tomasi TB. Host defense mechanisms at mucosal surfaces. Annu Rev Microbiol. 1981;35: 477–96.
9. Dowd FJ. Saliva and dental caries. Dent Clin North Am. 1999;43:579–97.
10. Matsuo R. Role of saliva in the maintenance of taste sensitivity. Crit Rev Oral Biol Med. 2000;11(2): 216–29.

11. Tabak LA, Levine MJ, Mandel ID, Ellison SA. Role of salivary mucins in the protection of the oral cavity. J Oral Pathol. 1982;11:1–17.
12. Saracco CG, Crabill EV. Anatomy of the human salivary glands. In: Dobrosielski-Vergona K, editor. Biology of the salivary glands. Boca Raton: CRC Press, Inc; 1993. p. 1–14.
13. Sreebny LM. Dry mouth and salivary gland hypofunction, part I: diagnosis. Compendium. 1988;9(7): 569–70. 573–4, 576 passim.
14. Nagato T, Yoshida H, Yoshida A, Uehara Y. A scanning electron microscope study of myoepithelial cells in exocrine glands. Cell Tissue Res. 1980;209(1): 1–10.
15. Nauntofte B. Regulation of electrolyte and fluid secretion in salivary acinar cells. Am J Physiol. 1992; 263(6):823–37.
16. Turner RJ, Sugiya H. Understanding salivary fluid and protein secretion. Oral Dis. 2002;8(1):3–11.
17. Catalán MA, Nakamoto T, Melvin JE. The salivary gland fluid secretion mechanism. J Med Invest. 2009;56(Suppl):192–6.
18. Petersen OH. Calcium-activated potassium channels and fluid secretion by exocrine glands. Am J Physiol. 1986;25:G1–13.
19. Hay DI, Smith DJ, Schluckebier SK, Moreno EC. Relationship between concentration of human salivary statherin and inhibition of calcium phosphate precipitation in stimulated human parotid saliva. J Dent Res. 1984;63(6):857–63.
20. García-Godoy F, Hicks MJ. Maintaining the integrity of the enamel surface. The role of dental biofilm, saliva and preventive agents in enamel demineralization and remineralization. JADA. 2008;139(2): 25S–34.
21. Fine DH, Furgang D, Beydouin F. Lactoferrin iron levels are reduced in saliva of patients with localized aggressive periodontitis. J Periodontol. 2002;73(6): 624–30.
22. Valenti P, Berlutti F, Conte MP, Longhi C, Seganti L. Lactoferrin functions: current status and perspectives. J Clin Gastroenterol. 2004;38(6):S127–9.
23. Walz A, Stühler K, Wattenberg A, Hawranke E, Meyer HE, Schmalz G, et al. Proteome analysis of glandular parotid and submandibular-sublingual saliva in comparison to whole human saliva by two-dimensional gel electrophoresis. Proteomics. 2006; 6(5):1631–9.
24. Yao Y, Berg EA, Costello CE, Troxler RF, Oppenheim FG. Identification of protein components in human acquired enamel pellicle and whole saliva using novel proteomics approaches. J Biol Chem. 2003;278(7): 5300–8. 14.
25. Malamud D, Abrams WR, Barber CA, Weissman D, Rehtanz M, Golub E. Antiviral activities in human saliva. Adv Dent Res. 2011;23(1):34–7.
26. Pfaffe T, Cooper-White J, Beyerlein P, Kostner K, Punyadeera C. Diagnostic potential of saliva: current state and future applications. Clin Chem. 2011;57(5): 675–87.

The History of Salivary Diagnostics

2

Kalu U.E. Ogbureke and Ezinne I. Ogbureke

Abstract

Within the last two-and-a-half decades, the area of salivary diagnostics continues to record significant and substantial activities on the radars of biomedical research and clinical diagnostics. Along with chronicling the highlight moments in the development and subsequent emergence of the field of salivary diagnostics to date, this chapter will discuss the concept of biomarkers and provide an overview of the advantages and disadvantages of saliva and serum as diagnostic media. Finally, the section on the *Legal Issues Related to Salivary Diagnostics* will provide ample speculations on potential legal scrutiny, pitfalls, and other legal tests anticipated along the path of development of salivary diagnostics.

The History of Salivary Diagnostics

The history of using saliva as an indicator of what is taking place within the human body dates back centuries. It is said that in ancient China that an individual's inability or perceived difficulty in swallowing a mouthful of dry rice was indicative of "guilt." The "Rice Test," as it consequently came to be known, was based on the notion that an accused's inability to form a bolus of dry rice results from anxiety and presumably guilt, which inhibited the saliva production necessary for the formation of a food bolus and swallowing [1–6]. Significantly, there are reports indicating that the parotid saliva flow rate appears to be dependent upon certain personality factors such as anxiety level, conscientiousness, shrewdness, and introversion [4, 7]. Thus, the pathophysiology of this folktale phenomenon is apparent from an age-long concept that an acutely innate feeling of guilt (as in an individual not telling the truth about a serious matter) has as one of its cardinal physical signs a manifestation of nervousness, often underscored by reduced saliva production and dry mouth. Heralding the twentieth century as the "modern age" of salivary diagnostics, conditions such as gout and rheumatism were subjects of cytochemical procedures, using saliva

K.U.E. Ogbureke, BDS, MSc, DMSc, JD, FDSRCS, FDSRCPS, FDSRCSEd, FRCPath, FACD (✉)
Department of Diagnostic and Biomedical Sciences, The University of Texas School of Dentistry at Houston, Houston, TX, USA
e-mail: Kalu.Ogbureke@uth.tmc.edu

E.I. Ogbureke, BDS, DMD
Department of General Dentistry and Dental Public Health, The University of Texas School of Dentistry at Houston, Houston, TX, USA

C.F. Streckfus (ed.), *Advances in Salivary Diagnostics*,
DOI 10.1007/978-3-662-45399-5_2, © Springer-Verlag Berlin Heidelberg 2015

samples to identify biomarkers and to better understand both disease processes [6].

Early attempts to use saliva for diagnostic purposes presumed the presence of specific biomarkers already known to be present in serum to also be present in saliva. Granted that this presumption appeared, and is now known, to be largely accurate, accounting for how biomarkers made their way into saliva remained confounding. Furthermore, limitations posed by the available technical methods of saliva collections, coupled with a lack of standardized parameters for collection and storage, sometimes translated into considerable difficulty with detection of low-level markers at the time [8–10]. The passage of time, of course, has seen our enhanced understanding of the salivary physiology, the standardization of salivary sample collection, and the development of more sensitive detection technologies such as enzyme-linked immunosorbent assay (ELISA) and quantitative reverse transcriptase-polymerase chain reaction (qRT-PCR) [10, 11].

The evolution of salivary diagnostics within the past two decades heralds a dynamic field now being incorporated as part of disease diagnosis, clinical monitoring, and important clinical decision-making for patient management and overall care. During this time span, notable advances in basic and translational sciences employing the "science of saliva" have been recorded [12–14]. Efforts along this path have been propelled by research investments by the National Institute of Dental Research (NIDCR) of the National Institutes of Health (NIH), Bethesda, Maryland, primarily directed at identifying and subsequently cataloging the human salivary proteome [12, 15–17].

The NIDCR-funded efforts in 2002 and 2006—dubbed "Development and Validation Technologies for Saliva Based Diagnostics"— mobilized collaborative research teams comprising engineers with skills in nanotechnology and microfluidic techniques and oral biology researchers [18]. This collaborative composite was charged with developing portable point-of-care (POC) diagnostic tools for the rapid detection and analysis of salivary biomarkers using advanced techniques [12, 18]. The teams comprised scientists from the University of California in Los Angeles (UCLA, led by Dr. David Wong) with focus on the detection of oral cancer, Tufts University (led by Dr. David Walt) with focus on the monitoring chronic obstructive pulmonary disease (COPD) and cystic fibrosis, Rice University (led by Dr. John McDevitt) to develop biomarkers for acute myocardial infarction, and New York University (led by Dr. Daniel Malamud) to develop a multiplexed test for human immunodeficiency virus (HIV), tuberculosis, and malaria [19–22]. As anticipated, outcomes of studies supported by these investments are translating to the development of POC technologies and clinical tests anticipated to increasingly benefit patients [12, 18–22].

One of the significant areas of projected benefits of salivary science is in clinical diagnosis of oral and systemic diseases. Although notable and inspiring gains have been made within the timeframe, these have, at best, helped to keep the field and the subject matter in research focus but still fall short of the threshold and indices justifying application in the definitive diagnosis of any specific human disease [12, 18]. Thus, to date, no salivary test is firmly established as a diagnostic criterion for any oral or systemic disease [12, 18]. The US Food and Drug Administration (FDA)-approved OraQuick ADVANCE Rapid HIV-1/2 Antibody Test (OraSure Technologies, Bethlehem, PA), for example, is not employed as a diagnostic test for HIV infection but as a *screening* tool for the presence of HIV-1 antibodies in saliva. Thus, a positive OraQuick ADVANCE Rapid HIV-1/2 Antibody Test suggests the *possibility* of HIV-1 infection short of a definitive proof (diagnosis) [12, 18]. In all cases therefore, western blot techniques (OraSure HIV-1 Western Blot, OraSure Technologies) are required to *confirm* the diagnosis of HIV-1. Similarly, there now are available salivary tests, such as the MyPerioPath (OralDNA Labs, Brentwood, Tenn.) that "confirm" the presence of infection [12].

Evolution of the Saliva "Omics"

We are familiar with the "omics" concepts that have so rapidly filtered into our biological science lexicon within the last two decades. They include "genomics," "proteomics," "epigenomics," "metabolomics," and "transcriptomics," defined as the "study of related sets of biologic molecules" [12, 18]. The emergence of "salivaomics," coined as recently as 2008, heralded the rapid development of knowledge about the various "omics" constituents of saliva [12, 15]. Since then, several subsets of salivaomics—"salivary proteome," "transcriptome," "microRNA" (miRNA), "metabolome," and "microbiome"—have expanded its scope [12, 19–22]. The salivary metabolome represents a complete set of small molecular metabolites in saliva sample and includes biochemical intermediates of carbohydrate, lipid, amino acid, and nucleic acid metabolism along with hormones and other signaling molecules [23]. Significantly, they now represent the "diagnostic alphabets" of saliva, and our emerging understanding of their significance (or lack thereof) underscores the potential relevance of saliva in translational research and in personalized medicine and dentistry utilizing omics-based tests [12]. The fact that disease states may be accompanied by detectable changes in one, but not all of the above five alphabets, is of substantial advantage. Informatics and statistical tools for the assessment of the most discriminatory combinations of salivary biomarkers for specific diseases are now available [23].

The salivary transcriptome was cataloged in 2004 as consisting of a core of 180 messenger RNAs (mRNAs), followed by documentation of the salivary proteome core consisting of 1,166 proteins between 2008 and 2009 via the combined efforts of several NIDCR-funded research groups [16, 19]. In 2009, documentation on the results of the salivary metabolome was published along with a demonstration of its utility for detection of oral and systemic diseases [12, 21]. In 2011, Farrell and colleagues reported findings indicating the utility of potential variation in salivary microbiome in the detection of resectable pancreatic cancer [12, 22]. The authors showed that in distinguishing patients with early-stage pancreatic cancer from participants without cancer, two

microbial markers, *Neisseria elongata* and *Streptococcus mitis*, showed a receiver operating characteristic plot area under the curve value of 0.90 (95 % confidence interval, 0.78–0.96; *P* < 0.001), with a 96.4 % sensitivity and an 82.1 % specificity [12, 22].

Utilizing the Salivaomics Database

In spite of the fact that high-throughput technologies have enabled the generation and storage of vast amounts of salivaomics data to date, impediments to their use by other researchers persist because of lack of "computationally accessible salivary data" coupled with difficulties in cross-referencing data sets from different studies [12, 24–27]. In recognition of these difficulties and the need to overcome them, researchers at the University of California at Los Angeles (UCLA) developed a data management system and Web resource they christened the Salivaomics Knowledge Base (SKB) [12, 23]. The SKB, predicated on the saliva ontology (SALO) and the BioMart data portal for salivary proteomic, transcriptomic, and metabolomic and microRNA data (SDxMart), functions with other omics databases to enhance the integration of data from various sources by employing a system biology approach [12].

The assays that constitute the omics-based tests stem from molecular measurements [12]. A fully specified computational model is paramount to interpreting the results in order for such results to be clinically "actionable" [12]. The SALO and SDxMart represent the prototype (in dentistry) of "standardized" vocabularies for the description of salivaomics data from varying sources and domains [12]. The SALO, created via cross-disciplinary interaction between several expertise (saliva, protein, diagnosticians, and ontologists), is optimized saliva ontology now available to clinicians in the course of diagnosis and to other omics researchers [12, 28, 29]. Characteristic of ontologies, the SALO aims to maintain sets of vocabularies to ensure consistency in the description of data from varying scientific domain and currently shares a framework with the gene ontology effort and with other disciplinary ontologies within the Open Biomedical Ontologies Foundry [2, 29].

The BioMart, a free, open-source database system, is cross-platform support for several popular database management systems, including MySQL (Oracle, Redwood Shores, Calif.), PostgreSQL (PostgreSQL Global Development Group), SQL Server (Microsoft, Redmond, Wash.), and DB2 (IBM, Armonk, N.Y.) [12, 30, 31]. The database of the BioMart software is pliable and therefore amenable to adaptation to existing data sets. Furthermore, it can be expanded and customized through plug-in system, and users are able to contribute to its development as an open-source system [12]. The system also allows databases at diverse geographic locations to be connected, thereby facilitating collaboration among groups at such diverse locations [12]. Furthermore, BioMart seamlessly can connect databases that are geographically disparate, thereby facilitating collaboration between groups and, consequently, the creation of the first-of-a-kind BioMart Central Portal [12, 32, 33]. In addition to contributing to the Portal, another salient advantage is the opportunity for the research community to share data easily, taking advantage of integrated tools that allows for sidestepping complicated steps that would otherwise be required for conventional cross-database search [12, 32, 33].

The SDxMart, a BioMart data portal, hosts salivary proteomic, transcriptomic, and metabolomic and miRNA data [12]. The SDxMart houses data from both oral and systemic disease studies, including oral cancer, Sjogren syndrome, pancreatic cancer, and breast cancer. It allows users to advance complex queries integrating genomic, clinical, and functional information in the process of salivary biomarker search and discovery [12]. The portal indexes sources for proteomic, transcriptomic, miRNA, and metabolomic data and is integrated with several public databases such as the Ensembl genome database (Ensembl release 37, Ensembl, a joint project of European Bioinformatics Institute and Wellcome Trust Sanger Institute, Hinxton, England) [34].

What Are Biomarkers?

A constellation of definitions for a "biomarker" (short form for biological marker) have been compiled. Most definitions are tailored along the identity of the category of disease or disease process of interest. For example, the National Cancer Institute (NCI) defines biomarkers in its dictionary of cancer terms as "a biological molecule found in blood, other body fluids, or tissues that is a sign of a normal or abnormal process, or of a condition or disease" [35, 36]. Other definitions have broadened the scope of the concept by incorporating biologic characteristics that are subject to objective assessment and evaluation as indicators of either normal biologic or pathogenic processes or as indicators of response to therapeutic (including pharmacologic) interventions [37–39]. Here are some of the examples:

- "A characteristic that is objectively measured as an indicator of normal biological processes, pathogenic processes, or a pharmacological response to a therapeutic intervention" [35].
- "Any substance, structure or process that can be measured in the body or its products and influences or predicts the incidence of outcome or disease" [40].
- "Physical, chemical, or biological agents accessible in body matrices that can be measured in body fluid or cells" [36]
- "Measurable phenotypic parameter that characterizes an organism's state of health or disease, or a response to a particular therapeutic intervention" [36]
- And as "cellular, biochemical or molecular alterations that are measurable in biological media such as human tissues, cells, or fluids" [37].

The latter category of definitions captures the salient elements of the concept of biomarkers and therefore represents a reasonable accommodation.

Utilizing various tools of emerging technology, the identification of biomarkers as aids to diagnoses, and for providing insight to the etiology, pathogenesis, prognosis, and treatment outcomes of specific diseases is increasingly gaining popularity. Although biomarkers are more often perceived as biologic entities—proteins, enzymes, and other biochemical elements or molecules identifiable via direct biologic assays of specific contents of tissues and body fluids (blood, urine, cerebrospinal, saliva)—they may be consistent and specific artifacts of procedures (e.g., imaging techniques) not involving direct sampling of biologic material [38]. In the latter instances, quantifiable changes in the composition or function of an organ/tissue discernible by imaging constitute biomarkers [39].

The application of biomarkers in the diagnosis and management of cardiovascular disease, infections, immunological, genetic disorders, and cancer is well known [37–41]. Biomarkers have the potential to provide a more direct measurement of exposures in the causal pathway of disease, free from recall bias, and with the potential for providing information on the absorption and metabolism of the exposures [39, 42]. The last two decades have seen sustained activities, including research resource allocations, toward the identification and understanding of the workings of biomarkers for specific diseases. These efforts are being facilitated by the equally advancing fields of molecular biology and novel laboratory techniques. The accruing gains so far suggest the imminence of the application of knowledge about certain biomarkers in diverse clinical settings, including diagnosis, disease management, analytic epidemiology, and clinical trials [43–45].

Classification of Biomarkers

Currently, biomarkers are, for all practical purposes, compartmentalized on the basis of disease-specific utility (e.g., cancer, heart disease, infection biomarkers). A recent proposal is to classify biomarkers into two major categories, namely, biomarkers of exposure and biomarkers of disease [39]. Biomarkers of exposure are used to predict risks, whereas biomarkers of disease are for the purposes of screening, diagnosis, prognosis, outcome determination, or any of these combinations [39]. Biomarkers for risk prediction, screening, and diagnosis are

well established [39]. The following subsections further illustrate biomarker classification in the context of cancer biomarkers.

Cancer Biomarkers

Some of the earliest, documented cancer biomarkers are the urinary *Bence Jones* protein in multiple myeloma and the tumor-specific antigen, *carcinoembryonic antigen* (CEA), in colon cancers [36, 46]. To date, the use of prostate-specific antigen (PSA) in the diagnosis index of prostate cancer, albeit controversial in recent times, appears to be the most standout use of human cancer biomarkers from a clinical utility standpoint [36, 47–57]. As in biomarkers in general, several classification models have been advanced for cancer biomarkers, particularly fuelled by recent explosion of technological development and knowledge in the biomedical sciences. Even then, there does not appear to be a consensus on a single operating model of classification [36].

In addition to classifications based on specific organ sites, biomolecules (DNA, RNA, proteins, carbohydrates, etc.) and cancer biomarkers have also been categorized variously as diagnostic, prognostic, and predictive biomarkers reflecting their specific point of clinical utility. However, this categorization appears to be redundant as most biomarkers will invariably be used at the stage of one or more of these diseases indices (diagnosis, prognosis, predictive) in all form of classification. As recently cautioned by Mishra and Verma, classifications should be considered contextual as identification of cancer biomarkers is one of the major multidisciplinary areas of the biomedical field [36]. Figure 2.1 offers a simplified, yet informative, classification of cancer biomarkers [36]. Regarding the role of bioinformatics in the identification of cancer biomarkers, Mishra and Verma provided an elegant summary of Web-based sources (including popular analytical tools) for some of the modern technologies combining clustering algorithms and visualization tools for the identification of cancer subtypes and related biomarkers [36].

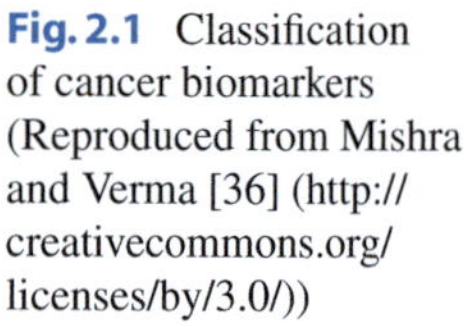

Fig. 2.1 Classification of cancer biomarkers (Reproduced from Mishra and Verma [36] (http://creativecommons.org/licenses/by/3.0/))

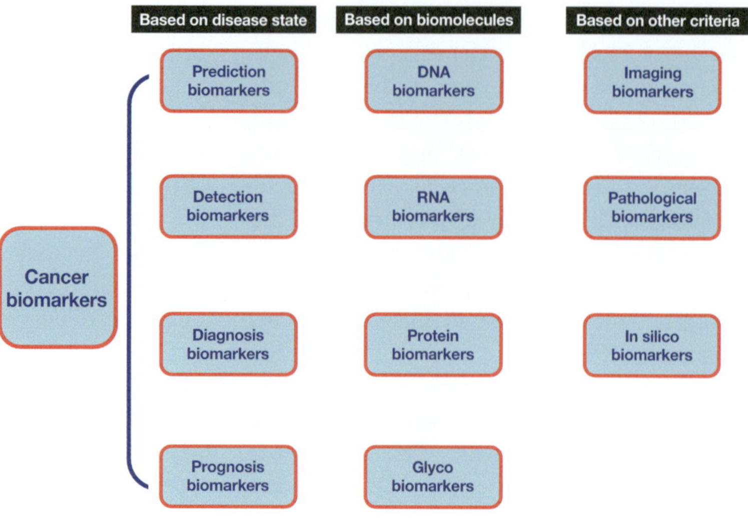

Organ-/Tissue-Based Cancer Biomarkers

Oral Head and Neck Cancers

Of the numerous signature changes emerging as candidate biomarker for oral/head and neck cancers in recent years, mutations in the tumor suppressor *p53* gene arguably stand out as the most studied to date. Protein of mutated p53 gene has been identified in saliva and in surgical margin analysis in head and neck squamous cell carcinoma (HNSCC) [47]. Recently, we reported the potential of MMP-9 and dentin sialophosphoprotein (DSPP) expressions at histologically negative resection margins of primary oral squamous cell carcinoma (OSCC) as predictive of primary site recurrence [48]. In an earlier report, DSPP expression in epithelial dysplasia of oral premalignant lesions indicated a fourfold increase in the likelihood of subsequent transition to invasive OSCC within 2 years compared to oral epithelial dysplasias lacking DSPP expression [49]. Loss of heterozygosity (LOH) and microsatellite instability at chromosome 3p, 9p, 17p, and 18q together with a hypermethylated promoter region of the *p16* gene also are frequently cited as signatories to oral/head and neck cancers [36, 50]. There is as yet, however, no potential biomarker for oral/head and neck cancers of a caliber (prognostic/predictive value) comparable to the likes of ER/HER2 for breast cancer or c-KIT

for gastrointestinal cancers. For this reason, it has been suggested that genomic profiling studies are needed to uncover head oral/head and neck cancer markers with prognostic/predictive values comparable to ER/HER2 or c-KIT for breast and GI cancers, respectively [36].

Lung Cancer

CEA is the most commonly used serum marker of lung cancers. Others are neuron-specific enolase (NSE), CA-125, cytokeratin fragment 21 (CYFR A 21–21), chromogranin A, retinol-binding protein (RBP), α(alpha) 1-antitrypsin, and α(alpha)1-antitrypsin [50]. Overexpression of *K-ras*, myc, *EGFR*, and *Met* oncogenes, or the inactivation of tumor suppressor genes, including *p53* and *Rb*, has been cited as biomarkers for lung cancers [52–56]. Other reports alluding to the amplification of *TTF-1*, *Pax9*, and *Nkx-8* at the DNA level as potential biomarkers of lung cancers have also been reported [36]. Within the last decade, it has been reported that hypermethylation of *p16*, *RARB*, and *DAPK* genes as detected in saliva and serum may predict the development of lung cancer [36, 57].

Uterine and Cervical Cancers

The role of high-risk HPV (HPV-16 and HPV-18) infection in the etiology and pathogenesis of cervical cancers has long been established. The E6 and E7 of the high-risk HPVs are the two oncoproteins whose cell cycle activity in the pathogenesis of cervical cancer has been extensively studied and fairly well understood and therefore pass muster test as uterine and cervical cancer markers [58]. Severely dysplastic uterine cervix lesions overexpress mini-chromosome maintenance (MCM) proteins, whereas overexpression of cycle protein 6 (CDC6) in malignant cervical cancer has been reported [59, 60]. The overexpression of p16^{INK4A} has emerged as a favorite surrogate marker of preneoplastic and neoplastic uterine cervix lesions [61]. In addition to serving as a screening marker of early disease, the ribosomal protein S12 gene has been suggested as holding promise as a potential target in cancer gene therapy trials [62, 63].

Breast Cancers

A large number of breast cancer biomarkers have emerged within the last three decades and more continue to be held as promising suspects. At the moment, the American Society for Clinical Oncology (ASCO) has cataloged about eight protein-related tumor markers for breast cancer: CA 15–13, CA 27–29, carcinoembryonic antigen, estrogen receptor (ER), progesterone receptor (PR), human epidermal growth factor receptor 2 (HER2), urokinase plasminogen activator (uPA), and plasminogen activator inhibitor (PAI)-1 [36, 64]. These subserve different aspects of breast cancer activities: monitoring (CA 15–13, CA 27–29 and CEA), treatment planning (ER, PR, and HER2), and recurrence/risk prediction (uPA and PAI-1) [64]. p53, cathepsin D, cyclin E, and kallikrein 14 have now been added to the list as protein-based potential biomarkers of breast cancer [36, 64, 65].

Messenger RNA (mRNA) expression-based platforms such as MapQuant Dx™ Genomic Grade (based on the expression of about 100 genes for breast cancer detection) and the RT-PCR-based assay system, BCtect™ with several genes for early detection, are now available [66]. There are also reports suggesting that a number of microRNAs (miRNA), including mir-125b, mir-145, mir-21, and mir-155, known to be dysregulated in breast cancers be considered among the list of candidate biomarkers for breast cancers [66, 67]. Indeed, reviews of the gene-expression signatures, namely, mRNA transcript expression patterns, have formed the bases for the classification of treatment modalities for breast cancer patients [36]. Hypermethylation of *BRCA1, p16, and 14-3-3 σ(sigma)* presents in about 95 % of sporadic breast cancers, and genes coding for *cyclin D2*, and *RAR-β(beta)* represent epigenetic biomarkers [68]. Other candidate and proposed biomarkers for breast cancer reported to date include: serum HER2; cytokeratins 8, 18, and 19; kallikrein; osteopontin; mutant p53; and crypto1. Effort to identify additional breast cancer biomarkers is being enhanced by the availability of nanotechnology [69].

Liver Cancer

To date, the frontrunner biomarkers for liver cancer (hepatocellular carcinoma) are alpha-fetoprotein (AFP) and its derivative, AFLP (*Lens culinaris*), and des-carboxy prothrombin (DCP) [70–72]. Proposed markers include plasma levels of transforming growth factor beta 1 (TGF-β1), I-6/10, IGF, and gamma-glutamyl transferase (GGT) enzymes [73, 74], while less established markers include levels of glypican-3 (GPC3) and golgi protein 73 (GP73) [36, 73, 74].

Prostate Cancer

In spite of the popularity and frontline status that PSA has enjoyed over many decades as a biomarker for prostate cancer, its validity has come under close scrutiny in recent years. This is because there is now increasing evidence, including data from the American College of Surgeons National Cancer Data Base (NCDB), showing that not all patients with previously acknowledged PSA levels associated with prostate cancer have cancer [36]. Furthermore, increasing knowledge of the interplay between ratios of the different PSA subtypes (fPSA, tPSA) in predicting such factors as the aggressiveness of prostate cancer has contributed the eroding the validity of PSA as a cancer biomarker [75]. This turn of events has served to refocus effort and attention to the investigation of other potential candidate biomarkers for prostate [36]. Candidate markers now touted include the overexpression of human kallikrein-related peptidase 2 (hK2), early prostate cancer antigen (EPCA), α(alpha)-methylacyl-coA racemase (AMACR), insulin-like growth factors and binding proteins (IGFBP-2 and IGFBP-3), and TGF-β(beta)1. Others are elevated circulating levels of interleukin-6 (IL-6) and its receptors, urokinase plasminogen activator (uPA) and receptor (uPAR), enhancer of zeste homolog 2 (EZH2), and prostate-specific membrane antigen (PSMA) [76–83].

Infectious Agent Cancer Markers

Viral Markers

The roles of infectious agents, notably viruses, in the etiology and/or pathogenesis of specific human cancers are fairly well established. Spanning over nearly half a century now, the link between Epstein-Barr virus (EBV) and a number of human malignancies, including nasopharyngeal carcinoma and Burkitt's lymphoma, is well documented [84, 85]. The established causative relationship between oncogenic HPVs (HPV-16, HPV-18) and uterine cervix cancer has already been discussed above, and similar potential etiologic relationship with a subset of oral/oropharyngeal cancers remains an area of intense investigation. Although HPV-16 (and to a lesser frequency HPV-18) is now easily demonstrable in a subset of oral cancers, proof of etiologic partnership between high-risk HPVs and oral cancer is less than concrete [86]. Hepatitis B virus (HBV) and hepatitis C virus (HCV) most probably have causal relationships with hepatocellular carcinoma [87]. Within the last three decades, the human herpes virus-8/Kaposi's sarcoma herpes virus (HHV-8/KSHV) has been firmly associated with Kaposi's sarcoma (KS), other sarcomas, and certain lymphoma [64]. The RNA virus, human T-cell lymphotropic virus type 1 (HTLV-1), is regarded as an etiological factor for certain types of leukemia [88].

Bacterial Markers

Helicobacter pylori is probably the only well-characterized bacterial pathogen associated with a specific human cancer. Although essentially an infectious agent whose primary pathogenic activity manifests by way of inflammation and ulceration of the upper gastrointestinal tract, including the stomach (gastrum), the last two decades have seen the apparent acceptance of *H. pylori* as a solid biomarker for gastric cancer [89, 90]. However, it is estimated that over 50 % of the world's population harbor *H. pylori* in their upper gastrointestinal tract with infection being more prevalent (80 %) in developing countries [36]. This certainly casts some shadow regarding the timeline significance of *H. pylori* detection in patients as well as its clinical utility and validity as a biomarker for gastric cancer. Either DNA polymorphisms or antibody-based technologies are used to detect *H. pylori* in patients [36]. The significance of *H. pylori* is perhaps more as a surrogate risk factor and therefore a surveillance parameter for monitoring potential disease progression, than it is a biomarker for gastric cancer.

Blood Versus Saliva as Diagnostic Medium

Serum and urine are still regarded as the gold standard body fluid for clinical investigations involving proteomics and the biochemical assays of other body fluid constituents. Even with advances in clinical proteomics providing the opportunity to identify disease biomarkers in biological fluids at reduced costs for early diagnosis of disease, most of the focus remains on the proteomics of serum or plasma. Predictably, the advent and rapid advances of the past two decades in the field of salivary diagnostics and the rising profile of saliva as a diagnostic medium are beginning to generate debates on a couple of fronts. The first questions whether saliva will ever be ready for "primetime" as a diagnostic body fluid; the second, and much more fundamental, is whether, aside from intellectual curiosity, there is a real need for a second (or third) diagnostic body fluid or the need to supplant serum/plasma at this time.

The Case for Saliva (Over Serum)

The attention toward other body fluids, such as saliva and urine, as attractive alternatives of potential sources of disease biomarkers, and as diagnostic fluid, is because of the noninvasive processes associated with these alternatives. The obvious attraction of saliva as a clinical tool in diagnostics is its availability (in the absence of xerostomia/dry mouth due to chronic disease state) as well as the relative ease of collection and storage compared to serum and urine [91, 92]. The process of saliva collection is relatively straightforward and convenient, particularly in multiple samples situation [91, 92]. In stark contrast to the "invasive" process of collecting blood/ serum from patients, the noninvasive process of saliva collection is near absolute. For example, patients who are phobic to needle pricks that invariably involved for blood draws will readily accede to the friendlier procedures for saliva collection, which is largely devoid of threatening maneuvers and also compatible with a stress-free appointment. Furthermore, the fact that, unlike blood, saliva lacks clotting ability simplifies the preservation steps and makes it easier to handle.

It is estimated that 20 % more Americans visit the dentists regularly than they do their physicians in any given time [12, 93]. This positions the dentist as an enhanced gateway opportunity for early detection systemic diseases, including life-threatening conditions [93]. Also the results of a survey by Greenberg and colleagues of 1,900 practicing dentists in the United States to determine their willingness to obtain saliva samples from patients and send same to a laboratory for diagnostic evaluation showed an 87 % "yes" response from respondents [93]. This result provides some evidence of the receptiveness of the dental profession to saliva-based diagnostic and risk-assessment technologies [12, 93]. From the perspective of dentistry as a profession, a full integration of salivary diagnostics into the practice of dentistry will enhance its profile and significance in the overall scheme of primary health care [12].

Given the present state of salivary diagnostics technology, it would appear that for routine clinical utility, the technology is currently expensive compared to the established serum technology. However, it is anticipated that as salivary diagnostics achieve a validity threshold, and subsequently becomes commonplace, its cost-effectiveness will become favorable. Recent development of room temperature analyte stabilization methods, nucleic acid pre-amplification techniques, and direct saliva transcriptomic analysis for accurate detection and quantification of saliva transcripts have already proven to be cost-effective [94]. Indeed, the lack of commercial success of serum-based markers have been deemed as presenting an opportunity for salivary diagnostics to thrive commercially, more so because several salivary biomarkers for oral and systemic diseases are poised for translational and clinical applications, and the market may well be ready for a "a new molecular-diagnostic product" [94]. For remote and impoverished regions and communities, salivary diagnostics offers affordable, yet highly accurate, alternative to the more expensive serum technology [94].

An anticipated utility, and therefore advantage, of salivary diagnostics technology is in the fight against bioterrorism [95]. Under these scenarios, a robust, fast, portable, and user-friendly technology with the capacity to screen for multiple agents simultaneously will offer a distinct advantage [95]. Saliva and other oral fluids collected for this purpose following defined forensic guidelines, including the necessary observation, will be less susceptible to adulteration [95]. In summary, the advantages of saliva as a clinical tool over serum are: the noninvasive procedures involved with obtaining sample, a smaller sample (aliquot) requirement, good patient psychology and cooperation, relative cost-effectiveness at the full turn of the requisite technology, ease of storage and transportation, greater sensitivity, and correlation of result analysis with that of serum.

The Case for Serum (Over Saliva)

While saliva diagnostics for detection of oral diseases (caries, periodontal disease, oral cancer, salivary gland disorders) makes natural sense to many, its reliability and utility in the diagnosis of systemic diseases remote from the oral cavity have been deemed as speculative by just as many [12, 95]. Among many others, a commonly adduced reason for the skepticism, and therefore the reluctant acceptance as an emerging field, is the absence of a clear mechanism providing the nexus between the expression of certain substances in salivary and a disease state at a remote organ or body site [12]. To address the mechanistic question, animal models are proposed with several investigators already exploring this using rodent tumor models [12, 95]. For example, one working hypothesis investigated via the animal models is that exosomes, which are microvesicular structures (30–100 nm in size) shed by tumors, transport tumor-specific contents to distant sites, including the salivary glands, accounting for their remote presence as "disease-discriminatory markers in saliva" [96].

Saliva as a diagnostic fluid is yet to achieve wide acceptance despite the gains and associated generous publicity of the last two decades. Although the same period of time has witnessed the approval of salivary diagnostics-related products by the FDA, such as the saliva HIV antibody detection kits and a number of saliva-based kits for detection of hormones, clinical test application remains quite minimal [3, 12]. It has been suggested recently to be partly attributable to the portrayal of saliva in a negative light in some quarters and culture where social, cultural, and psychological stigmas are associated with saliva [3]. Therefore, it is conceivable that in such cultures, the collection of saliva in even in a clinical setting may be equated to "spitting in public" [95].

Relative to the current state of technological and infrastructural support for salivary diagnostics, the infrastructure of clinical laboratories and blood-serum detection assays are already well established to argue against any need for an equivalent whose competitiveness, viability, and validity are yet to be fully assessed [3]. It is further contented that, unlike the well-established serum technologies that already offer reliable tests for early detection and diagnosis of diseases such as cancer, the current stage of development of salivary diagnostic technology is still years from attaining the same level of reliability [3, 12]. In summary, further in-depth understanding of the nexus between biomarker of systemic diseases and the salivary gland and the validation of

current salivary diagnostics technology via multiplex assay are hurdles on the path of universal acceptance of saliva as a diagnostic fluid. This fact also suggests that, because of the need to substantiate the scientific rationale of salivary biomarkers for systemic diseases, that the pace of acceptance of saliva as a diagnostic medium by physicians may be slower than that of dentists for oral diseases [3].

Legal Issues Related to Salivary Diagnostics

There does not appear to be available as yet an established legal framework specifically focused on salivary diagnostics, even though the use of saliva (and oral fluids in general) for forensic and drugs of abuse investigations is fairly well established. In this section, an attempt is made to summarize and speculate on potential areas of legal ramifications that may arise from the use of saliva for clinical diagnosis of human diseases. Some of the anticipated bases for challenges include: the mode of saliva sample collection, accuracy/reliability/validity questions regarding saliva test outcomes, challenges to suitability of test site, specimen integrity (including chain of custody), and interpretation of test results.

Scientific Evidence in the Legal System

A primary hurdle that scientific evidence in the US legal system must cross is satisfying the legal requirements for "admissibility." Essentially, admissibility speaks to the full "evidentiary value" of any scientific evidence via a process of determining whether or not the evidence is reliable enough to be entertained by the court and subsequently admitted as part of the court record for the issue at stake. On admission, the "weight" to be ascribed to the evidence in the context of the matter is assessed. The standards of evidentiary proof are hardly consistent and will depend on whether the proceeding is adversarial/non-adversarial. In adversarial proceedings, for

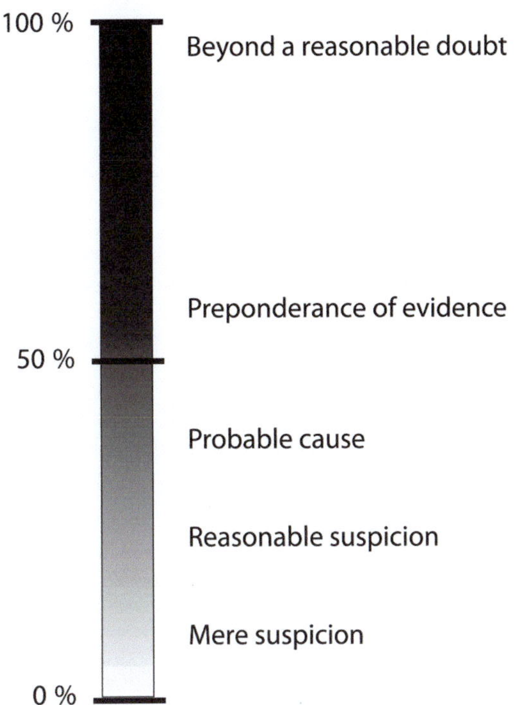

Fig. 2.2 Hierarchy of legal decision-making (Modified from Kadehjian [4] with permission from Elsevier)

example, evidentiary proof ranges from "beyond a reasonable doubt" in criminal cases to "preponderance of the evidence" in civil matters or probation hearings. Lower standards of proof, such as "probable cause" and "reasonable suspicion," are occasionally entertained. Thus, the scientific certainty of test results is subject to different levels of scrutiny depending upon the nature of legal proceedings as indicated above. Figure 2.2 summarizes estimates of percent accuracies used for various legal decision-making [4].

Admissibility of scientific evidence in the US federal courts is governed by the 1975 Federal Rules of Evidence [4, 97]. In 1993, the US Supreme Court used the opportunity of the Daubert v. Merrell Dow Pharmaceuticals Inc., 509 U.S. 579 [98] (and other cases that followed shortly) to elaborate and provide guidance on the criteria for determining the admissibility of scientific evidence [97]. In assessing the admissibility of scientific evidence, the US Supreme Court, via the Daubert case, enumerated the following factors that could be considered by a judge

in answering admissibility questions related to scientific evidence: testing, peer review or publication, known or potential rate of error, standards controlling operation, and general acceptance [98]. Currently, about two-thirds of the US states have adopted the Federal Rules of Evidence as it pertains to scientific evidence [4]. Although the use of saliva and other oral fluid tests for drugs of abuse appears to routinely meet the requirements, it is unclear how well salivary diagnostics will fair, particularly with respect to the factors enumerated in the Daubert case. At least, it is reasonable to anticipate the courts to accord deference comparable with that in saliva tests in drug abuse cases to legal challenges of equivalent aspects of salivary diagnostics testing.

Potential Legal Challenges to Salivary Diagnostics

The acceptability of saliva as a specimen for analysis is borne out by both history and a record of acceptability [4]. Saliva tests are now commonplace in forensic investigations when samples may be obtained from drinking glasses, cigarette butts, envelopes, and other sources to detect blood-group substances, salivary genetic proteins, and many other substances [3, 4]. However, as is characteristics of formative stage projects, part of the uncharted waters of salivary diagnostic are potential legal landmines that may accompany its increasing relevance. It is prudent to anticipate that with stronger footholds of salivary diagnostics comes the likelihood of legal challenges, particularly if sanctions are a possible outcome of legal resolution. Although it is impossible to see all the facets of potential legal questions to be generated by salivary diagnostics from our current vantage, likely areas include challenges to: insurance claims related to positive/negative saliva tests, methods of saliva sample collection, accuracy and reliability of laboratory test results, and interpretation of test results.

Challenges to *insurance claims* (post-treatment or preapproval for therapy) based, for example, on positive or negative results of salivary diagnostic tests are foreseeable. Insurance companies may deem saliva test results and diagnosis unacceptable for reimbursement purposes or to approve therapy and may insist on verifications with a "gold standard"—presumably serum. In litigation, questions also may arise regarding specific methods of collection. A method of collection must be consistent with preservation of the integrity of the specimen before tests. As an illustration, if the use of citrate to stimulate saliva flow could be proven to, even remotely, interfere with assayed substances, results of such tests may prove *unreliable* [4, 99]. The FDA approval/validation of both methods of saliva collection and laboratory procedures for assays is likely to be a requirement for insurance reimbursement. Even when the saliva tests are deemed *accurate*, challenges may be focused on *interpretation of the results* [4]. For example, while the presence of a particular substance in serum may be "diagnostic" of the disease in question, its presence in saliva (outside the serum evidence) may not necessarily meet the required diagnostic threshold for the same disease.

In summary, consistent with the standards for established body fluid collected for biologic analyses, saliva for diagnostic purposes will invariably face legal challenges, scrutiny, and questions as the science and technology matures. However, with the current state of the science of salivary diagnostics and the success of the antecedent application of saliva tests to areas such drug detection, analyses, and in forensic investigations, level of optimism regarding the ability of salivary diagnostics to survive the rigors of legal should be very high.

References

1. Michael P. Saliva as an aid in the detection of diathetic diseases. Dent Diag. 1901;7:105–10.
2. Kirk EC. Saliva as an index of faulty metabolism. Dent Diag. 1903;9:1126–38.
3. Hensen B, Zentz R, Wong DT. A primer of salivary diagnostics. American Dental Association 1995–2009. www.ada.org/.../Science%20and%20Research/Files/saliva_diagnostics.ashx
4. Kadehjian L. Legal issues in oral fluid testing. Forensic Sci Int. 2005;150(2–3):151–60.
5. Tabak LA. A revolution in biomedical assessment: the development of salivary diagnostics. J Dent Educ. 2001;65:1335–9.
6. Malamud D, Tabak LA, editors. Saliva as a diagnostic fluid, vol. 694. New York: Annals of the New York Academy of Sciences; 1993.
7. Costa Jr PT, Chauncey HH, Rose CL, Kapur KK. Relationship of parotid saliva flow rate and composition with personality traits in healthy men. See comment in PubMed Commons below. Oral Surg Oral Med Oral Pathol. 1980;50(5):416–22.
8. Garrett JR. Changing attitudes on salivary secretion—a short history on spit. Proc R Soc Med. 1975;68:553.
9. Mandel ID. A contemporary view of salivary research. Crit Rev Oral Biol Med. 1993;4:599.
10. Schipper RG, Silletti E, Vingerhoeds MH. Saliva as research material: biochemical, physicochemical and practical aspects. Arch Oral Biol. 2007;52(12):1114–35.
11. Jaedicke KM, Taylor JJ, Preshaw PM. Validation and quality control of ELISAs for the use with human saliva samples. See comment in PubMed Commons below. J Immunol Methods. 2012;377(1–2):62–5. doi:10.1016/j.jim.2012.01.010. Epub 2012 Jan 28.
12. Wong DT. Salivaomics. J Am Dent Assoc. 2012;143(10 Suppl):19S–24.
13. Brinkmann O, Wong DT. Salivary transcriptome biomarkers in oral squamous cell cancer detection. Adv Clin Chem. 2011;55:21–34.
14. Urdea MS, Neuwald PD, Greenberg BL, Glick M, Galloway J, Williams D, Wong DT. Saliva, diagnostics, and dentistry. Adv Dent Res. 2011;23(4):353–9. doi:10.1177/0022034511420432.
15. Yan W, Yu W, Than S, Hu Z, Zhou H, Wong DT. Salivaomics knowledge base (SKB) (abstract 1179). Presented at the 37th annual meeting and exhibition of the American Association for Dental Research; 5 Apr 2008; Dallas.
16. Li Y, Elashoff D, Oh M, et al. Serum circulating human mRNA profiling and its utility for oral cancer detection. J Clin Oncol. 2006;24(11):1754–60. doi:10.1200/JCO.2005.03.7598 [Published online ahead of print 27 Feb 2006].
17. Li Y, St John MA, Zhou X, et al. Salivary transcriptome diagnostics for oral cancer detection. Clin Cancer Res. 2004;10(24):8442–50.
18. Wong DT, Segal A. Salivary diagnostics: enhancing disease detection and making medicine better. Eur J Dent Res. 2008;12(S1):22–9.
19. Denny P, Hagen FK, Hardt M, et al. The proteomes of human parotid and submandibular/sublingual gland salivas collected as the ductal secretions. J Proteome Res. 2008;7(5):1994–2006. doi:10.1021/pr700764j [Published online ahead of print 25 Mar 2008].
20. Yan W, Apweiler R, Balgley BM, et al. Systematic comparison of the human saliva and plasma proteomes. Proteomics Clin Appl. 2009;3(1):116–34.
21. Sugimoto M, Wong DT, Hirayama A, Soga T, Tomita M. Capillary electrophoresis mass spectrometry-based saliva metabolomics identified oral, breast and pancreatic cancer-specific profiles. Metabolomics. 2010;6(1):78–95. doi:10.1007/s11306-009-0178-y [Published online ahead of print 10 Sept 2009].

22. Farrell JJ, Zhang L, Zhou H, et al. Variations of oral microbiota are associated with pancreatic diseases including pancreatic cancer. Gut. 2012;61(4):582–8. doi:10.1136/gutjnl-2011-300784 [Published online ahead of print 12 Oct 2011].
23. Salivaomics Knowledge Base. www.skb.ucla.edu. Accessed 19 Aug 2012.
24. Hu S, Li Y, Wang J, et al. Human saliva proteome and transcriptome. J Dent Res. 2006;85(12):1129–33.
25. Huang CM, Zhu W. Profiling human saliva endogenous peptidome via a high throughput MALDI-TOF-TOF mass spectrometry. Comb Chem High Throughput Screen. 2009;12(5):521–31.
26. Takeda I, Stretch C, Barnaby P, et al. Understanding the human salivary metabolome. NMR Biomed. 2009;22(6):577–84.
27. Ng DP, Koh D, Choo S, Chia KS. Saliva as a viable alternative source of human genomic DNA in genetic epidemiology. Clin Chim Acta. 2006;367(1–2):81–5. doi:10.1016/j.cca.2005.11.024 [Published online ahead of print 4 Jan 2006].
28. Ai J, Smith B, Wong DT. Saliva ontology: an ontology-based framework for a salivaomics knowledge base. BMC Bioinforma. 2010;11:302.
29. Ashburner M, Ball CA, Blake JA, et al. Gene ontology: tool for the unification of biology. Nat Genet. 2000;25(1):25–9.
30. Kasprzyk A. BioMart: driving a paradigm change in biological data management. Database (Oxford). 2011;2011:bar049. doi:10.1093/database/bar049 [Published online before print 12 Nov 2011].
31. Zhang J, Haider S, Baran J, et al. BioMart: a data federation framework for large collaborative projects. Database (Oxford). 2011;2011:bar038. doi:10.1093/database/bar038 [Published online before print 19 Sept 2011].
32. Guberman JM, Ai J, Arnaiz O, et al. BioMart Central Portal: an open database network for the biological community. Database (Oxford). 2011;2011: bar041. doi:10.1093/database//bar041 [Published online ahead of print 16 Sept 2011].
33. Haider S, Ballester B, Smedley D, et al. BioMart Central Portal: unified access to biological data. Nucleic Acids Res. 2009;37(Web Server issue): W23–7. doi:10.1093/nar/gkp/265 [Published online ahead of print 6 May 2009].
34. Birney E, Andrews TD, Bevan P, et al. An overview of Ensembl. Genome Res. 2004;14(5):925–8. doi:10.1101/gr.1860604 [Published online ahead of print 12 Apr 2004].
35. National Institutes of Health (NIH) Working Group and the Biomarker Consortium. http://www.biomarkersconsortium.org
36. Mishra A, Verma M. Cancer biomarkers: are we ready for the prime time? Cancer. 2010;2:190–208.
37. Hulka BS. Overview of biological markers. In: Hulka BS, Griffith JD, Wilcosky TC, editors. Biological markers in epidemiology. New York: Oxford University Press; 1990. p. 3–15.
38. Naylor S. Biomarkers: current perspectives and future prospects. Expert Rev Mol Diagn. 2003;3:525–9.
39. Mayeux R. Biomarkers: potential uses and limitations. NeuroRx. 2004;1(2):182–8.
40. Biomarkers in risk assessment: validity and validation, environmental health criteria series, No. 222, WHO. http://apps.who.int/bookorders/anglais/detart1.jsp?codlan=1&codcol=16&codcch=222
41. Perera FP, Weinstein IB. Molecular epidemiology: recent advances and future directions. Carcinogenesis. 2000;21:517–24.
42. Verbeek MM, De Jong D, Kremer HP. Brain-specific proteins in cerebrospinal fluid for the diagnosis of neurodegenerative diseases. Ann Clin Biochem. 2003;40:25–40.
43. Galasko D. New approaches to diagnose and treat Alzheimer's disease: a glimpse of the future. Clin Geriatr Med. 2001;17:393–410.
44. Rohlff C. Proteomics in neuropsychiatric disorders. Int J Neuropsychopharmacol. 2001;4:93–102.
45. Reiber H, Peter JB. Cerebrospinal fluid analysis: disease-related data patterns and evaluation programs. J Neurol Sci. 2001;184:101–22.
46. Golub TR, Slonim DK, Tamayo P, Huard C, Gaasenbeek M, Mesirov JP, Coller H, Loh ML, Downing JR, Caligiuri MA, Bloomfield CD, Lander ES. Molecular classification of cancer: class discovery and class prediction by gene expression monitoring. Science. 1999;286:531–7.
47. van Houten VM, Tabor MP, van den Brekel MW, Denkers F, Wishaupt RG, Kummer JA, Snow GB, Brakenhoff RH. Molecular assays for the diagnosis of minimal residual head-and- neck cancer: methods, reliability, pitfalls, and solutions. Clin Cancer Res. 2000;6:3803–16.
48. Ogbureke KU, Weinberger PM, Looney SW, Li L, Fisher LW. Expressions of matrix metalloproteinase-9 (MMP-9), dentin sialophosphoprotein (DSPP), and osteopontin (OPN) at histologically negative surgical margins may predict recurrence of oral squamous cell carcinoma. Oncotarget. 2012;3(3):286–98.
49. Ogbureke KU, Abdelsayed RA, Kushner H, Li L, Fisher LW. Two members of the SIBLING family of proteins, DSPP and BSP, may predict the transition of oral epithelial dysplasia to oral squamous cell carcinoma. Cancer. 2010;116(7):1709–17. doi:10.1002/cncr.24938.
50. Nunes DN, Kowalski LP, Simpson AJ. Detection of oral and oropharyngeal cancer by microsatellite analysis in mouth washes and lesion brushings. Oral Oncol. 2000;36:525–8.
51. Buccheri G, Ferrigno D. Lung tumour markers in oncology practice: a study of TPA and CA125. Br J Cancer. 2002;87:1112–8.
52. Slebos RJ, Kibbelaar RE, Dalesio O, Kooistra A, Stam J, Meijer CJ, Wagenaar SS, Vanderschueren RG, van Zandwijk N, Mooi WJ. K-ras oncogene activation as a prognostic marker in adenocarcinoma of the lung. N Engl J Med. 1990;323:561–5.
53. Hirsch FR, Varella-Garcia M, Bunn Jr PA, Di Maria MV, Veve R, Bremmes RM, Barón AE, Zeng C, Franklin WA. Epidermal growth factor receptor in

non-small-cell lung carcinomas: correlation between gene copy number and protein expression and impact on prognosis. J Clin Oncol. 2003;21:3798–807.

54. Christensen JG, Burrows J, Salgia R. c-Met as a target for human cancer and characterization of inhibitors for therapeutic intervention. Cancer Lett. 2005;225:1–26.

55. Steels E, Paesmans M, Berghmans T, Branle F, Lemaitre F, Mascaux C, Meert AP, Vallot F, Lafitte JJ, Sculier JP. Role of p53 as a prognostic factor for survival in lung cancer: a systematic review of the literature with a meta-analysis. Eur Respir J. 2001;18:705–19.

56. Salgia R, Skarin AT. Molecular abnormalities in lung cancer. J Clin Oncol. 1998;16:1207–17.

57. Belinsky SA, Klinge DM, Dekker JD, Smith MW, Bocklage TJ, Gilliland FD, Crowell RE, Karp DD, Stidley CA, Picchi MA. Gene promoter methylation in plasma and sputum increases with lung cancer risk. Clin Cancer Res. 2005;11:6505–11.

58. zur Hausen H. Papillomaviruses and cancer: from basic studies to clinical application. Nat Rev Cancer. 2002;2:342–50.

59. Ishimi Y, Okayasu I, Kato C, Kwon HJ, Kimura H, Yamada K, Song SY. Enhanced expression of Mcm proteins in cancer cells derived from uterine cervix. Eur J Biochem. 2003;270:1089–101.

60. Murphy N, Ring M, Heffron CC, King B, Killalea AG, Hughes C, Martin CM, McGuinness E, Sheils O, O'Leary JJ. p16INK4A, CDC6, and MCM5: predictive biomarkers in cervical preinvasive neoplasia and cervical cancer. J Clin Pathol. 2005;58:525–34.

61. Murphy N, Ring M, Killalea AG, Uhlmann V, O'Donovan M, Mulcahy F, Turner M, McGuinness E, Griffin M, Martin C, Sheils O, O'Leary JJ. p16INK4A as a marker for cervical dyskaryosis: CIN and cGIN in cervical biopsies and ThinPrep smears. J Clin Pathol. 2003;56:56–63.

62. Kumar D, Verma M. Molecular markers of cervical squamous cell carcinoma. CME J Gynecol Oncol. 2006;11:41–60.

63. Cheng Q, Lau WM, Chew SH, Ho TH, Tay SK, Hui KM. Identification of molecular markers for the early detection of human squamous cell carcinoma of the uterine cervix. Br J Cancer. 2002;86:274–81.

64. Harris L, Fritsche H, Mennel R, Norton L, Ravdin P, Taube S, Somerfield MR, Hayes DF, Bast Jr RC. American Society of Clinical Oncology. American society of clinical oncology 2007 update of recommendations for the use of tumor markers in breast cancer. J Clin Oncol. 2007;25:5287–312.

65. Borgoño CA, Grass L, Soosaipillai A, Yousef GM, Petraki CD, Howarth DH, Fracchioli S, Katsaros D, Diamandis EP. Human kallikrein 14: a new potential biomarker for ovarian and breast cancer. Cancer Res. 2003;63:9032–41.

66. Iorio MV, Ferracin M, Liu CG, Veronese A, Spizzo R, Sabbioni S, Magri E, Pedriali M, Fabbri M, Campiglio M, Ménard S, Palazzo JP, Rosenberg A, Musiani P, Volinia S, Nenci I, Calin GA, Querzoli P, Negrini M, Croce CM. MicroRNA gene expression deregulation in human breast cancer. Cancer Res. 2005;65:7065–70.

67. Sotiriou C, Pusztai L. Gene-expression signatures in breast cancer. N Engl J Med. 2009;360:790–800.

68. Jing F, Zhang J, Tao J, Zhou Y, Jun L, Tang X, Wang Y, Hai H. Hypermethylation of tumor suppressor genes BRCA1, p16 and 14-3-3sigma in serum of sporadic breast cancer patients. Onkologie. 2007;30:14–9.

69. Banerjee HN, Verma M. Use of nanotechnology for the development of novel cancer biomarkers. Expert Rev Mol Diagn. 2006;6:679–83.

70. Gupta S, Bent S, Kohlwes J. Test characteristics of alpha-fetoprotein for detecting hepatocellular carcinoma in patients with hepatitis C. A systematic review and critical analysis. Ann Intern Med. 2003;139:46–50.

71. Liebman HA, Furie BC, Tong MJ, Blanchard RA, Lo KJ, Lee SD, Coleman MS, Furie B. Des-gamma-carboxy (abnormal) prothrombin as a serum marker of primary hepatocellular carcinoma. N Engl J Med. 1984;310:1427–31.

72. Wang SS, Lu RH, Lee FY, Chao Y, Huang YS, Chen CC, Lee SD. Utility of lentil lectin affinity of alpha-fetoprotein in the diagnosis of hepatocellular carcinoma. J Hepatol. 1996;25:66–71.

73. Block TM, Comunale MA, Lowman M, Steel LF, Romano PR, Fimmel C, Tennant BC, London WT, Evans AA, Blumberg BS, Dwek RA, Mattu TS, Mehta AS. Use of targeted glycoproteomics to identify serum glycoproteins that correlate with liver cancer in woodchucks and humans. Proc Natl Acad Sci U S A. 2005;102:779–84.

74. Zhu ZW, Friess H, Wang L, Abou-Shady M, Zimmermann A, Lander AD, Korc M, Kleeff J, Büchler MW. Enhanced glypican-3 expression differentiates the majority of hepatocellular carcinomas from benign hepatic disorders. Gut. 2001;48:558–64.

75. Catalona WJ, Partin AW, Slawin KM, Brawer MK, Flanigan RC, Patel A, Richie JP, deKernion JB, Walsh PC, Scardino PT, Lange PH, Subong EN, Parson RE, Gasior GH, Loveland KG, Southwick PC. Use of the percentage of free prostate-specific antigen to enhance differentiation of prostate cancer from benign prostatic disease: a prospective multicenter clinical trial. JAMA. 1998;279:1542–7.

76. Gaylis FD, Keer HN, Wilson MJ, Kwaan HC, Sinha AA, Kozlowski JM. Plasminogen activators in human prostate cancer cell lines and tumors: correlation with the aggressive phenotype. J Urol. 1989;142:193–8.

77. Ivanovic V, Melman A, Davis-Joseph B, Valcic M, Geliebter J. Elevated plasma levels of TGF-beta 1 in patients with invasive prostate cancer. Nat Med. 1995;1:282–4.

78. Kattan MW, Shariat SF, Andrews B, Zhu K, Canto E, Matsumoto K, Muramoto M, Scardino PT, Ohori M, Wheeler TM, Slawin KM. The addition of interleukin-6 soluble receptor and transforming growth factor beta1 improves a preoperative nomogram for predicting biochemical progression in patients with clinically localized prostate cancer. J Clin Oncol. 2003;21:3573–9.

79. Paul B, Dhir R, Landsittel D, Hitchens MR, Getzenberg RH. Detection of prostate cancer with a blood-based assay for early prostate cancer antigen. Cancer Res. 2005;65:4097–100.

80. Reiter RE, Gu Z, Watabe T, Thomas G, Szigeti K, Davis E, Wahl M, Nisitani S, Yamashiro J, Le Beau MM, Loda M, Witte ON. Prostate stem cell antigen: a cell surface marker overexpressed in prostate cancer. Proc Natl Acad Sci U S A. 1998;95:1735–40.

81. Rhodes DR, Barrette TR, Rubin MA, Ghosh D, Chinnaiyan AM. Meta-analysis of microarrays: inter-study validation of gene expression profiles reveals pathway dysregulation in prostate cancer. Cancer Res. 2002;62:4427–33.

82. Shariat SF, Lamb DJ, Kattan MW, Nguyen C, Kim J, Beck J, Wheeler TM, Slawin KM. Association of pre-operative plasma levels of insulin-like growth factor I and insulin-like growth factor binding proteins-2 and -3 with prostate cancer invasion, progression, and metastasis. J Clin Oncol. 2002;20:833–41.

83. Varambally S, Dhanasekaran SM, Zhou M, Barrette TR, Kumar-Sinha C, Sanda MG, Ghosh D, Pienta KJ, Sewalt RG, Otte AP, Rubin MA, Chinnaiyan AM. The polycomb group protein EZH2 is involved in progression of prostate cancer. Nature. 2002;419:624–9.

84. Srivastava S, Verma M, Gopal-Srivastava R. Proteomic maps of the cancer-associated infectious agents. J Proteome Res. 2005;4:1171–80.

85. McLaughlin-Drubin ME, Munger K. Viruses associated with human cancer. Biochim Biophys Acta. 2008;1782:127–50.

86. Zaravinos A. An updated overview of HPV-associated head and neck carcinomas. Oncotarget. 2014;5(12):3956–69.

87. Taneja S, Sen S, Gupta VK, Aggarwal R, Jameel S. Plasma and urine biomarkers in acute viral hepatitis E. Proteome Sci. 2009;7:39–40.

88. Boxus M, Willems L. Mechanisms of HTLV-1 persistence and transformation. Br J Cancer. 2009;101:1497–501.

89. Yin M, Hu Z, Tan D, Ajani JA, Wei Q. Molecular epidemiology of genetic susceptibility to gastric cancer: focus on single nucleotide polymorphisms in gastric carcinogenesis. Am J Transl Res. 2009;1:44–54.

90. Suerbaum S, Michetti P. Helicobacter pylori infection. N Engl J Med. 2002;347:1175–86.

91. Streckfus CF, Bigler LR. Saliva as a diagnostic fluid. Oral Dis. 2002;8:69–76.

92. Malathi N, Mythili S, Vasanthi HR. Salivary diagnostics: a brief review. ISRN Dentistry 201. http://dx.doi.org/10.1155/2014/158786.

93. Greenberg BL, Glick M, Frantsve-Hawley J, Kantor ML. Dentists' attitudes toward chairside screening for medical conditions. JADA. 2010;141(1):52–62.

94. Bonne NJ, Wong DTW. Salivary biomarker development using genomic, proteomic and metabolomics approaches. Genome Med. 2012;4(10):82.

95. Gao K, Zhou H, Zhang L, et al. Systemic disease-induced salivary biomarker profiles in mouse models of melanoma and non-small cell lung cancer. PLoS One. 2009;4(6):e5875. doi:10.1371/journal.pone.0005875.

96. Lau CS, Wong DT. Breast cancer exosomes-like microvesicles and salivary gland cells interplay alters salivary gland cell-derived exosome-like microvesicles in vivo. PLoS One. 2012;7(3):e33o37. doi:10.1371/journal.pone.0033037.

97. Federal Rules of Evidence, Pub. L. 93–593, 88 Stat. 1926, 28 U.S.C. app. 1976.

98. Daubert v. Merrell Dow Pharmaceuticals Inc., 509 U.S. 579, 1993.

99. Knott C, Reynolds F. Citrate and salivary drug measurement. Lancet. 1987;1:97.

Saliva Collection Devices and Diagnostic Platforms

Paul Desmond Slowey

Abstract

Over the last few years, there has been a tremendous growth in less invasive diagnostic testing as a replacement for painful and expensive blood draws. The role of saliva in this growth trend has been enormous, and this has been driven in part by a growing awareness of the broad utility of saliva as a diagnostic medium and reinforced by a rapidly growing number of publications supporting new and varied applications for saliva. The aim of this chapter is to highlight some of the tools now available that are responsible for this growth trend and provide a glimpse into the future for salivary diagnostics in the research and clinical environments.

Salivary Diagnostics: The Future of Diagnostic Testing

Over the last few years, there has been a tremendous growth in less invasive diagnostic testing as a replacement for painful and expensive blood draws. The role of saliva in this growth trend has been enormous, and this has been driven in part by a growing awareness of the broad utility of saliva as a diagnostic medium and reinforced by a rapidly growing number of publications supporting new and varied applications for saliva. The aim of this chapter is to highlight some of the tools now available that are responsible for this growth trend and provide a glimpse into the future for salivary diagnostics in the research and clinical environments.

Over the last decade, the opportunity to use saliva as a noninvasive testing option has been reinforced by a number of high-profile organizations including the National Institutes of Health (NIH) [1], National Institute of Dental and Craniofacial Research (NIDCR) [2, 3], American Dental Association [4], American Association of Dental Research [5], and the Federation Dentale Internationale (FDI, World Dental Federation) [6], among others, who have endorsed approaches using salivary diagnostics. Some of these institutions have also provided valuable funding that has resulted in new technologies that overcome many of the barriers that slowed down the earlier development of oral fluid-based diagnostics.

Funded by the NIH, the Salivary Proteome Project [7] was a "landmark" undertaking that led to the characterization of 1,166 proteins in saliva

P.D. Slowey, BSc (Hons), PhD
Department of Corporate Management, Oasis Diagnostics® Corporation, Vancouver, WA, USA
e-mail: pds@4saliva.com

C.F. Streckfus (ed.), *Advances in Salivary Diagnostics,*
DOI 10.1007/978-3-662-45399-5_3, © Springer-Verlag Berlin Heidelberg 2015

and elucidation of the roles of many of these proteins in disease and disease progression. This initiative provided the impetus and foundation for a future generation of oral tools. In this groundbreaking initiative, data was collected from 23 adults from both sexes and multiple races. Using salivary diagnostics, the research team was able to detect and monitor changes in the individual proteome as a means of accurately and painlessly identifying the onset of a particular disease at the molecular level, which has obvious implications in disease identification at an earlier time point leading to the saving of lives. The legacy of the Salivary Proteome Project is that it has spurred a significant amount of activity and new research in this area.

The Streckfus group at Mississippi provided early evidence of the potential role of saliva in studies looking at a number of malignancies, particularly breast cancer using salivary c-erbB-2 (also known as Her-2/neu) and other biomarkers [8–10], and these studies provided an essential building block that formed a solid foundation for others to follow.

A "landmark meeting" in Lanier Lakes, near Atlanta Georgia in 2006, entitled "Oral Diagnostics," was attended by many of the world's leading minds in the saliva area and culminated in the publication of a successful monograph of the same name [11]. This "coming together" of many of the world's "leading lights" in a single focused event also moved the field forward by a significant margin.

Early in 2013, the State of Massachusetts provided significant funding ($4.1 million) to the Forsyth Institute for Salivary Diagnostics in Cambridge Massachusetts, an affiliate of the Harvard School of Dental Medicine, to build a center devoted entirely to research, development, and commercialization of saliva-based diagnostic tests [12], a move that clearly signals an expanding interest in providing answers through saliva.

The aforementioned examples simply illustrate some of the factors pointing to the immediate and growing interest in salivary diagnostics. Many others exist. The reader is referred to a number of important reviews on salivary diagnostics, which will serve to provide excellent background information (see [11, 13–21]). Many other good reviews on salivary diagnostics exist, so these are just a selection of what the reader may wish to view in order to understand this subject in greater detail.

Typically levels of analytes in saliva/oral fluids are significantly lower than in serum/blood, so the current growth in the development of oral fluid technologies has coincided with improvements in detection sensitivities, which now allow low-level quantification of biomarkers in lateral flow, lab-on-a-chip, polymerase chain reaction (PCR), enzyme-linked immunosorbent assay (ELISA), microarrays, mass spectrometry, and multiple other technologies. As a result, the number of new oral fluid diagnostics in the development pipeline or commercially available has increased exponentially. Add to this significant technological advances in the manufacturing of oral-based devices, which are now produced with much greater precision on a lot-to-lot basis, and clear cost efficiencies and you have three of the major factors that are contributing to the salivary diagnostics "success story" and are responsible for the growth in oral fluid technologies.

Saliva is an "ultra-filtrate" of blood and as such acts as a "mirror of the body's health" [4] offering many unique advantages over other bodily fluids. Most analytes, biomarkers of disease, and drugs appear in the saliva through passive diffusion and other mechanisms. Saliva offers several advantages for downstream diagnostic work-up. These include the fact that saliva is the easiest sample to collect, offering considerable cost and disposal advantages to the user; specimens can be collected in observed fashion by minimally trained individuals, eliminating the need for costly phlebotomists and additional processing steps once the sample has arrived at the laboratory or alternate testing site. In addition, saliva samples are noninfectious and may be readily disposed with minimal cost or the need for biohazardous waste containment during transportation. When required, sample transportation is also significantly cheaper, and saliva also eliminates certain cultural "taboos" associated with blood collection prevalent in certain international cultures.

An additional contributing factor to the growth of oral-based technologies is the availability of *standardized* saliva collection methodologies offering the ability to successfully and *consistently* collect and test for a rapidly growing number of diseases and biomarkers from small quantities of saliva. Examples now abound in the literature and include infectious diseases, drugs of abuse, hormones for general wellness, oncology markers, DNA, RNA, and multiple proteins among others.

The subject topic is very broad, so this chapter will focus on four key areas, which are intended to provide a snapshot in time of current and future saliva collection tools and platform systems that are likely to positively impact salivary diagnostics over the next few years.

Following an illustrated history of salivary diagnostics and factors influencing the future impact of saliva as a bodily fluid for diagnosis, this chapter will cover the following major subtopic areas:

1. Whole versus glandular saliva secretions
2. Collection devices for whole saliva and various salivary gland secretions
3. Preservation of saliva specimens
4. Saliva diagnostic platforms

Note: Salivary diagnostics is a highly dynamic area that is in a major growth spurt, so while the author makes every effort to include all technologies of relevance, it may be that certain newer technologies may not be included. Readers are encouraged to review a number of excellent review and scientific articles cited here [11, 13–21].

History

The modern history of salivary diagnostics is fairly recent (1990s); however, saliva actually has a much longer and quite "checkered" history. In ancient Chinese times, for instance, authorities conceived the world's first "lie detector" test using the properties of saliva. At that time, those suspected of a crime were asked to chew rice, while being questioned for a suspected misdemeanor. After question time was over, if the rice was dry, the suspect was assumed to be guilty.

Authorities believed then, which is now supported by recent evidence, that nervous tension created by falsifying statements slows or blocks the flow of saliva from the glands leading to a dry mouth condition and hence dryer than normal saliva. Under such circumstances, suspects are unable to moisten the rice and found guilty of the charges.

Saliva still has a very important role to play in traditional Chinese medicine. Saliva is considered a "precious" fluid, and this comes from a Chinese theory known as the "Fluids of the Five Organs." There are five critical fluids that support healthy life, according to ancient Chinese medicine, and of these, saliva is the "fluid of the spleen and the kidneys." Since these organs are particularly important for a long and active life, saliva as the bodily fluid that maintains the spleen and kidneys has become a highly precious fluid. Taoists in particular believe that chewing, producing saliva, and swallowing saliva are important contributory factors to a healthy mind and body. The manuscript Huangdineijing Lingshu [22] is considered the "Bible" of traditional Chinese medicine books, and in that text saliva is considered the "spiritual fluid" implying a relationship between the mind, brain function, and saliva. Taoists firmly believe that in order to have longevity in life, saliva should not be expectorated, but instead kept in the mouth then swallowed. According to belief, the net effect of this is a clear mind and moist skin.

In the Middle Ages, spitting was an accepted practice and was commonplace in normal life in the Western world. At that time swallowing one's spit was considered rude, but, obviously, things have changed since then. Public spitting was outlawed in the 1700s when officials introduced legislation prohibiting the practice. It was at that time that public spittoons appeared, providing a place for the public to discard unwanted "oral material."

The military has always had a use for saliva in "spit shining" boots, but this practice was eventually replaced by warm water instead of the more traditional saliva, to create the optimum boot shine.

Irwin Mandel [23], well-renowned saliva researcher and noted historian on salivary matters, recounts that many centuries ago early physicians believed that the salivary glands were "lowly excretory organs" functioning to rid the body of toxins and evil spirits from the brain. During those times "doctors" would carry out strange acts, including administering poisonous mercury chloride to patients, causing saliva to ooze from the mouth. In Mandel's mind "saliva is a latecomer," and he commented that scientists in general only began to seriously look at saliva after they had looked at other (more) traditional bodily fluids, particularly blood. Mandel's now well-known statement "saliva doesn't have the drama of blood, it doesn't have the integrity of sweat and it doesn't have the emotional appeal of tears" captured the moment of the time, but from the 1950s onward, this statement became less and less accurate as many scientists, including Mandel, went on to provide evidence and new discoveries in the field, including the important observation that human saliva is actually bursting with hundreds of useful chemical components mixed in with millions of bacteria, viruses, yeasts, and skin cells in a concoction now known to provide excellent protection to the oral cavity. Many salivary proteins have since been characterized that are absolutely critical for the maintenance of good oral health and work in the proteomics area continues to be a burgeoning field where many new and fascinating discoveries are made on a daily basis.

Some recent historical milestones belong to OraSure Technologies (formerly Epitope, USA, http://www.orasure.com) and a former rival Company Saliva Diagnostic Systems (SDS, USA, now StatSure Diagnostics, http://www.statsurediagnostics.com), which led the race for early superiority in the commercial end of the salivary diagnostics arena in the early 1990s. In the end, history shows that it was OraSure who succeeded in producing both the first laboratory oral human immunodeficiency virus (HIV) test kit to gain US Food and Drug Administration (FDA) approval (OraSure HIV-1) and the first and only *rapid, oral point-of-care* (POC) test to gain marketing approval through the FDA Pre Market Approval (PMA) process (OraQuick HIV 1/2).

In 1994, Epitope, Inc. obtained FDA approval to collect oral fluid and reflex to an ELISA test (the Vironostika HIV MicroElisa test kit from Organon Teknika). This remained the only laboratory test that processed oral fluid specimens for HIV diagnosis until a few years ago when the company Avioq, Inc. successfully gained FDA approval for a second oral HIV ELISA test. OraSure Technologies' rapid oral POC test, OraQuick HIV 1/2 later successfully passed FDA scrutiny through an arduous Biological License Application (BLA) process and is now sold directly to consumers, who can purchase the OraQuick HIV 1/2 test in certain pharmacies to test themselves in the privacy of their own homes for $39.99.

Saliva Diagnostic Systems was later able to gain FDA clearance for its Saliva•Sampler® Oral Fluid Collection device, but the limited regulatory approval was for saliva collection only. Despite the lack of approvals for clinical applications, the device found widespread use in the research community.

Perhaps one of the most important areas where saliva can play a role is in the collection of nucleic acids. The harvesting of nucleic acids from bodily fluids and tissue is a rapidly growing area, particularly in life science research and more recently in the clinical realm. A major milestone was reached in 2011 when DNA Genotek (Canada, http://www.dnagenotek.com) successfully obtained FDA clearance for its Oragene DNA Collection Device when used in conjunction with the GenMark Diagnostics e-Sensor Warfarin Sensitivity polymerase chain reaction (PCR) Assay. Although the FDA status is confined to a single application, this clearly opens up the door for other clinical tests to be validated for saliva/orally collected specimens.

The major history of saliva diagnostics remains to be written, but all signs point to a major role to play for this underutilized fluid.

Factors Likely to Positively Impact the Role of Salivary Diagnostics in the Future

The importance of saliva as a bodily fluid for diagnosis of diseases is finally rising rapidly in significance due to a number of important contributing factors. There has never been any doubt on the ease of use of saliva as a diagnostic specimen, or the fact that it is noninvasive, is considered a "safe" sample, or may be readily transported at lower cost than traditional blood, urine, or serum specimens. Very few dispute the fact that when offered the option of providing a blood or saliva sample, most people opt to provide a saliva specimen. It is also an easy specimen to dispose of, without the need for biohazardous waste management, and contains many of the important components of blood that are relevant to disease detection. So, why has saliva not been the ideal medium for test developers in the past and what are the reasons for the current "exploding" demand for "salivary diagnostics"? Opinions may vary, but in this author's opinion, there are a number of reasons for this change, and these may be broken down into specific categories. Some of these are described as follows:

1. *Technological Developments*: Briefly discussed above, one of the most fundamental changes over the last 20 years has been the development of newer saliva specimen collection technologies as well as downstream testing technologies with enhanced sensitivity and specificity characteristics, which now allow very small concentrations of analytes to be detected and quantified in saliva, with high precision. Typically, analytes in saliva are present in much lower quantities than in blood (1/100th to 1/2000th the concentration) so the advent of technologies such as PCR for detection of nucleic acids, tandem mass spectrometry to detect small concentrations of proteins and chemiluminescence, fluorescence, and magnetic bead technologies to detect small- and medium-sized molecules in lateral flow immunochromatographic platforms are just some of the reasons for the rapid growth in oral specimen testing. Specifically in the point of care area, improvements in manufacturing technology and knowledge of how lateral flow test strips are carefully assembled have resulted in more consistent products, which result in much less variability from strip lot to strip lot.

   Another contributory factor is a historical use of collection materials that were not totally appropriate for the collection of saliva. Certain absorbent materials that were used in a multitude of early studies as the vehicle for saliva collection have been shown to bind specific molecules tightly, leading to poor recoveries of target analyte and inferior correlation with serum or whole blood assays. Multiple publications have confirmed that various cotton-based products and, to a lesser extent, certain cellulose products can have less-than-desirable effects on recovered concentrations from oral specimens. While a number of publications [24–27] now highlight this phenomenon, it has taken many years to overcome this negative "perception" of saliva, and even now further education is necessary to inform potential users tainted by earlier negative reports. Due caution should always be observed when choosing the most appropriate tools for collection of saliva for analysis or disease diagnosis.

2. *External Forces*: A number of key organizations now put their weight behind the movement for more and better salivary diagnostics, and the reasons behind this and some important details have already been discussed. NIH, ADA, AADR, FDI, and NIDCR are just some of the organizations that have made policy statements supporting the development and implementation of salivary diagnostic tools. In addition to these contributions, several external "market forces" come into play that make oral diagnostic systems even more attractive:

   The *in vitro diagnostics* (IVD) market into which all diagnostic products fit was estimated to be worth $46 billion USD in 2012 according to Frost and Sullivan [28] and growing at an annual rate of 7 %, leading to an estimated market of $65 billion by 2017. Within the overall market, there are multiple segments; however, as a general rule, diagnostics typically fit into one of the three broad categories: laboratory-based diagnostics, molecular diagnostics (MDx), and point-of-care (POC) systems. Certain products could fit into one or more categories, but for the purposes of looking at broad diagnostic areas, these three sectors define the overall market well. If each of these sectors is looked at independently, there is significant growth in all three areas;

however, the areas of greatest growth are in the fields of MDx and POC diagnostics. Multiple factors affect the commercial markets for diagnostic tests, and some of these factors impact individual sectors more than others. As an example, cost plays an important role in the decision of laboratorians, medical directors of testing organizations, public health departments, and other healthcare decision makers involved in choosing tests for implementation. Reimbursement for those tests from Medicare, Medicaid, or private insurance companies also plays a key role.

Turnaround time (TAT) is now a much more important consideration for stakeholders as testing laboratories look to provide results "quicker, faster, and better" than the competition. Decentralization of testing over the last 10 years or so has also changed the landscape for diagnostics as customers look to options for testing in outpatient centers, clinics, and less traditional settings to move testing out of the laboratory and closer to the patient.

Since the introduction of molecular diagnostics with the advent of polymerase chain reaction, the role of traditional immunoassays has continued to grow but is now supported by an ever-expanding demand for molecular assays that can provide new and valuable information on genetic susceptibility, genotype, phenotype, familial traits, origins of our species, and many other pieces of fundamental information relevant to gaining a complete picture of disease and disease processes. It is estimated that 500 million MDx tests were performed in 2010, and this number is expected to climb to 750 million in 2015 [28]. Although the costs of MDx tests are typically higher than traditional immunoassays, the additional information on disease processes provided by such tests outweighs any cost implications. Saliva as a convenient and cost-effective bodily fluid for diagnostic use has probably found its greatest potential in the MDx field, but applications in traditional diagnostics and point of care are now appearing in greater numbers. These aspects will be covered in greater detail in the section devoted to saliva collection tools.

3. *Market Trends*: There has been a lot of focus in the medical literature on "personalized medicine" and the tailoring of therapeutics to each individual. Certain medicines have been found to be ineffective in people who possess certain genotypes/phenotypes, which has resulted in greater levels of testing to identify patients who will benefit from new therapeutics, those who will remain unaffected, and those who might even suffer adverse effects by being enrolled on such a treatment. Various drugs prove not only to be ineffective in certain patients with known genotype/phenotype, but have been shown to have adverse effects on patient outcomes, so this important finding ensures that greater levels of testing will need to be done in the future prior to enrollment in treatment regimens.

Another phrase that is used liberally in the therapeutic/diagnostic area is the term "companion diagnostics" (CDx). This terminology generally refers to the requirement to have a diagnostic test available at the same time as the market entry for any new drug entity likely to require some degree of monitoring. Specific companion diagnostic tests will typically be recommended on labeling by the FDA during the approval process for the drug and will be used to test all candidate patients to ensure that only those patients who will benefit from a given new drug are treated. Particularly, if it is known that patients with certain genetic profiles will benefit from a therapeutic and others will not, or patients with a specific genetic profile will suffer adverse effects by taking a new drug, the FDA will exert its authority to mandate that a diagnostic test be available to screen patients prior to enrollment in treatment regimens.

The development of a companion diagnostic is a cooperative effort where pharmaceutical companies and diagnostics manufacturers enter into some sort of "partnering agreement" and work together to develop a test that will be cleared or approved for marketing in the United States at the same time as the medicine. One of the first examples of this was the combination of therapeutics for colorectal cancer from Amgen (cetuximab) and Bristol Myers Squibb (Erbitux), with the "Scorpions" KRAS PCR diagnostic test from DxS (now part of Qiagen Corporation, Germany).

There are a number of CDx tests in development, and this number is forecast to grow rapidly in the years ahead. Saliva is an ideal matrix for CDx testing.

Another market, which is experiencing significant growth, is noninvasive prenatal testing. A number of companies now offer tests for prenatal screening. Examples include the Panorama test from Natera, Inc., the Harmony test from Ariosa Diagnostics, Verifi from Verinata Health (an Illumina Company), and the MaterniT21 test from Sequenom that use cell-free DNA (cfDNA) to look for various chromosomal abnormalities in the DNA of the maternal blood that has been passed to the mother by the fetus while still in the womb. Some of the conditions that can be detected from defects in the chromosomal order are Down syndrome, Edwards syndrome, Patau syndrome, and certain sex chromosome trisomies.

While these tests use blood (which in the author's opinion is not truly "noninvasive"), the attention focused on these tests brings greater awareness for the need for less intrusive forms of testing, including urine, finger stick blood, tears, and saliva.

4. *Milestones*: There are a number of events in the history of salivary diagnostics that will be seen in the future very much as landmark events that put oral testing "on the map." Two of the most recent occurrences have been even more effective in capturing the imagination and interest of the consumer market in general and have led to a new generation of diagnostics under development.

The approval of the OraSure HIV-1 Oral Specimen Collection Device and the Organon Teknika Vironostika HIV-1 ELISA Test Kit in 1994 was a major achievement at the time, and this paved the way for the subsequent approval of the first rapid, oral HIV test 10 years later. Again OraSure Technologies was responsible for developing the OraQuick

HIV 1/2 initially for sale to healthcare professionals only. In retrospect these were both highly significant events, but even more "powerful" was the subsequent approval of the OraQuick HIV 1/2 test for consumer/over-the-counter use in 2012. This milestone signaled the first ever oral test for a potentially high-risk infectious disease to be sold directly to consumers through independent pharmacies throughout the nation.

In the molecular area, DNA Genotek (Ottawa, Canada) was successful in obtaining an FDA clearance for its oral DNA specimen collection device (OraGene) when used with the GenMark Diagnostics e-Sensor Warfarin Sensitivity Tests. During the FDA regulatory process, DNA Genotek was able to demonstrate that saliva proved equivalent in performance to blood and as a result users of the e-Sensor Warfarin Test can now opt to use either saliva or blood. The clearance for the OraGene device has since opened up the door for many other potential clinical applications for saliva and the use of salivary samples for nucleic acid testing. At this point in time, this single application remains the only test cleared by the FDA for clinical use, but many companies now see saliva as a viable fluid and are proceeding with the development of orally based clinical tests.

5. *Funding for Salivary Diagnostics*: The topic of endorsement by key organizations and the availability of funding for research has been covered in some depth above, but some other recent funding events have brought increased attention to salivary diagnostics.

In August 2013, the NIH, through its National Center for Advancing Translational Services, provided $17 million in funding for 24 projects under a new "Extracellular RNA Communication Program."

A significant share ($5.5 million) of the $17 million went to UCLA Dentistry to study biological markers in saliva in order to develop functional tools for the detection of pancreatic cancer. According to a press release from UCLA, "the study will create a new paradigm in the field of salivary diagnostics, and it could supply concrete evidence that saliva can be used in the detection of life threatening diseases, including diabetes and cancers of the pancreas, breasts, ovaries and stomach" [29].

In 2010, NIH through the NIDCR (National Institute for Dental and Craniofacial Research) funded two important studies entitled "salivary biomarkers for early oral cancer detection" and "salivary proteomic and genomic biomarkers for primary Sjögren's syndrome." Scientists have now identified the genes and proteins that are expressed in the salivary glands, so using the vast accumulated information as their guide, they will define the patterns and certain conditions under which these genes and proteins are expressed in the salivary glands and how these parts function as a fully integrated biological system.

Back in 2002, NIDCR provided funding for the development of new salivary POC testing platforms. At that time, seven research groups received funding to develop tools focused on the use of microfluidics and micromechanical systems. The projects were directed at detection and analysis of the constituents of saliva, including miRNA, mRNA, proteins, DNA, electrolytes, and others. Second round funding was provided to four of the seven, and NIDCR has recently reported that each is on the way to completing development of a platform based upon oral specimens.

Whole Versus Glandular Saliva Secretions

The word "saliva" has been used in widespread fashion in the published literature to describe secretions in the oral cavity; however, a number of different subcomponents exist in saliva, and various terms may be used to describe fluids collected from the mouth, including the broad term saliva, oral fluids, gingival crevicular fluid (GCF), and others. It is important, therefore, to provide brief definitions of the most important terms used when discussing salivary tools with potential diagnostic or investigative applications:

Saliva – this is a watery substance located in the mouth of organisms, secreted by the three main salivary glands (the submandibular, the parotid, and sublingual), as well as hundreds of other minor salivary glands and gingival crevicular fluid. Human saliva is composed of 95 % water, but also electrolytes, mucus, antibacterial compounds, and enzymes, and performs many normal functions including food digestion, lubrication, taste facilitation, and bolus formation.

Oral Fluids – this is a term often used interchangeably with "saliva" and used very often in forensic toxicology and, in particular, the drug testing world.

Gingival Crevicular Fluid – a fluid occurring in minute amounts in the gingival crevices, believed by some authorities to be an inflammatory exudate and by others to cleanse material from the crevices. GCF contains sticky plasma proteins, which improve adhesion of the epithelial attachment, has antimicrobial properties, and exerts antibody activity[1]. Definitions of other oral secretions are included below in the text.

Saliva is produced in the salivary glands and secreted from there as clusters of cells known as acini. The acini secrete fluids containing a mixture of enzymes, water, mucinous material, and various electrolytes. This concoction is collected from the acinus into specific collection ducts, where the composition of the fluid may be altered. These ducts lead into much larger ducts that eventually form a single duct that delivers the saliva mixture into the oral cavity.

Humans have three pairs of salivary glands that each delivers different secretions. The parotid gland produces a serous watery secretion, the submaxillary (mandibular) glands empty a mixed serous and mucous containing secretion, and the sublingual glands secrete a fluid that is essentially mucinous in character. The basis for the different compositions of saliva secreted by each of the various gland types has been proven histologically, and early studies by oral biologists

---

[1] Definition from Jablonski S. *Illustrated Dictionary of Dentistry*, W B Saunders Co. July 1982.

have shown that the composition of certain components can vary significantly from one type of salivary gland to another. For this reason it is important that the differences are understood and that the proper mouth location for appropriate sample collection is consistently used. This is also the reason that tools exist to collect whole saliva and also for various glandular types that may provide different and additional informative information on events happening in the oral cavity and in general disease processes.

Collection Devices for Whole Saliva and Various Salivary Gland Secretions

Tools for Collection of Whole Saliva

Nonmolecular Tools

The modern history of salivary collection tools with high commercialization potential can be traced back to the early 1990s when two companies based in the Pacific Northwest of the United States—Epitope Inc. (Beaverton, OR) and Saliva Diagnostics Systems (Vancouver WA)—vied for early market supremacy. The first "entrées" for each of these companies were unique, and distinct saliva collection devices that two decades later have gone on to become the most successful salivary collection tools so far produced. Epitope Inc. (which became OraSure Technologies www.orasure.com following the acquisition of Solar Technologies Corporation, STC in 2000) is the most successful saliva diagnostic company in the world with revenues of just under $88 million in 2012. Epitope originally developed the OraSure® Oral Fluid Collection Device for general purpose saliva collection, but did not realize the full potential for the device until it successfully partnered with a Dutch Company (Organon Teknika, Boxtel, Netherlands) to enable the use of the device for collection of salivary samples for HIV diagnosis. By linking the OraSure device to an HIV-1 ELISA test from Organon Teknika, the OraSure device would become a component of the first FDA-approved oral test for detection of the HIV virus. The major market applications for the OraSure

HIV-1 product include public health screening, surveillance, life insurance risk assessment, and outreach programs. The OraSure device consists of a rectangular cellulose pad attached to a detachable blue plastic stem. The pad material is rubbed across the surfaces of the cheeks adjacent to the gum line for a period of time then left in the gap in the oral cavity between the teeth and gum line to absorb a salivary sample. The current manufacturer, OraSure, describes this sample as "oral mucosal transudate." The pad material is pretreated with certain proprietary salts designed to facilitate more rapid sample collection. The average specimen collection time is between 2 and 5 min, after which the OraSure device is placed into a collection tube containing a buffer and transported to a laboratory. Prior to analysis the sample must be centrifuged. Following centrifugation, the specimen is assay ready.

OraSure's expertise extends into drugs of abuse testing, so in order to capitalize on this core competency, the company developed a very similar device (using the Intercept® brand name) specifically for substance abuse testing for the main NIDA-5 accepted panel of drug entities (THC/marijuana, cocaine, opiates, methamphetamines, and PCP) and other abused drugs. The Intercept® device features an identical specimen collection device to the OraSure HIV-1 product, but differs in the proprietary buffer used to dilute the collected specimen and also the unique packaging used to brand the product. Intercept® is currently used in many areas of abused drug testing including workplace testing, drug courts, forensic toxicology, and various criminal justice settings. In the case of both OraSure HIV-1 and Intercept®, samples collected using the devices are processed in the laboratory.

Across the Columbia River from Epitope in Washington State was another emerging company in oral diagnostics, Saliva Diagnostics Systems (SDS, Vancouver, WA), now StatSure Diagnostic Systems (New York, NY, www.statsurediagnostics.com). SDS was the original developer and manufacturer of the Saliva•Sampler® Collection Device, which was also known in other countries around the world as Omni•SAL®.

The Saliva•Sampler®/Omni•SAL® device was used for general purpose standardized saliva collection and received 510(k) marketing clearance from the FDA strictly for saliva collection only. At the time, SDS chose to market the collection tool as a collection tool only and did not "pair" the device to any specific diagnostic (e.g., HIV) or abused drug tests as its rival Epitope/OraSure had done. Later, the manufacturer transferred the rights to the product to California-based Immunalysis Corporation (Pomona, www.Immunalysis.com), a company with an existing presence in the drugs of abuse testing market through strong sales of urine-based ELISA tests. Immunalysis subsequently rebranded the product as Quantisal™ and validated saliva collection to a series of their ELISA-based drug test assays, which have received FDA clearance and are now routinely sold for workplace testing, forensics, criminal justice, and other applications.

The Quantisal™ Saliva Collection Device also uses a cellulosic (paper-based) material attached to a stem to harvest saliva from the mouth. An absorbent pad is placed in the mouth and saliva collected until a sample volume indicator built into the device changes color from white to blue (usually approximately 2 min) indicating sufficient saliva (1.0 mL + or –10 %) has been collected to perform any subsequent analysis. The absorbent pad has a series for perforations near the top of the cellulose pad, which allows easy detachment of the pad into a transportation tube containing a stabilizing buffer to ensure safe delivery of the sample to the laboratory for testing.

A third early saliva innovator in the saliva collection area was Sarstedt (Germany, www.sarstedt.com), which introduced "Salivette" to the commercial market in 1987. This device has been used extensively by the research community for a wide assortment of applications ranging from detection of steroid hormones from saliva, HIV antibody detection, markers of oxidative stress, and others. Salivette does not have any regulatory clearances from the FDA but is CE marked in the EU.

The Salivette device is available as either cotton or polyester rolls or sponges, and each configuration includes a sample transport tube. To collect a sample, the Salivette is placed in the mouth and chewed for approximately 2 min then placed into the transport tube for dispatch to a testing laboratory. The device does not incorporate any means of sample sufficiency, and the specimen must be centrifuged prior to analysis.

Note: As mentioned earlier, there are now a number of published articles that caution against the use of salivary collection devices that use cotton as the collection media, including Salivette, for certain applications, particularly the detection and quantification of steroid hormones, marijuana, and others. In such cases, use of cotton-based collection media can lead to an over- or underestimation of actual concentrations of target analyte in oral fluids. A few examples are cited here as references [24–27].

Neogen Corporation (Lexington, USA, www.neogen.com) purchased International Diagnostic Systems (IDS, St Joseph, MI) in 2009 and at that time gained the rights to the UltraSal-2™ Saliva Collection Device, manufactured by IDS. UltraSal-2™ is a large-volume saliva collection device that provides a capability to "split" the collected sample into two mutually distinct samples collected simultaneously. The device includes two collection tubes connected to a single mouthpiece into which the user expectorates. The mouthpiece can be tilted/rotated during collection to direct saliva into one or the other of the two tubes. In this way, sufficient sample can be collected into both tubes for subsequent analysis in the laboratory. In total, this device can collect up to 24 mL of whole saliva by the drool technique. UltraSal-2™ is used mainly for drug testing purposes.

The SalivaBio Saliva Collection Aid was originally developed by SalivaBio LLC (USA, www.salivabio.com) in collaboration with researchers at the Center for Interdisciplinary Salivary Bioscience Research at the Johns Hopkins School of Nursing for Hormonal Analysis, but this device has been shown to have broader applicability and may be used for most applications where saliva is required. The device works by expectorating/spitting saliva into the Saliva Collection Aid, a plastic funnel-type device. The "plastic funnel" component is connected directly to a transport tube provided by the manufacturer, so when sample collection is finished, the tube is capped and sent to a laboratory for processing. The manufacturer has ensured that the device is compatible with multiple cryovials so samples may be collected directly into Wheaton, Sarstedt, Nalgene, or Greiner cryovials for ready storage in a freezer. SalivaBio is now also available through Salimetrics (State College, PA, www. salimetrics.com), a leading manufacturer of salivary tests for steroid hormones, neurotransmitters, and others.

In addition to marketing the SalivaBio device, Salimetrics also produces the Salimetrics Oral Swab (SOS) Device. The SOS device uses a 10×30 mm "interference free" pad as the collection medium. This is fabricated from an inert polymer material that is used as part of a kit that includes a conical tube storage box, storage tube, and bar-coded labels. The sample is collected by placing the absorbent pad in the mouth of pediatric patients for between 1 and 5 min, after which the pad is placed into the conical tube provided, labeled, and shipped to a laboratory or frozen for storage purposes.

The British Company Malvern Medical Developments (www.malmed.co.uk) developed the ORACOL Collection Kit that uses an absorbent foam material in a swab format to collect up to 1 mL of whole saliva. The ORACOL Collection Kit consists of an absorbent foam swab, centrifuge tube, and cap. To collect saliva, the ORACOL swab is placed in the mouth and allowed to absorb saliva for a period of time. The sample is removed from the swab by centrifugation using a tube provided in the kit. The processed specimen is typically used for infectious disease testing particularly measles, HIV, hepatitis A and B, mumps, syphilis, and rubella, but has also been used for substance abuse testing.

Greiner Bio-One (Kremsmünster, Austria, www.gbo.com) is the manufacturer of the SCS Saliva Collection System, a device for the collection of whole saliva by trained professional users that incorporates a series of tubes, reagents, and a sample cup for general purpose saliva collection. The first step in a series of steps with the SCS system is to rinse the mouth with a safe and proprietary reagent provided by Greiner. The second step involves taking a sample of 4 mL of a tartrazine solution in the mouth for 2 min then spitting the entire contents into a clean tube containing preservative agents that stabilize the saliva sample for long periods of time. A separate evacuated tube is used to take the collected specimen from one container into the final transportation tube. Once filled, the sample is stable for analysis or for transportation to a laboratory. An advantage of the Greiner system is that the internal colored dye (tartrazine) is used as a means of calculating the exact saliva quantity present in the total solution using colorimetric analysis.

Oasis Diagnostics® Corporation (Vancouver WA USA, www.4saliva.com) is involved in the manufacture of a series of oral-based tools. Historically the first device to be introduced by the company was Versi•SAL®, a device for standardized whole saliva collection. Versi•SAL® uses an absorbent pad made out of noncellulosic pad material to collect saliva from under the tongue until a sample volume adequacy indicator in the device changes, signifying sample sufficiency. Typical collection time using the device is approximately 1–2 min. Saliva is separated from the absorbent collection pad by expressing the sample through a plastic compression tube provided and into a standard delivery tube (2 mL Eppendorf or 1.5 mL microfuge tube). Various configurations of the device can provide between 0.5 and 1.4 mL of whole saliva, with the option to obtain two samples from the same patient using a modified compression tube. The Versi•SAL® Oral Fluid Collection Device is currently used for general purpose saliva collection for downstream testing in the laboratory. Applications include hormone testing for general wellness, substance abuse testing, cotinine (nicotine), infectious diseases, and others.

Oasis also recently introduced a second device, Super•SAL™, for standardized saliva collection with medium to large volume saliva collection capability. Super•SAL™ collects saliva using a cylindrical absorbent pad along the side of the tongue between the tongue and gum line. This device also includes a sample sufficiency indicator, which changes once an adequate sample has been obtained for subsequent analysis.

Super•SAL™ has a shorter collection time due to the higher surface area of pad material exposed to fluid in the oral cavity. In this case, the sample is expressed through a compression tube resembling a syringe barrel and into a standard receptacle (2 mL Eppendorf tube or 1.5 mL microfuge tube). A sample of 1.0 mL is typically collected in approximately 1–3 min.

The area of drug testing from oral fluids is a significant business in the United States and other parts of the world, and a number of devices exist for rapid drug testing at the point of care. Similarly, a number of oral collection devices exist that use absorbent materials to collect salivary specimens. In both cases, many of these have suffered from poor recoveries of marijuana (THC) caused by the binding of the "sticky" THC molecule to the collection matrix. The Accu•SAL™ Oral Fluid Collection Device (Oasis Diagnostics®) was designed to overcome this particular problem. A proprietary collection strip attached to a handle is placed in the mouth until the strip is saturated (as indicated by the change in the sample volume adequacy indicator incorporated as part of the device, approximately 1 min). Upon saturation the collection strip is placed in a tube containing a predetermined quantity of a reagent buffer that stabilizes the sample during transportation to the laboratory. Upon receipt at the laboratory, the handle and collection strip are removed, and the tube containing the sample can be immediately used for ELISA, homogeneous immunoassays, or GC-MS as required without further dilution. An added feature of this device is that in cases of insufficient saliva collection, there is a procedure that can be followed to provide an accurate dilution of the saliva obtained. This device may be used for multiple applications including steroid hormones for general wellness, therapeutic drug monitoring, workplace testing, and forensic applications.

In 2011, two of the IVD industry leaders, Quest Diagnostics (USA, www.Questdiagnostics.com), the largest reference testing laboratory in the United States, and Thermo Fisher Scientific (USA, www.thermofisher.com), a major *in vitro* diagnostics manufacturer, formed a partnership and sought FDA clearance for a series of homogeneous immunoassays for abused drugs produced by ThermoFisher under the CEDIA® brand. Sample collection is performed using the Quest Diagnostics Oral-Eze® Device. According to the summary of the FDA (510 K) regulatory clearance documentation, samples collected using the Oral-Eze® device may be used in the ThermoFisher assays for the NIDA-5 drugs (amphetamines, cannabinoids [THC], opiates, cocaine, methamphetamines, and phencyclidine [PCP]). Quest similarly promotes a list of drugs including the NIDA-5 series of drugs that have been validated to the Oral-Eze® collection tool in its marketing literature and Website. Quest also performs analytical testing for various drugs in its laboratory facilities at several locations around the United States.

To collect samples using the Oral-Eze®, the donor inserts the pad of the device into the mouth between the lower cheek and gum line. Collection is complete when a white indicator in a viewing window changes to a blue color. Time of collection is suggested to be up to 10 min, but four out of five collections are complete within 5 min. The saturated collection pad is then ejected from the handle of the device using pressure on a series of ridges on the side of the plastic housing, into a collection tube containing a stabilizing buffer. A cap is placed on the tube, which is then protected with a "tamper proof" seal across the top of the specimen vial. The sealed collection tube is then shipped in a specimen bag to a laboratory for subsequent testing. Quest promotional materials suggest that the main areas of application for Oral-Eze® are in preemployment, random, reasonable decision, return to duty, and postaccident testing.

Another new drug collection system, the Wolfe Reality CHECK Premium Oral Fluid System, is available through Wolfe Workplace Protection (Ashville, NC, www.wolfeinc.com). This device collects a neat oral fluid specimen by expectoration through a plastic mouthpiece into a connected transport tube. A fill line on the transport tube provides an indication of the quantity of saliva required for downstream drug analysis. After collection the mouthpiece is removed and the sample capped and sealed for protection, then shipped to the laboratory, where ELISA, homogeneous immunoassays, or GC-MS among others may be ran on the samples.

In addition, there are a number of other "specialized" collection tools for salivary hormone detection developed by manufacturers of microplate ELISA kits as "companion tools" for collection that are sold in conjunction with various test kits. Examples include DiaMetra (Italy), IBL (Germany), Salimetrics (USA), DRG International (USA), and others.

Molecular Tools

The growth in molecular technologies (PCR, genotyping, microarrays, genome-wide association studies, sequencing, and others) has coincided with the expanding interest in saliva as a specimen, which in turn has spawned a number of very important commercial tools for salivary collection of nucleic acids. This area of salivary diagnostics is probably growing faster than any other market sector at the present time. The reasons have a common thread with those for general saliva collection, particularly that it has been proven that salivary samples are equivalent in performance to blood sampling and more cost-effective, convenient, and simpler to use.

In the molecular diagnostics space, DNA Genotek was the early market leader introducing salivary collection technologies for DNA and RNA and today continues to hold that position. DNA Genotek (Ottawa, Canada) was acquired by OraSure Technologies in 2011 but continues to operate as a wholly owned subsidiary of OraSure. DNA Genotek now offers several tools for nucleic collection from salivary samples. Originally the company launched the OraGene® DNA device in two formats, which simplified the collection and stabilization of DNA from saliva samples, and these two configurations are sold widely in the life sciences research area as well as in the personal genomics field. In December 2011, the OraGene® DNA device became the first salivary collection tool for nucleic acids cleared by the FDA for *clinical* use when used in conjunction with the GenMark Diagnostics eSensor test for warfarin sensitivity. To date this remains the only cleared device for clinical use. FDA regulatory clearance is currently restricted to collection of

oral fluids and application for clinical testing with the GenMark eSensor test only.

The OraGene® DNA device is set up for home collection and has been used by a number of the early adopters of "consumer genomics" (i.e., 23andMe, Navigenics, now part of Life Technologies, Pathway Genomics and others). An OraGene® DNA specimen is collected when a subject expectorates into the OraGene collection tube until a fill line on the OraGene® device is reached. The volume is set at 2 mL, and the collection time ranges from 2 to 30 min, depending upon the subject. Once sample collection is complete, a special cap, prefilled with a proprietary and patented buffer, is attached to the OraGene® collection tube and screwed into place, resulting in the release of the buffer into the saliva specimen. The buffer has the effect of immediately stabilizing the DNA present in the sample. OraGene® DNA collects a large quantity of DNA, for a range of downstream applications. DNA Genotek also supplies reagents for the isolation of DNA and RNA from the sample and works with other reagent suppliers to offer multiple options for nucleic acid isolation.

Following up on their success with OraGene DNA, DNA Genotek has launched a series of other devices for molecular fragments including the OraGene® RNA device, the ORAcollect™, and the OMNIgene™ DISCOVER.

OraGene® RNA is described by DNA Genotek as "an all in one system for the collection, stabilization, transportation of RNA from human saliva." OraGene® RNA is basically a plastic collection vial that donors use to spit into until a specific volume of saliva (2 mL) is collected. The cap of the collection vial conceals an RNA preservative liquid that is released when the cap is placed on the vial and sealed. The RNA-preserving liquid confers several months of stability on the sample at room temperature. In order to isolate RNA from the sample, DNA Genotek supplies reagent kits. Alternately kits from outside suppliers, such as Qiagen (Germany), Norgen Biotek (Canada), or Mo Bio Laboratories (USA), may be used.

ORAcollect™ is another innovation for the collection of DNA from oral fluids. ORAcollect™

comprises a swab-shaped sponge attached to a cap that screws into a transportation tube containing buffer. Prior to use, the sponge end of the device is on the outside of the transport tube and is used to rub the lower gums ten times back and forth in one direction then a further ten times in the opposite direction. After sample collection is complete, the screw cap containing the sponge is unscrewed and inverted and into the bacteriostatic buffer solution to stabilize and transport the sample. After shaking vigorously ten times, the sample is ready for shipment to a laboratory or immediate DNA isolation. DNA Genotek promotes this particular device as an affordable alternative to buccal swabs.

A similar device, called PERFORMAGENE™-LIVESTOCK is sold into the large animal veterinary area. PERFORMAGENE™-LIVESTOCK™ collects DNA from the nasal passages of cattle and other livestock. The device uses a similar or identical sponge to the ORAcollect™ device, but in this case, the sponge is rubbed inside the nostrils of the animal for up to 5 s in order to collect an adequate specimen. The remaining procedure is identical to that of the ORAcollect™ tool, and the resulting DNA collected may be immediately purified or taken directly to downstream testing (PCR, genotyping, etc.).

OMNIgene™ DISCOVER is a specific saliva collection kit for harvesting and stabilizing *microbial* DNA. The device is in fact a tube identical or very similar to the OraGene® DNA Device that subjects spit into (through a funnel-shaped head) until a fill line marked on the device is reached. The sample is then capped, releasing a stabilizing agent into the saliva that preserves bacterial DNA in the specimen. The funnel-shaped lid may be removed by unscrewing a complete section of the device, then the lower section of the tube is capped and the mixed sample shaken then processed using off-the-shelf kits capable of isolation of microbial DNA.

According to OraSure Technologies' public financial statements, its DNA Genotek subsidiary had revenues for OraGene® DNA and other devices of $14.3 million in fiscal year 2012.

Oasis Diagnostics® uses a different approach to collection of nucleic acids from saliva. Its first market entry in 2011 was the DNA•SAL™ Salivary DNA Collection Device. DNA•SAL™ is an ergonomically correct device that has a collection "head" connected to a detachable handle. The collection head has a series of sharp edges that are rubbed across the surfaces of the inside of the cheek area, gently, for 30 s. This action captures buccal cells on the device head but also causes a significant number of detached cells to remain free flowing in the oral cavity. The loose cells are "harvested" using a small quantity of a safe stabilizing solution that is "swished" around in the mouth for 15 s then retransferred back into the same sample tube by spitting. The stabilizing rinse solution present in the sample tube confers long-term stability on the sample. DNA can then be immediately processed or transported to the laboratory for extraction followed by downstream analysis (PCR, genotyping, etc.).

Oasis provides a method for *immediate* downstream testing *without DNA isolation* with a simple sample manipulation and also supplies DNA isolation kits specifically optimized to samples collected using the DNA•SAL™ Device (which are not strictly saliva but a more complex mixture of stabilizing solution, cells, and saliva).

A new tool, RNAPro•SAL™, was recently launched by Oasis Diagnostics® for the isolation of RNA and/or proteins from saliva. This device integrates certain elements from the Oasis Super•SAL™ Universal Saliva Collection Device (for whole saliva) with components necessary to separate and independently stabilize both RNA and proteins for downstream research or clinical studies. RNAPro•SAL™ incorporates a proprietary secondary filtration unit, which functions to provide cell-free saliva. The procedure involves placing a cylindrical pad in the inside of the mouth along the gum line next to the teeth and collecting saliva until a sample volume adequacy indicator changes appearance, confirming that sufficient sample has been collected (minimum 1.0 mL, typical collection time approximately 1–2 min). The absorbent pad used to collect the salivary specimen is then placed in a compression tube that is connected to the secondary "splitting unit" that in turn connects to two collection tubes (Eppendorf or microfuge tubes). The saturated saliva collection pad is pushed through the compression tube and through the secondary filtration unit and the eluted sample subsequently separated into two distinct fractions. The secondary filter may contain variable media, but each acts to remove cells from the sample, allowing two samples of purified saliva to be received in the sample collection tubes. These two fractions are stabilized independently with specific reagents provided with the RNAPro•SAL™ Device to yield long shelf-life fragments of RNA and proteins that are assay ready.

The last 2–3 years has seen a number of new oral nucleic acid collection tools based on expectoration (spitting) that are beginning to find application in research studies. For instance, Norgen Biotek, a Canadian company based in Thorold, Ontario (www.norgenbiotek.com), introduced a "convenient saliva collection and preservation device" as a kit known simply as the "Saliva DNA Collection, Preservation, and Isolation Kit." The kit provides an "all-in-one" procedure for the collection, preservation, and isolation of salivary DNA at ambient temperature. The technology resembles the OraGene® DNA technology, where the sample is collected by spitting into a collection tube (with a funnel connected to the top of the tube to direct the sample) until a sample fill line is attained. The funnel piece is removed and in this case a preservative is added directly from an ampoule provided. The preservative has a dual function to lyse the cells as well as preserve DNA in the sample. One positive feature of the device is that each device is uniquely numbered for positive sample identification.

Another similar device is the SalivaGene Collector from Stratec Molecular (Berlin, Germany, www.stratec.com). As for the OraGene® DNA and Saliva DNA Collection and Preservation Device from Norgen Biotek, the SalivaGene device connects a basic funnel to a collection and transport tube. Saliva is expectorated through the funnel and into the tube until a minimum saliva volume is collected, then detached and capped. One distinct feature of SalivaGene is that the buffer is pre-dispensed into the collection tubes in a lyophilized format.

Devices for Collection of Oral Specimens from Salivary Gland Secretions

There are three major salivary glands (submandibular, sublingual, and parotid) that contribute to 90 % of total (whole) saliva. The remaining 10 % comes from a number of smaller (minor) glands, particularly the buccal, lingual, labial, and palatal glands. The composition and quantities of saliva secreted by each of the different glands differ, so in order to evaluate individual salivary gland function, it is important to use tools specifically designed for collection from each of the glands. A good account of saliva composition and quantities can be found in the work of Mese and Matsuo [30]. Saliva can be collected from these individual salivary glands using a number of available tools. These tools are not used routinely, so none of them are commercialized on a widespread basis and are typically used for research studies only. Due to the limited application for these devices, innovation in this area is limited; nevertheless, these tools find application in research protocols around the world.

Parotid Gland Collection Methods

Parotid gland collections are the easiest of the individual glandular secretions to collect and may be accomplished by modifications to a device known as the Carlson-Crittenden collector, originally reported in 1910, but still in use due to the reliability and accuracy of the device. Although the Carlson-Crittenden Collector (also known as the Lashley cup) is a robust system, it needs to be expertly fitted by a skilled person. The device is used sterile, fitted with polyvinyl chloride (PVC) tubing. The inner portion of the device is connected to a bulb or a suction pump, and the device is placed over the main parotid excretory duct (Stensen's duct) in the oral cavity. Samples are collected via suction onto ice using an induced stimulation (typically a sterile aqueous citric acid solution applied to the tongue by means of a cotton swab at periodic intervals). Samples can be collected bilaterally, allowing for simultaneous collection from both parotid glands to increase yield and shorten collection times.

Cannulation is also used to obtain parotid saliva specimens. In this case, a thin tube is placed directly at the outlet of the main parotid excretory duct (Stensen's duct). This method suffers from certain drawbacks including discomfort and requires a skilled operator. In some cases, application of a local anesthetic is required.

Submandibular/Sublingual Gland Collection Devices

The most widely used device for submandibular (SM) and sublingual (SL) saliva collection is the device invented by Wolff and Davis [31], which may be used to collect either specimen type (SM or SL) using slightly modified procedures. The "Wolff" device consists of four components: tubing for collection (cellulose acetate butyrate), a polycarbonate buffering chamber (to avoid saliva being sucked into the suction device and to also remove bubbles from the collected sample), a storage tube, and a vacuum device to produce suction. The device produces pure saliva and appears to be efficient, reportedly collecting 90 % of the fluid that enters the device into the storage chamber [32]. As for parotid saliva collection, some sort of stimulus is required (usually 2 % citric acid applied directly to the tongue) with this device.

To collect saliva from the submandibular gland, the openings to each of the two parotid glands are typically blocked using $2'' \times 2''$ cotton gauze. The floor of the mouth is then dried, and the openings to the sublingual glands on both sides of the mouth are also blocked. The subject/patient is required to raise their tongue into an elevated position allowing access to the submandibular gland. At that point, collection using the Wolff device can successfully begin. To collect saliva from the sublingual gland only, a similar procedure is used, except in this case access to the submandibular gland is blocked in preference to the sublingual gland.

A 1998 study from Chile by Morales et al. reported new devices for the collection of saliva from both the parotid and major salivary glands producing on average 1.0–1.5 mL of saliva in a 10–15 min period [33]. Although the devices were not described in detail, they were used repeatedly by the Chilean authors in subsequent studies

[34, 35]. Flow rates obtained from submandibular/sublingual glands were on average 180 µl per minute and from the parotid gland 80 µl per minute. One advantage of the reported devices is that collection of both parotid and submandibular/sublingual saliva may be achieved simultaneously under the supervision of a solo healthcare professional. As for other similar devices, artificial saliva stimulation using citric acid is required and samples must be collected on ice.

More recently, researchers in New Zealand have reported a custom fabricated device for the collection of submandibular saliva that is less invasive than those previously available [36]. Although the device collects a lower quantity of saliva than that collected by expectoration (spitting), the stimulated saliva specimen has a pH close to that of unstimulated saliva. The authors suggest that the device minimizes sample contamination due to the fact that the unit is a sealed device. Validation experiments performed on the device compared to saliva collected by expectoration (spitting). In each case, samples were collected over 5 min. In the case of expectoration, samples were collected by "forcible expectoration" every 30 s, and using the device, by inserting the device in the mouth and directing a tube so that saliva flowed freely from Wharton's duct into the collection cup provided. The customization element of this device requires that an accurate impression of the mouth cavity is taken, which uses a modification of the altered cast technique for lower Kennedy Class I impressions [37].

Older research from Sweden [38], published online for the first time in 2007, describes a device for submandibular/sublingual saliva using a modified Block-Brotman device, a tool originally described in 1962 [39]. The study compared the results of submandibular/sublingual collection versus collection of parotid saliva by means of standard Carlson-Crittenden cups, and results indicate that the device successfully provided higher flow rates of saliva than parotid collection at two time points throughout the day.

A more invasive option for submandibular collection is cannulation via Wharton's duct. This may be carried out using one of a number of available metal cannulae including blunt hypodermic syringe needles, catheters with a metal tip, and a device known as the Schaitkin Salivary Duct Cannula from Hood Laboratories (Pembroke, MA), which is designed for short-term intubation of the salivary ductal system and for holding open the ductal tissue. The Walvekar Salivary Duct Stent (also Hood Laboratories) has also been used to hold open salivary ductal tissue to allow the flow of fluids from the glands and collection into a suitable receptacle.

For more in-depth information on devices for submandibular and sublingual collection, see reference [40].

Devices for Collection from the Minor Salivary Glands

There are many minor glands that make up the remainder of salivary gland secretions, including the labial, buccal, lingual, and (glosso) palatine glands. Typically, minor gland salivary secretions are less useful in providing meaningful information for diagnostic purposes, so the number of available devices for collection from these glands is limited. Samples from the minor glands are more viscous in nature, so this has also hampered studies using minor gland secretions. A variety of qualitative methods have been tried, including filter papers, capillary tubes, sponges, and micropipettes. In addition, semiquantitative assessment has been done using weight measurements, and methods involving measurement of colored spots on chromatography paper have been used to determine flow rate.

The most widely used method in current practice is an electronic device known as the Periotron® from Pro-Flow, Inc. (Amityville, NY), which has made quantitative assessment of minor salivary gland secretion much more accurate and precise. The Periotron® method uses a piece of blotting paper to harvest moisture from the mucosa. The blotting paper is subsequently placed between two plates on the Periotron® measuring instrument across which a voltage is applied. The dielectric properties of the saliva are used to calculate the volume of moisture absorbed by the blotting paper. The moisture collected is recovered, and then the blotting paper is once again returned to the instrument. A standard curve constructed from known volumes of water added to blotting papers is finally used to back calculate the amount of moisture originally present on the paper.

Interestingly, minor salivary gland secretions are reported to be less likely to respond to stimulation than the major gland secretions, although additional data confirms that mechanical stimulation of a denture "base plate" adjacent to the palatal mucosa can induce increased salivary secretions from the minor glands.

Preservation of Saliva Specimens

Saliva is a complex mixture of electrolytes, proteins, bacteria, various glycoproteins, mucins, and aqueous material, among others. While some molecules in the saliva (certain drugs, drug metabolites, steroids, cancer markers, and others) remain relatively stable in oral fluids, others, for example, RNA and proteins, are notoriously unstable and require the addition of validated stabilization reagents in order to preserve the integrity of the sample, prior to the analysis phase.

The science of sample stabilization, and in particular salivary sample stabilization, is a growth area, and a number of commercial companies have active strategies to support saliva stabilization for genomics, proteomics, and transcriptomics. Without the activity in this area, the salivary diagnostics area would stagnate.

Stabilization of Analytes in Saliva

With the appearance of new and better tools for saliva collection and clean up, opportunities to use saliva as the ideal specimen are increasing. In order to capitalize on this growth trend, adequate methods of saliva stabilization were needed and have recently been developed. Multiple strategies now exist for sample stabilization, and the number of companies offering suitable products is growing rapidly to the benefit of the entire salivary diagnostics space, another small sign that saliva is attracting greater attention from companies supporting the *in vitro diagnostics* market.

Stabilization of Nucleic Acids

RNA

Commercial sources of RNA protection are designed to halt RNA degradation at the time of salivary specimen collection until the time of analysis, which may be one of a number of downstream applications such as PCR, RT-PCR, qRT-PCR, RNA sequencing, or others. From a user standpoint, such reagents should be capable of stabilization of saliva at ambient temperature, be relatively simple to use, and remain cost-effective in comparison to the downstream technology applied.

The stability of RNA often depends upon the method of collection, pre-analytical steps taken to clean up the specimen prior to analysis, and the absolute purity of RNA. For this reason, there are multiple literature reports claiming RNA to be highly unstable, whereas others report longer shelf life, even at ambient temperature. This is clearly an area where new approaches are leading to better solutions. Due to the conflicting reports, precautionary measures are usually taken to stabilize RNA in bodily fluids, including saliva.

A number of manufacturers have introduced reagents targeting this area, and each competes for a growing market share. Reagents for the stabilization of RNA appear to be broadly applicable to the stabilization of RNA in multiple bodily fluids, including saliva, and may not be specific to application with oral specimens. Some of the most widely used are described as follows:

Qiagen, Inc. (Germany, www.qiagen.com) now provides a number of reagents for protection of transcriptomic elements from human specimens, including the RNAlater® and RNAprotect® systems for tissue and bacteria. For saliva samples particularly, the RNAprotect™ reagent [41, 42] has been commonly used. According to the manufacturer, the RNeasy® Protect Saliva Micro Kit (which includes RNAprotect® Saliva Reagent) "stabilizes RNA in saliva samples to preserve gene expression profiles." The RNeasy® Micro Kit purifies and concentrates total RNA using a spin column technique. Stabilized saliva samples can be shipped at 37 °C for 1 day, for 14 days at 15–25 °C, or for 4 weeks at 2–8 °C, prior to RNA purification. The kit provides sufficient reagents for 50 preparations. The current cost of the RNAprotect® saliva reagent and RNeasy® Micro Kit (sold together) is approximately US $660.

Qiagen also supplies the RNAlater® RNA stabilizing reagent for the immediate stabilization of RNA from multiple bodily fluids. Originally developed for tissue samples, Qiagen supports a modified protocol for adaptation to saliva. RNAlater® is sold in 50 mL or 250 mL bottles for $73.10 and $302.00, respectively. The stability of samples reported using RNAlater® is the same as for RNAprotect®/RNeasy®.

Life Technologies (USA, www.lifetechnologies.com) also markets the same RNAlater® brand in a number of kits that have been validated with Life Technologies' own RNA isolation kits from the Ambion® company (owned by Life Technologies). Pricing and sample sizes for the RNAlater® stabilizing solution from Life Technologies is $116.00 for 100 mL and $363.00 for 500 mL. Life Technologies also offers a second option for RNA stabilization, known as SUPERase•In™ RNase Inhibitor at a concentration of 20U/μ(mu)L. SUPERase•In™ Inhibitor is a nonhuman protein-based inhibitor that binds the interfering RNases including RNase A,B,C,1, and T1. The company promotes this product as "a reagent for the removal of RNases in any application where RNase contamination can be problematic." The material itself is shipped on dry ice but is conveniently priced at $125.00 for 2,500 units. Other reagents available from Life Technologies include RNaseOUT™ Recombinant Ribonuclease Inhibitor, RNase Inhibitor, and RNAsecure™.

A 2006 publication by Wong et al. [42] reported a side-by-side evaluation of the stability conferring properties of SUPERase•In™, RNAlater®, and RNAprotect® Saliva Reagent and concluded that RNAprotect® Saliva was the "optimal room temperature stabilization reagent for the salivary transcriptome." A later publication by Andreas Kurth from the Center of Biological Safety at the Robert Koch Institute in Berlin, Germany, looked at the stability of samples stabilized with RNAlater® and cautioned that samples so treated can still harbor viral infectivity and should be treated as potentially hazardous and capable of transmitting disease, if handled inappropriately [43]. This study was somewhat limited in that it did not investigate any other RNA protective agents, so caution should be observed when looking at similar reagents, as these may or may not harbor similar properties.

Later work on RNAprotect™ Saliva Reagent has reinforced the applicability of this product for long-term stabilization of the salivary transcriptome. Jiang et al. reported 10 week stability on salivary DNA/RNA specimens, as well as 6 days stability on salivary proteins in a saliva filtrate, all carried out at ambient temperature [41].

Biomatrica (USA, www.biomatrica.com) now offers RNAstable® for the preservation of RNA at room temperature without degradation. RNAstable® is available either in liquid form, or as a dried reagent, which can be added directly to RNA samples in tubes, multi-well plates, or other suitable containers. The Biomatrica Website provides support information describing the protection of total RNA, messenger RNA (mRNA), and microRNA (miRNA) for 12 years at ambient temperature without degradation. RNAstable® is available in various sizes and specifications depending upon customer requirements. Pricing information is not immediately available.

US Company Zymo Research (www.zymoresearch.com) is now commercializing a dual function reagent that effectively stabilizes DNA and/or RNA upon contact, allowing shipping of stabilized nucleic acids at ambient temperatures with long shelf life. DNA/RNA Shield™ preserves genetic integrity and expression profiles of samples (including cells, blood, tissue, saliva, urine, and others) at ambient temperatures. In addition, DNA and RNA can be isolated directly without precipitation or reagent removal and have been shown to be compatible with most DNA and RNA purification kits. DNA/RNA™ Shield, which also inactivates infectious agents (viruses), is sold in units of 50 mL for $62.00, or 250 units for $221.00. DNA/RNA Shield™ is also sold as part of a "Mini-Prep Kit" for RNA Isolation for $239.00 (50 mL/50 preps).

The ClonTech division (www.clontech.com) of Takara Bio (Japan, www.takara-bio.com) offers the Takara RNase Inhibitor, a ribonuclease inhibitor material, expressed in *E. coli* and purified by affinity chromatography. This inhibitor is available in two sizes of 5,000 units for $112.00 and 25,000 units for $450.00. This product can be used in most applications where protection of RNA is critical.

Creative Biogene Biotechnology (USA, www.creative-biogene.com) also offers a similar "RNase Inhibitor," which is an acidic 52 kDa protein that is a potent inhibitor of pancreatic-type ribonucleases such as RNases A, B, and C. This product is offered as a 20,000 unit size, described more fully as an enzyme, which is a fusion of the RNase Inhibitor gene with a 22.5 kDa protein tag attached. This reagent must be stored at −15 to −25 °C.

OraGene RNA (DNA Genotek, Canada, www.dnagenotek.com) reagent has also been used successfully for the stabilization and rapid isolation of RNA from saliva in the OraGene RNA Self Collection Device. RNA collected using OraGene RNA is stable "for months" according to the manufacturer and may be used for human mRNA expression profiling.

At the time of this writing, the author learned of a new RNA-stabilizing agent from Norgen Biotek (Canada, www.norgenbiotek.com), a supplier of multiple kits for DNA and RNA isolation and stabilization from multiple sources and specimen types. The new reagent from Norgen is available only in liquid format and additional details on the product were unavailable at the time of writing.

For each of the aforementioned commercial RNA stabilization reagents, the actual compositions of the stabilization reagent are not reported in detail.

Finally, early methods for stabilization of RNA included "snap-freezing" saliva samples at −80 °C until analysis. This method is still commonly used in the area of transcriptomic research.

DNA

Like RNA, similar stabilization processes are carried out on crude DNA samples in saliva, until DNA isolation can provide highly stable DNA free from impurities in an assay ready format for downstream processing. The number of manufacturers and commercially available salivary collection devices for DNA is increasing, and each supplier typically provides reagents for oral DNA stabilization, either with the collection tool or as standalone isolation kits that can be purchased as optional components.

Salivary DNA collected using the popular Oragene Device (DNA Genotek, Canada, www.dnagenotek.com) is protected by an addition of proprietary reagents including a bacteriostatic compound to inhibit the growth of the bacteria. This is introduced into the sample immediately after collection. The protected sample is said to be stable for a minimum of 1 year.

The DNA•SAL™ Salivary DNA Collection Device (Oasis Diagnostics®, USA, www.4saliva.com) includes a stabilizing solution containing alcohol and glycerol that also acts to prevent bacterial growth. Again the stabilizing agent is introduced immediately after sample collection, minimizing any potential for DNA degradation. The sample is stable for a minimum of 30 days. Additional stabilizing agents are available for longer-term storage.

DNA/RNA Shield™ from Zymo Research (USA, www.zymoresearch.com) is a reagent that enables prolonged nucleic acid stability during sample storage/transport at ambient temperatures. The DNA/RNA Shield™ reagent works efficiently for both RNA and DNA, acting to effectively lyse cells and inactivate nucleases and viral activity. Zymo has validated DNA/RNA Shield™ to a number of collection and storage devices including oral fluid collection tools.

The SalivaGene collection device from Stratec Molecular (Germany, www.stratec.com) includes a lyophilized stabilizing reagent, which is reconstituted upon sample collection. According to the same manufacturer, the PSP SalivaGene DNA Kit [44] is intended for genomic, mitochondrial, and bacterial DNA isolation from stabilized saliva samples. SalivaGene DNA includes a proprietary buffer, which acts to immediately stabilize saliva samples on contact, by effecting inactivation of DNases. It also acts to preserve the microorganism titer and pre-lyses bacteria. The stability of the sample is 12 months at room temperature and several years at −20 °C.

Norgen Biotek provides a device known simply as the "Norgen Saliva DNA Collection and Preservative Device." In this device, whole saliva is stabilized by addition of an "aqueous storage buffer," which, according to the manufacturer, is designed for rapid cellular lysis and subsequent preservation of DNA. The buffer prevents growth of gram-negative and gram-positive bacteria and fungi and also inactivates viruses [45].

Salimetrics Corporation (USA), a leader in salivary hormone ELISA test kit production, has partnered with DNA Genotek (Canada) to offer opportunities to carry out genotyping and hormone measurement on the same saliva sample [46]. In this case, whole saliva is collected by the passive drool technique into cryovials that are held on ice. Samples may be collected using the Salimetrics Saliva Collection Aid, then are rapidly frozen at −20 °C.

Biomatrica (USA, www.biomatrica.com) has developed the DNAguard™ Saliva Reagent for preservation of the integrity of genomic DNA both at ambient and elevated temperatures. The company claims that the product is based upon "an innovative technology platform applied to the chemical design of a long term saliva preservative that protects DNA in saliva with high yield and quality in comparison to cold-stored samples, but at ambient temperatures." DNAguard™ Saliva is one of the products from Biomatrica that is said to "disrupt the cellular membranes, penetrate immediately other cellular structures and inhibit nuclease activity as well as free radical activity." Further specified attributes include "protection of nucleic acids in the biosample specimen from hydrolysis such as depurination."

There are a number of other commercial sources of DNA stabilization reagents that are too numerous to mention within this brief review, so the reader is encouraged to review this subject further when trying to identify the most efficient reagents for DNA stabilization.

Proteins

Knowing that proteomics has become a major area of study, it is perhaps difficult to understand why relatively little work has been done on the stability and stabilization of salivary proteins.

Saliva has been shown to consist of 1,166 proteins [7], so the salivary proteome is a valuable tool to investigate ongoing disease processes. Evidence exists to show that the salivary proteome is very easily degraded, so methods capable of stabilizing saliva samples to protect the integrity of the salivary proteome are necessary. A compelling overview on the subject of "whole saliva proteolysis" by Oppenheim et al. [47] provides excellent background on this subject and also describes valuable solutions to slow down proteolytic activity in saliva, allowing effective downstream testing of saliva to take place. This body of work also provides strong evidence to support the hypothesis that the addition of suitable stabilizing agents to protein moieties is critical to successful salivary testing. A number of suitable stabilization cocktails are discussed by the authors, particularly the development and implementation of protease inhibitors. In all, Oppenheimer et al. tested 19 potential inhibitor cocktails and showed that a mixture of AEBSF, aprotinin, pancreatic trypsin inhibitor, leupeptin, and antipain (serine protease inhibitors) supplemented with EDTA, prevented noticeable degradation in synthetic substitutes for the proteins histatin 5, statherin, and PRP1. The authors were also able to eliminate degradation by reducing the pH of the saliva to 3.0.

Xiao et al. published a method for stabilization of the salivary proteome using ethanol [48]. Using reference proteins (beta-actin and interleukin 1-ß[beta]), the authors were able to show that the salivary proteome was stable if held at 4 °C for up to 2 weeks and using ethanol as a stabilizing agent, proteins were stable for up to 2 weeks at ambient temperature.

Sample stability and protein composition were evaluated extensively by Dutch researchers Esser et al. who examined protein stability at room temperature in freshly collected whole saliva, with and without protease inhibitors and inhibitors of bacterial metabolism, using Surface Enhanced Laser Desorption/Ionization (SELDI) [49]. Degradation was evaluated using gels followed by liquid chromatography tandem mass spectrometry (LC-MS/MS). The results confirmed rapid protein degradation within 30 min with decomposition beginning immediately after sample collection. Improved stability was observed using a cocktail of phenylmethylsulfonyl fluoride (PMSF) and leupeptin (both serine and cysteine protease inhibitors) and EDTA, a metalloprotease inhibitor, but protein breakdown was still noticeable. Addition of sodium azide, on the other hand, did not confer any stability on protein samples, indicating that bacterial metabolism is not contributing significantly to protein breakdown. This study also postulates at least six proteases are at work to potentially degrade saliva specimens.

A standard method of protein stabilization that has been used routinely in the research laboratory involves the addition of a cocktail consisting of aprotinin (1 µ[mu]L, 10 mg/mL solution), sodium orthovanadate (Na3OV4, 3 µ[mu]L, 400 mM solution), and PMSF (10 µ[mu]L, 10 mg/mL). This cocktail is added to the supernatant fraction obtained from 1.0 mL of centrifuged whole saliva and preserves saliva samples for extended time periods (up to 2 weeks).

A similar mixture comprising of sodium orthovanadate (1 mM) and a commercially available protease inhibitor cocktail (Sigma, 1 mg/mL of whole saliva) was incorporated in pioneering work on saliva protein profiling for breast cancer detection in women by Streckfus et al. [8]. Even with the stabilizing cocktail present, the researchers kept samples on ice throughout the process, then aliquoted their samples and froze them at −80 °C for long-term storage.

A "universal" stabilizing agent capable of stabilizing nucleic acids (DNA and RNA) *and* proteins would be highly advantageous for research and clinical protocols, so the 2009 finding by Jiang et al. [41] that RNAprotect™ Saliva Reagent (Qiagen, Germany) functions not only to stabilize RNA and DNA for up to 10 weeks at ambient temperature but also stabilizes proteins in saliva filtrates for 6 days, was a valuable contribution to the field. Despite this, the use of RNAprotect™ Saliva Reagent has not been broadly adopted for the protection of the integrity of proteins, mainly due to the requirement for a high dilution relative to the saliva sample (reagent must be added in a ratio of 5:1 versus saliva), resulting in a less-than-desirable solution from a cost standpoint.

Most other reported methods for protein stabilization require low temperatures, which only serve to minimize the attractiveness of salivary testing, so it is clear that there are opportunities for more effective protective agents for the salivary proteome. Recently the activity in this area of research has increased considerably.

Saliva Diagnostic Platforms

The early success of companies like Epitope (OraSure), SDS (StatSure), Sarstedt, and others has paved the way for a much broader array of integrated saliva diagnostic platforms that are now available targeting two main areas of the IVD and life sciences markets. In addition to nonmolecular saliva platform devices targeting proteins, infectious disease antigens, and antibodies, on which most of the current technologies are based, a new area has emerged from the combination of non- and minimally invasive specimen collection with point of care molecular testing platforms that incorporate on board nucleic acid purification, hybridization, and amplification. This newly emerging market segment, which we will refer to as point of care molecular diagnostics (POC MDx), offers up the perfect combination of rapid diagnostic results with immediate diagnosis for most, if not all, diseases or conditions, so this particular segment of the IVD business could rapidly become the fastest growth area in oral diagnostics.

In the remainder of this section, some of the tools/devices that have already made an impact in the aforementioned important areas of the *in vitro* diagnostic industry will be described:

Nonmolecular Platforms

Most of the current oral point-of-care tests combine the ability to collect saliva specimens in standardized fashion with functional lateral flow immunochromatographic (LFT) test strips to deliver real-time results in 20 min or less. The number of commercially available targets is still relatively few, but platforms now exist to significantly increase the number of disease targets over the next few years. Areas that have seen the most significant growth include substance abuse detection and HIV diagnosis, but newer targets aimed at salivary hormone detection, other infectious diseases and more recently systemic diseases are now emerging.

Of all the salivary diagnostics on the market today, there is no doubt that OraSure Technologies' OraQuick Advance HIV 1/2® rapid, oral fluid test for the HIV virus has made the greatest impact. This product was launched in the year 2000 internationally. Since then the device has received FDA approval and has changed the whole paradigm for clinical testing for HIV in the United States. OraQuick Advance® HIV 1/2 has been adopted widely by governmental public health organizations including the Centers for Disease Control (CDC), Substance Abuse Mental Health Services Administration (SAMHSA), and WHO overseas as a tool to identify HIV-infected individuals in nontraditional settings including mobile vans, bathhouses, and emergency room situations and in publicly funded screening programs.

The OraQuick Advance® HIV 1/2 consists of a fairly rigid pad connected to a lateral flow immunochromatographic (LFT) test strip. The user swabs the area under the lips and around the top of the gum line for a few seconds in order to collect an adequate specimen. The sample device is then immersed in a buffer/reagent solution in a tube provided by OraSure and the buffer allowed to migrate up and onto the LTF test strip embedded in the device. After 20 min the results of the (qualitative) test are read. If a single line is observed, the sample is negative. If two lines appear, the result is classified as a "preliminary positive" result until the result can be confirmed by a more accurate test (usually Western blot analysis). The performance of OraQuick Advance® is equivalent or better than many FDA-approved ELISA tests for the HIV virus and has become a standard for diagnosis in the industry.

In 2012, the FDA-approved OraSure Technologies' Biological License Application

(BLA) submission allowing for the first time home users to purchase the OraQuick Advance® kit to test themselves for HIV in the privacy of their own homes. The over-the-counter approval for OraQuick Advance® HIV 1/2 has catalyzed new activity in the oral diagnostics arena, which eventually will result in the development and commercialization of a new generation of saliva-based lateral flow (LTF) assays that "piggyback" on a number of available enabling technology platforms.

Chembio Diagnostics, Inc. (Long Island, NY, www.chembio.com) followed OraSure becoming only the second company to achieve FDA approval status for a rapid HIV diagnostic test using oral fluid samples. At the beginning of 2013, Chembio obtained FDA approval for its "Dual Path Platform (DPP)" point-of-care HIV antibody test. This device accepts a number of sample types including saliva, serum, fingerstick whole blood, venous whole blood, or plasma specimens. In the case of oral fluid specimens, a swab is used to capture saliva from under the lips around the gum line top and bottom. It is recommended that the swabbing action is done four times around the outside of the gums on the top and bottom of the mouth. The swab is inserted into a buffer tube called a SampleTainer containing a proprietary buffer and the handle of the swab removed by snapping off the head at a carefully positioned notch. Two drops of the saliva buffer mixture is then added to a well (Well 1) on the DPP Oral Fluid HIV 1/2 Device. After 5 min, a secondary buffer reagent is added to a second well (Well 2) and the reaction allowed to proceed to completion. The visual read on the qualitative test is 25–40 min. A positive result is considered presumptively positive for either HIV-1 or HIV-2 and should be confirmed by a secondary method.

Ahead of the anticipated emergence of new oral fluid tests, the author notes the existence of a number of other rapid oral LTF tests. Microimmune in the United Kingdom and its partner at the Public Health Laboratory Branch at Colindale in London (UK) have introduced an oral-based test for measles IgM [50] that may be used for either saliva or serum specimens. The microimmune measles IgM test is a qualitative test that requires oral specimen collection using the ORACOL Oral Swab (Malvern Medical Developments, UK) followed by analysis using LTF strips. Samples are extracted from the ORACOL device and placed on the microimmune IgM LTF strips and incubated for a period of 20 min. The signal line is evaluated relative to a control line. If two lines are present, the test is positive for measles IgM antibodies.

Researchers from the University of Queensland [51] have developed a "one-step homogeneous C-reactive protein assay from saliva." This assay is a bead-based assay using streptavidin-coated donor beads that bind to anti-CRP antibody conjugated to acceptor beads. The assay time is approximately 15 min and the sample required is unstimulated whole saliva. At the time of writing, this assay has not reached the commercialization stage.

Foresite Diagnostics (UK) is now commercializing a rapid saliva kit for the detection of cortisol levels in pigs to determine stress levels [52]. The Foresite kit, developed at the Central Science Laboratory in York (UK), requires four drops (70 µ[mu]L) of pig saliva, collected using a large cotton bud that the pig chews until the pad is saturated. The saliva-soaked pad is then separated from the bud with scissors and placed in a plastic plunging unit (resembling a syringe), which expels up to 1.0 mL of saliva ready for analysis. Results are available in 5 min and read visually as a qualitative test. The device can also be used in a semiquantitative manner using a bench top reader, for instance, a Biodot reader connected to a PC, or alternately one of a number of generic handheld readers capable of quantifying signals on LTF strips.

In August 2013, Oasis Diagnostics® [53] was awarded a Phase II Small Business Innovation and Research grant to complete the development of a test for *human* salivary cortisol levels in its VerOFy® rapid POC platform. VerOFy® is another LTF device that uses an absorbent pad to collect saliva from under the tongue until a sample volume adequacy indicator built into the device changes its appearance (pale yellow-green to dark blue). The test device is removed from the mouth and allowed to sit while the test runs for an additional 10–15 min, after which results are available. VerOFy® may be configured for visual or instrument readout, but in the case of the VerOFy® cortisol test, levels of the hormone are quantified using fluorescently labeled particles that are read by a small, portable reading device known as LIAM™ (Light Image Analysis Module). Results may be downloaded to a Smartphone or PC. The VerOFy® platform may be configured to evaluate multiple biomarkers simultaneously in quantitative fashion.

A team at Rice University headed by Dr. John McDevitt has been pioneering the development of next-generation Lab-on-a-Chip (LOC) systems for oral-based cardiac diagnostics, under a project funded by the NIH/NIDCR through a long-term (U01) grant, among others. The unique approach of the McDevitt group has resulted in the development of the "Texas Bio Nano-chip (NBC)" sensor system [54] that is based upon the use of micro-bead arrays. Using microfabrication tools, McDevitt et al. have been able to micro-etch pits within silicon wafers that have on them a variety of chemically sensitized bead "micro-reactors." The Rice group describes these as "chemical processing units." The NBC has ultra-sensitive multi-analyte detection capabilities in a miniaturized format and has already been adapted to diagnostic tests for cardiac surveillance, electrolytes, sugars, proteins, toxins, antibodies, and others. Tools from the McDevitt initiative are available through a company formed by McDevitt called LabNow, Inc. Other applications in development include tests for periodontitis, C-reactive protein (CRP), CD4 counts in HIV-infected individuals, and oral cancer.

Washington-based Seattle Sensors is working with surface plasmon resonance (SPR) technology and has developed an alternate instrument-based system for the detection of cortisol in saliva [55]. The portable instrument from Seattle Biosensors is based upon the technology developed in the laboratory of Dr. Clement Furlong at the University of Washington using a competitive assay and cortisol-specific monoclonal antibodies, with a six channel (portable) SPR biosensor. The technology is built upon Texas Instruments' Spreeta 2,000 sensor chips and has a published detection limit of 0.36 ng/mL. A pre-purification step in the instrument separates small molecules from larger macromolecules in saliva, prior to sample presentation to the sensor resulting in enhanced sensitivity. The system is reported to be useful for a wide range of applications, particularly detection of small molecules in complex mixtures. Results are available using the technology in 10–20 min, but require a separate (whole) saliva collection process using one of a number of commercially available saliva collection tools.

Drug testing is one particular area where saliva testing has gained a strong foothold, and this may be attributed to the convenience factor of being able to collect samples noninvasively from would-be "drugged" drivers and employees under workplace conditions, for example. Over the last 10 years, many companies have emerged with new innovations, each providing unique methods for detecting the NIDA-5 series of drugs (THC/marijuana, opiates, cocaine, amphetamine/methamphetamine, and PCP), but most still rely on an approach that includes the application of (stalwart) lateral flow technology. A number of companies have had some commercial success, and this may in part be due to the large number of drug tests that are performed in the United States each year. It is estimated that between 50 and 60 million drug tests are performed annually in the United States alone, so even a small fraction of this represents strong revenues for commercial suppliers. There are still technological challenges to be overcome, most notably the ability to detect marijuana effectively in saliva samples at low levels, but despite this, many oral drug tests are processed on a daily basis.

The early leaders in the oral drug testing field were Cozart Biosciences (UK www.concateno.com now Alere, Inc.), Securetec (Germany, www.securetec.net), Branan Medical (www.brananmedical.com), and Mavand (Germany, www.mavand.com).

Cozart/Concateno's early versions of the RapiScan Drug Testing Unit combined saliva collection using the Saliva Diagnostic Systems Omni•SAL® Device with rapid lateral flow test strips that were immediately read on a handheld reading unit (RapiScan). Test results were delivered in 10–15 min for a series of six abused substances. Cozart/Concateno's parent Company (Alere, Inc.) now market an upgraded version of the RapiScan Device, called DDS2, which uses an absorbent pad-based system to collect oral fluids. Once collected the sample is immediately transferred onto a test cartridge on board the DDS2 instrument. Oral fluids mix with buffers in the device and then flow along LTF test strips in the unit. The DDS2 analyzes for five drug classes in 5 min. The results of a recent study [56] are encouraging; however, in 24 % of cases, the DDS2 unit failed to provide a valid result. Cozart's systems have been employed successfully in Europe and Australia in particular.

Securetec AG's DrugWipe 5 S (Germany) is a 10 min test that detects the NIDA-5 panel of drugs following a very rapid collection of specimen. The DrugWipe Device cassette itself houses a unique saliva collection pad that is removed from the cassette and then used to collect saliva by wiping the insides of the moistened cheeks. An indicator dye on the pad changes color from red to yellow signifying that an adequate sample has been collected. The collection pad is placed back in the device cassette, and results are read visually on the test strip in 8 min.

Branan Medical markets the OraTect III as the "first single step" oral fluid drug test. Collection on the OraTect is by means of an absorbent pad connected to the Branan test cassette. The subject rubs the absorbent pad across each cheek 15–20 times, then rubs the tongue 15–20 times then places the absorbent pad under the tongue until a series of blue lines begin to flow and are visible in the test cassette. Results are available for up to six drugs in 5–30 min using the OraTect device.

Mavand offers a multidrug screen known as RapidStat that can detect up to eight drugs in about 6–8 min. Collection of saliva is easy (less than 30 s) using a swab. Once collected the saliva is transferred to sample wells on the Mavand RapidStat Device, which are connected directly to lateral flow test strips embedded in the device.

There are many other devices in the marketplace that successfully test saliva for drugs of abuse, so two additional resources are provided that will enable the reader to learn more about this field.

The European body known as ROSITA (ROadSIde Testing Assessment, www.ROSITA.org) is an independent body responsible for evaluation and validation of tools for drug testing at the roadside, so for further information on salivary devices with applicability in law enforcement screening, the reader is referred to the ROSITA Website.

In addition, Table 3.1 includes Websites for a number of companies marketing other handheld drug tests that are commonly used for substance abuse drug testing in forensics, employment screening, workplace testing, and criminal justice. This list is not comprehensive, but provided as a reference resource only.

Table 3.1 List of representative rapid oral drugs of abuse tests/manufacturers

Manufacturer	Website	Product name
Confirm Biosciences	www.confirmbiosciences.com	SalivaConfirm
Drug Testing America/others	www.drugtestingamerica.com	i-Screen
ASC	www.americanscreeningcorp.com	Discover
American Biomedica Corporation	www.abmc.com	OralStat
JAJ Scientific	www.jajinternational.com	QikTech
Innovacon (Alere)	www.innovaconinc.com	OrALert
Mavand	www.mavand.com	RapidSTAT
Envitec	www.envitec.com	SmartClip
Branan Medical	www.brananmedical.com	Oratect XP
Ulti-med	www.ultimed.org	SalivaScreen
Varian	www.varian.com	OraLab 6
Securetec	www.securetec.net	DrugWipe 6
Express Diagnostics	www.drugcheck.com	SalivaScan

While rapid POC saliva tests are definitely growing in significance and certain tools have made a clear impact, point-of-care diagnosis using oral samples is still in the embryonic phase.

Molecular Platforms

Since the discovery of PCR and other molecular techniques, the use of DNA as a building block for diagnostics has grown rapidly. Market sources estimate that more than 500 million molecular tests are done annually in the United States (2010 numbers) and that this number will grow to 750 million by 2015 [28, 57].

Other statistical reports estimate that the worldwide market for molecular diagnostics was $5.5 billion in 2013 and on a growth curve [58]. Already a small fraction of the estimated 500–750 million tests use saliva as a sample source, particularly in the research and life sciences environments, but trends indicate that as current studies are published confirming the efficacy of saliva as an ideal specimen, the proportion of oral-based tests will rise sharply. In addition, new high-profile research projects targeting salivary RNA (including mRNA and miRNA) and proteins (proteomics) will magnify the interest in oral testing, resulting in new diagnostic areas where saliva will be a specimen of choice. A significant example of this is the recent grant award of more than $5 million to the Wong group at UCLA to examine extracellular RNA in exosomes and other microvesicles in gastric cancer [29].

A recent publication by Gallo et al. [59] has surprisingly shown that the majority of microR-NAs detectable in serum and saliva are concentrated in exosomes, so this is likely to lead to a focus in this area of salivary research.

The literature supports the widespread use of saliva as an ideal medium for SNPs, genotyping, microarrays, genome-wide association studies (GWAS), and other molecular technologies; however, most of the current applications are confined to the life sciences research area. At this time the only clinical test using saliva specimens on an automated platform is the eSensor Warfarin Sensitivity Test, which uses samples collected using the OraGene Saliva DNA Device. Saliva samples are pipetted into a cartridge that fits into the eSensor XT8 multiplex PCR system. Microfluidic chambers in the cartridge deliver diluted specimens to the PCR reaction site. The eSensor XT8 delivers results for multiple genetic mutations (in this case VCORC-1 and CYP2C19) in 30 min.

A number of other tests have been validated to saliva and are available as Lab Developed Tests (LDTs) in the United States. These tests are run in CLIA (Clinical Lab Implementation Amendments Act 1988) certified laboratories, who perform internal validations and obtain state approvals to begin running the tests. This list is not exhaustive, but some of the tests/platforms validated to saliva specimens include human papillomavirus (HPV) and periodontal disease detection at Oral DNA Laboratories (Brentwood TN, now part of Access Genetics), personal genomic profiling at 23andMe (Mountain View, CA), and whole genome sequencing at the Personalized Genome Project (PGP) headed by Dr. George Church at Harvard University. The Mayo Clinic now runs a series of genotyping tests including CYP2C19, CYP2D6, HLA B1502, HLA B5701, UGT1A1, and many others using a single saliva sample. Samples are analyzed using sequencing and single gene/gene mutation techniques.

The literature abounds with new applications for saliva, too many to provide an exhaustive list, but some of the newer molecular tests to be validated to saliva include the InPlex Cystic Fibrosis Test from Hologic (Bedford MA), which simultaneously detects 23 mutations in the cystic fibrosis transmembrane receptor (CFTR) gene and the IVS8/5T/7T/9T markers, the Asuragen AmplideX FMR1 Gene test for Fragile X Syndrome in autism and the multiparameter Affymetrix GeneChip Scanner 3,000 Targeted Genotyping System, capable of detecting close to 3,000 SNPs. In this latter example, saliva was shown to be equivalent or better than blood for genotyping 2,918 SNPs from Human Ch12 (developed during the HapMap Project). Positive results for saliva were also observed with the Affymetrix Drug Metabolism Enzymes and Transporters (DMET) Microarray system. In this example, simultaneous genotyping of a large number of known markers (1,936 markers in 225 genes) was carried out. Earlier work validated the use of saliva on the Illumina Hap370 Microarray technology [60], as well as across two genotyping platforms (the Applied Biosystems Taqman™ and Illumina BeadChip™ genome-wide arrays [61], so it is hoped that over the course of the next few years, some of these and the many other research applications published translate into future clinically relevant tests.

The advent of point-of-care devices for nucleic acid testing (POCMDx) from companies such as TwistDx, Biohelix, Rheonix, Douglas Scientific, Alere, and others could also offer up new opportunities for oral testing in the future. Currently these devices are based upon blood sampling technologies and would clearly benefit from validated noninvasive protocols using saliva.

Conclusion

In summary, the future of saliva testing is extremely bright with a number of exciting and functional techniques offering up noninvasive and cost-effective solutions for diagnosis that will find value in disease diagnosis all over our planet. The number of companies involved in salivary diagnostics has risen sharply over the last 2–3 years, and the industry now looks favorably at opportunities to look at clinically relevant biomarkers in saliva samples. Later in 2014, the first annual North American Saliva Symposium is planned, and it is hoped that this landmark meeting will bring together the greatest minds in the saliva world to share ideas on research and clinical diagnosis. The NIH has embraced saliva as a biologically important specimen, and the FDA has already cleared tests through the 510(k) and PMA processes. The "ice has been broken," and in the eyes of this author, the time of saliva as a mature body fluid has arrived!

References

1. NIH Public Health Service Document "Healthy People 2010". Available at: http://www.healthy.gov/healthypeople/. Accessed 31 May 2014.
2. NIH Budget Proposal for the NIDCR 2006 Lawrence A Tabak DDS, PhD: Presentation to the House Sub-Committee March 9th 2005.
3. Tabak LA. The revolution in biomedical assessment: the development of salivary diagnostics. J Dent Educ. 2001;65(12):1335–9.
4. American Dental Association Position Statement on Oral Fluid Diagnostics. Available at: http://www.ada.org/prof/resources/positions/statements/fluid_diagnostics.asp. Accessed 31 May 2014.
5. International Association of Dental Research [IADR]. http://www.iadr.com/i4a/search.cfm#.UqTeSfRDtrp. Accessed 31 May 2014.
6. FDI Policy Statement on Salivary Diagnostics, Adopted by the General Assembly, Istanbul, Aug 2013. Accessible at: http://www.fdiworlddental.org/media/31116/salivary_diagnostics-2013.pdf. Accessed 31 May 2014.
7. Hu S, Li Y, Wang J, Xie Y, Tjon K, Wolinsky L, Loo RRO, Loo JA, Wong DT, et al. Human salivary proteome and transcriptome. J Dent Res. 2006;85:1129–33.
8. Streckfus CF, Bigler L, Tucci M, Thigpen JT. A Preliminary Study of CA 15-3, c-erbB-2, Epidermal growth factor, Cathepsin D and p53 in saliva of women with breast carcinoma. Cancer Invest. 2000;18(2): 101–9.
9. Streckfus CF, Bigler L. The use of soluble, salivary c-erb-b2 for the detection and post-operative follow-up of breast cancer in women: the results of a five-year translational research study. Adv Dent Res. 2005;18(1):17–24.
10. Streckfus CF, Bigler L, Dellinger TD, Dai X, Kingman A, Thigpen JT. The presence of soluble c-erbB-2 in saliva and serum of women with breast carcinoma: a preliminary study. Clin Cancer Res. 2000;6(6):2363–70.
11. Oral Diagnostics Symposium, Lanier Lakes [Atlanta] 2006. Oral-based diagnostics. Ann N Y Acad Sci. 2007;1098.
12. Boston Business Journal Bioflash, March 18th 2013. Available at: http://www.bizjournals.com/boston/blog/bioflash/2013/03/state-gives-41m-grant-to-build.html. Accessed 31 May 2014.
13. Malamud, Rodriguez-Chavez IR. Saliva as a diagnostic fluid. Dent Clin North Am. 2011;55(1):159–78.
14. Punyadeera C, Slowey PD. Chapter 22: Saliva as an emerging biofluid for clinical diagnosis and applications of MEMS/NEMS in salivary diagnostics. In: Subramani K, Ahmed A, Hartsfield JK, Eds. Nanobiomaterials in clinical dentistry. New York: Elsevier; 2013. p. 453–75. ISBN 978-1-4557-3127-5.
15. Streckfus C, Bigler L. Saliva as a diagnostic fluid. Oral Dis. 2002;8:69–76.
16. Slowey PD. Commercial saliva collections tools. J Calif Dent. 2013;41(2):97–105.
17. Malamud D, Tabak LA, editors. Saliva as a diagnostic fluid, vol. 694. New York: Annals of New York Academy of Sciences; 1992.
18. Samaranayake LP. Saliva tells the body's health. In: Moss S, editor. The benefits of chewing. 2006. p. 24–35.
19. Rollins G. Saliva tests: ready to spit? Clinical Laboratory News. 2008;34(8).

20. Hofman LF. Human saliva as a diagnostic specimen. Am Soc Nutr Sci. 2001;131:1621S–5.
21. Punyadeera C. An often forgotten, but convenient diagnostic fluid. Clinical Laboratory News. 2013;39(1).
22. Why Your Saliva May be the Real Reason You Have Digestive Issues. http://taoofmedicine.com/category/mind-body-medicine/. Accessed 31 May 2014.
23. Mandel ID. A contemporary view of salivary research. Clin Rev Oral Biol Med. 1993;4:599.
24. Kozaki T, Lee S, Nishimura T, Katsuura T, Yasukouchi A. Effects of saliva collection using cotton swabs on melatonin enzyme immunoassay. J Circadian Rhythms. 2011;9:1.
25. Gleeson M, Li T-L. The cotton swab method for human saliva collection: effect on measurements of saliva flow rate and concentration of protein, secretory immunoglobulin A, amylase and cortisol. In: Proceedings of the Physiological Society, Human and Exercise Physiology abstracts, University College London. J Physiol. 2003;547P, PC5.
26. Mohamed R, Campbell J-L, Cooper White J, Dimeski G, Punyadeera C. The impact of saliva collection and processing methods on CRP, IgE and myoglobin immunoassays. Clin Transl Med. 2012;1:19.
27. Shirtcliff EA, Granger DA, Schwartz E, Curran MJ. Use of salivary biomarkers in behavioral research: cotton-based sample collection methods can interfere with salivary immunoassay results. Psychoneuroendocrinology. 2001;26:165–73.
28. Frost and Sullivan report: globalization of IVD companies, summarized in Genetic Engineering News. 1 May 2013;33(9). Available at http://www.slideshare.net/FrostandSullivan/the-globalization-of-in-vitro-diagnostics-markets. Accessed 31 May 2014.
29. http://newsroom.ucla.edu/portal/ucla/ucla-dentistry-receives-5-million246826.aspx. Accessed 31 May 2014.
30. Mese H, Matsuo R. Salivary secretion, taste and hyposalivation. J Oral Rehabil. 2007;34:711–23.
31. Wolff A, Davis RL. Universal collector for submandibular and sublingual saliva. US Patent Number 5,050,616.
32. Wolff A, Begleiter A, Moskona D. A novel system of human submandibular and sublingual saliva collection. J Dent Res. 1997;76(11):1782–6.
33. Morales I, Dominguez P, López RO. Devices for saliva collection from the major salivary glands. Results in normal subjects. Rev Med Chil. 1998;126(5):538–47.
34. Morales I, Urzūa-Orellana B, Aguilera S, Dominguez P, López RO. Patterns and variability of in electrophoretic polypeptide profiles of human saliva in a healthy population. J Physiol Biochem. 2006;62(3):179–88.
35. Morales I, Urzūa-Orellana B, Dominguez P, Retamales P. Available at: http://www.captura.uchile.cl/bitstream/handle/2250/7027/MoralesB_Irene.pdf?sequence=1. Accessed 31 May 2014.
36. Hanning S, Motio L, Medlicott NJ, Swindells S. A device for the collection of submandibular saliva. N Z Dent J. 2012;108(1):4–8.
37. Bauman R, DeBoer J. A modification of the altered cast technique. J Prosthet Dent. 1982;47:212–3.
38. Nederfors T, Dahlöf C. A modified device for collection and flow rate measurement of submandibular and sublingual saliva. Eur J Oral Sci. 1993;101(4):210–4.
39. Block P, Brotman SA. A method of submaxillary saliva without cannulization. N Y State Dent J. 1962;28:116–9.
40. Wong DT. Salivary diagnostics. Ames: Wiley-Blackwell; 2008. ISBN 978-0-8138-1333-2.
41. Jiang J, Park NJ, Hu S, Wong DT. A universal pre-analytic solution for concurrent stabilization of salivary proteins, RNA and DNA at ambient temperature. Arch Oral Biol. 2009;54:268–73.
42. Park NJ, Yu T, Nabili V, Brinkman BMN, Henry S, Wang J, Wong DT. RNAprotect saliva: an optimal room temperature stabilization reagent for the salivary transcriptome. Clin Chem. 2006;52(12):2303–4.
43. Kurth A. Potential biohazard risk from infectious tissue and culture cells preserved with RNAlater™. Clin Chem. 2007;53(7):1389–90.
44. http://www.invitek.de/products_and_service/products. Accessed 31 May 2014.
45. http://www.norgenbiotek.com/display-product.php?ID=385. Accessed 31 May 2014.
46. http://www.salimetrics.com/articles/print/collecting-and-handling-saliva-for-dna-samples. Accessed 31 May 2014.
47. Thomadaki K, Helmerhorst EJ, Tian N, Sun X, Siqueira WL, Walt DR, Oppenheim FG. Whole-saliva proteolysis and its impact on salivary diagnostics. J Dent Res. 2011;90(11):1325–30.
48. Xiao H, Wong DT. Proteomic analysis of microvesicles in human saliva by gel electrophoresis with liquid chromatography-mass spectrometry. Anal Chim Acta. 2012;722:63–9.
49. Esser D, Alvarez-Llamas G, Dr Vries MP, Weening D, Vonk RJ, Roelofsen H. Sample stability and protein composition of saliva: implications for its use as a diagnostic fluid. Biomark Insights. 2008;3:25–37.
50. Warrener L, Slibinskas R, Chua KB, Brown KE, Nigatu W, Sasnauskas K, Samuel D, Brown D. A point-of-care test for measles diagnosis: detection of measles-specific IgM antibodies and viral nucleic acid. Bull World Health Organ. 2011;89:675–82.
51. Punyadeera C, Domeski G, Kostner K, Beyerlein P, Cooper-White J. One-step homogeneous C-reactive protein assay for saliva. J Immunol Methods. 2011;373:19–25.
52. Lane J, Flint J, Danks C. The development of a rapid diagnostic test for cortisol in the saliva of pigs. Report for the UK Government Department of the Environment Food and Rural Affairs [DEFRA]; London, England: 2010.
53. NIH Awarded Grant [NCCAM, 2R44AT006634-04]. VerOFy®, a new tool to improve productivity and reduce costs for stress research. Oasis Diagnostics Corporation, Aug 2013.

54. Weigum SE, Floriano PN, Cristodoulides N, McDevitt JT. Toward the development of a lab-on-a-chip dual function leucocyte and C-reactive protein analysis method for the assessment of inflammation and cardiac risk. Lab-on-a-Chip. 2007;7:995–1003.
55. Stevens RC, Soelberg SD, Near S, Furlong CE. Detection of cortisol in saliva with a flow-filtered, portable surface resonance biosensor system. Anal Chem. 2008;80(17):6747–51.
56. Moore C, Kelley-Baker T, Lacey J. Field testing of the Alere DDS2 mobile test system for drugs in oral fluid. J Anal Toxicol. 2013;37:305–7.
57. Molecular Diagnostics Market Report 2009 Research and Markets Limited Report. Available at: http://www.researchandmarkets.com/product/65f2db/molecular_diagnostics_markets. Accessed 31 May 2014.
58. Kalorama Information Market Report: World Molecular Diagnostics Market Update. Available at: http://www.kalroamainformation.com/Molecular-Diagnostics-Month-7969379/. Accessed 31 May 2014.
59. Gallo A, Tandon M, Alevizos I, Illie GG. The majority of microRNAs detectable in serum and saliva is concentrated in exosomes. PLoS One. 2012;7(3):e30679. www.Plosone.org.
60. Bahlo M, Stankovich J, Danoy P, Hickey PF, Taylor BV, Browning SR, et al. Saliva-derived DNA performs well in large-scale, high-density, single-nucleotide polymorphism microarray studies. Cancer Epidemiol Biomarkers Prev. 2010;19:794–8.
61. Abraham JE, Maranian MJ, Spiteri I, Russell R, Ingle S, Luccarini C, et al. Saliva samples are a viable alternative to blood samples as a source of DNA for high throughput genotyping. BMC Genomics. 2012;5(19):1–6.

Salivary Omics

4

Marta Alexandra Mendonça Nóbrega Cova,
Massimo Castagnola, Irene Messana,
Tiziana Cabras, Rita Maria Pinho Ferreira,
Francisco Manuel Lemos Amado,
and Rui Miguel Pinheiro Vitorino

Abstract

Salivary diagnostics has become an attractive research field to assess physiological and pathological states from prognosis, condition onset, and diagnosis to monitoring and therapeutic outcomes. Saliva, as a diagnostic biofluid, besides being a noninvasive method, offers a cost-effective approach to healthcare providers and also can be used for the screening of large populations. The advancements and discovery of high-throughput techniques for the identification and quantification of several types of biomarkers, including salivary DNA, RNA, proteins, and metabolites, were essential for salivary diagnostics development. In this review we explored the biomedical applications of saliva summarizing the salivary candidate biomarkers found using genomic, transcriptomic, and proteomic approaches for oral and systemic diseases. Despite all achievements obtained so far using saliva as diagnostic fluid, which strengthen its position as an alternative diagnostic fluid, a cooperative effort must be performed in the next decade in order to optimize and standardize the methodological protocols and validate the potential salivary biomarkers through long-term longitudinal and cohort studies in large-scale population.

M.A.M.N. Cova, MSc (✉) • R.M.P. Ferreira, PhD
F.M.L. Amado, PhD
Department of Chemistry,
University of Aveiro,
Aveiro, Portugal
e-mail: marta.cova@ua.pt

M. Castagnola, PhD
Istituto di Biochimica e di Biochimica Clinica,
Università Cattolica, Rome, Italy

I. Messana, PhD
Department of Life and Environmental Sciences,
University of Cagliari, Monserrato, Italy

T. Cabras, PhD
Dipartimento di Scienza della Vita e dell'Ambiente,
Università degli Studi di Cagliari, Cagliari, Italy

R.M.P. Vitorino, PhD
QOPNA, Mass Spectrometry Center, Department
of Chemistry, University of Aveiro, Aveiro, Portugal

C.F. Streckfus (ed.), *Advances in Salivary Diagnostics*,
DOI 10.1007/978-3-662-45399-5_4, © Springer-Verlag Berlin Heidelberg 2015

Introduction

The most life-threatening diseases are diagnosed at advanced stages due to the presence of clinical features with poor diagnostic value that do not distinguish well between other diseases with similar signs and symptoms (nonspecific pathologic features), and in some cases, comorbidity is associated. In this last possibility, one condition may alter the presentation of another or may provide an explanation for the presenting symptoms. The more promptly the disease is diagnosed, the more likelihood the patient has to be successfully cured or controlled, improving the patient's quality of life. Therefore, several efforts and researches have been focused on enhancing diagnostic methods and its accuracy. The search for a noninvasive approach to assess physiological states, detect disease initiation and progression, or monitor therapeutic outcomes became a growing trend in healthcare research since it offers financial advantages to healthcare providers and embraces a greater number of outpatients [1]. In this field, saliva appears as an attractive biofluid for surveillance of general health status and diseases because it is easily available in a noninvasive and painless manner [2].

Saliva is a hypotonic fluid found in the oral cavity, composed of water (99 %), a complex mixture of secretory products (organic and inorganic) from the salivary glands, and other substances coming from the oropharynx, upper airway, gastrointestinal reflux, gingival sulcus fluid, food deposits, and blood-derived compounds [3]. Saliva is essential for the accomplishment of multiple physiological functions encompassing lubrication, buffering action, maintenance of tooth integrity, chewing, initial digestion of some foods, swallowing, tissue hydration and lubrication, speech, wound healing, and antibacterial and antifungal activity [4]. To accomplish these functions, saliva harbors an extensive spectrum of proteins, peptides, nucleic acids, electrolytes, and hormones that originate from multiple local and systemic sources. So, it is not surprising that scientific and clinical interest nowadays has been given to saliva envisioning its potential screening value and risk assessment of several oral and systemic diseases.

Achievements on Salivary Diagnostics

The field of salivary diagnostics arose in the early 1900s, through Michael's [5] and Kirk's [6] evaluation of saliva samples to identify biomarkers for rheumatism and gout (Fig. 4.1). After that, Irwin Mandel [7], in 1967, reported increased salivary calcium concentrations in cystic fibrosis patients, emphasizing saliva as an important diagnostic fluid. In addition, Oppenheim [8] in 1970 identified for the first time serum components in saliva. In the following decades, saliva-based diagnostics increased dramatically due to achievements of high-throughput approaches afforded by mass spectrometry innovations and bioinformatics [9].

In 2002, the application of salivary diagnostics for oral and systemic diseases received a major boost as a result of funding support by the National Institute of Dental and Craniofacial Research (NIDCR). This initiative was designed to establish collaborative research between engineers and scientists to develop point-of-care diagnosis platforms for rapid detection and analysis of salivary biomarkers [10]. Therefore, to support clinical applications of saliva, efforts have been conducted in the development of five salivary areas: genomics, transcriptomics, proteomics, metabolomics, and microbiomics [11]. Salivary metabolome offers a promising clinical strategy by characterizing the association between salivary analytes and a particular disease. In 2010, Sugimoto et al. [12] identified oral, breast, and pancreatic cancer-specific profiles using capillary electrophoresis time-of-flight mass spectrometry (CE-TOF-MS). Regarding salivary microbiome, in 2012, Farrell et al. [13] observed variations of salivary microbiota related to pancreatic cancer and chronic pancreatitis. As a result of the advancements in novel technological means (e.g., quantitative real-time polymerase chain reaction (qRT-PCR), mass spectrometry approaches, bioinformatics tools, and microfluidic techniques), point-of-care (POC) devices and rapid tests for saliva have been integrated as part of disease diagnosis, clinical monitoring, and patient care management [14]. There are

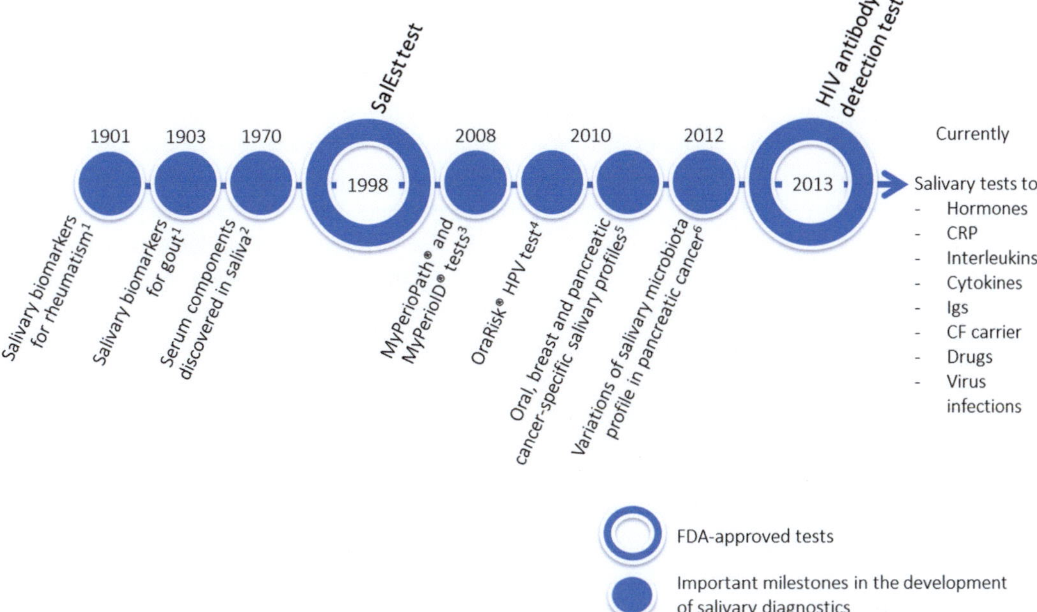

Fig. 4.1 The landmarks in the development of salivary diagnostics. (*1*) Salivary rheumatoid-specific antibody test is used for rheumatism diagnosis, whereas salivary uric acid test is used for gout diagnosis and monitoring. (*2*) The disclosure of serum components in saliva opened doors to the development of diagnostic test for oral and systemic diseases through saliva specimen. (*3*) MyPerioPath® is a salivary test that identifies the type and concentration of specific perio-pathogenic bacteria that are known to cause periodontal disease. MyPerioID® salivary test identifies individual genetic susceptibility to periodontal disease. (*4*) OraRisk® HPV test recognizes in saliva the type(s) of oral HPV that could potentially lead to oral cancer. (*5*) Salivary tumor marker panels were developed to aid in specific cancer diagnosis. (*6*) There is a specific salivary DNA test for a set of bacteria that correlates with pancreatic cancer. *CF* cystic fibrosis, *CRP* C-reactive protein, *Igs* immunoglobulins, *HIV* human immunodeficiency virus, *HPV* human papillomavirus, *SalEst test* salivary estradiol test

already two US Food and Drug Administration (FDA)-approved products (Fig. 4.1) that use saliva for diagnostic purposes: for human immunodeficiency virus (HIV) antibody detection (OraQuick ADVANCE Rapid HIV-1/2 Antibody Test, OraSure Technologies) and for the measurement of estradiol (SalEst, Biex Inc.) for the prediction of premature birth [11]. In addition, several saliva laboratory-based tests are available to assess the presence of drugs, hormones, viruses, and other microbial components (Fig. 4.1). For instance, to assess periodontal status of a patient in a periodontitis setting, there are tests for periodontal pathogens (MyPerioPath, OralDNA Labs, Brentwood, Tenn.) and for assessing the patient's genetic risk of developing the disease (MyPerioID PST, OralDNA Labs). Another important salivary test is the OraRisk HPV test (OralDNA Labs), which identifies the type or types of oral human papillomavirus (HPV), a mucosal virus that may give rise to oral cancers [3, 15].

The importance of salivary proteome, transcriptome, and genome in the discovery, development, and validation of disease biomarkers will be critically analyzed in more detail as follows.

Genomics and Transcriptomics: DNA and RNA Analysis

Salivary genomics and transcriptomics arise as interesting research fields once saliva provides a convenient source of microbial and human DNA and RNA, owning highly informative and discriminatory evidences of physiological and pathological conditions. This awareness coupled with the ability to harness genomic and transcriptomic information by high-throughput technology platforms, such as microarrays and next-generation sequencing, positions salivary genomics and transcriptomics in the detection of specific disease states [16, 17].

Methodologies Used in Salivary Genomics and Transcriptomics

The starting point in the genomic and transcriptomic analysis of human saliva is sample collection followed by the extraction of salivary RNA or DNA. The extraction of the nucleic acids comprises cell disruption with a buffer that includes a nonionic detergent, and the resultant lysate is used for the isolation of DNA or RNA—most often by organic and/or solid-phase extraction. There are several kits available that allow this extraction (e.g., Oragene self-collection and QIAamp viral RNA kits), and more interestingly, there already exist kits that perform the RNA and DNA co-extraction (e.g., Promega DNA IQ™ System) [18–21]. The co-extraction of the two nucleic acids minimizes sample requirements and can eliminate the need for two separate extractions when the aim of the study is genomic and transcriptomic analysis [18]. For RNA profiling, the supernatant phase of saliva (CFS) is typically used instead of whole saliva (WS) since saliva naturally contains microorganisms, oral epithelial cells, and extraneous substances that are minimized in CFS samples [22, 23]. Salivary DNA or RNA often contains large amounts of bacterial nucleic acids, and the relative proportion of human DNA or RNA might be difficult to determine [24].

After the isolation of the nucleic acids, it is important to assess the integrity and quality of the sample—typically by reverse transcription followed by polymerase chain reaction (PCR) or quantitative PCR (RT-PCR or RT-qPCR) [20, 25]. This step also allows the amplification of DNA and RNA, which is important for further studies. In order to identify the genome or transcriptome profile of the isolated samples, two major technologies are employed: next-generation sequencing (NGS) or microarray platforms [24, 26–28]. NGS is a term used to describe a number of different modern sequencing technologies (e.g., Roche 454 sequencing) that grant the sequence of DNA and RNA more quickly and economically than the previously used Sanger sequencing. Moreover, the recent advances in NGS technologies engender an exhaustive analysis of genomes and transcriptomes [29].

In the last years, efforts have been made to improve the current standard operating procedures either on salivary genomics or salivary transcriptomics. One of the promising advances relies in a streamlined direct saliva transcriptome analysis (DSTA), which is characterized by the use of CFS instead of isolated mRNA for saliva transcriptomic detection. All the following procedures (including processing, stabilization, and storage of samples) are performed at ambient temperature without a stabilizing reagent [30]. With these new technologies available, the salivary DNA and RNA became interesting samples for biomarker researches and biomedical applications.

Biomedical Applications of Salivary Genomics

DNA holding the information of an individual's genome, oral microbiota, and infecting DNA viruses are present in saliva and also reflect the presence or absence of specific gene mutations and methylation status. Thus, salivary genome analysis can provide insights into the presence of pathogens and alterations in gene profiles that directly reflect pathological conditions such as cancer [31]. Over the last decade, it has been proved that genomic DNA extracted from saliva may be used in a clinical and research environment since salivary DNA is equivalent in quantity and purity to those obtained from blood [32–34].

Salivary DNA has been investigated to assist clinicians in the early diagnosis of patients with a family history of diseases such as Parkinson's and other life-threatening diseases, including certain types of cancer and cystic fibrosis [35]. One of the major aims of salivary genomics is to find a gene or a gene mutation or another type of alteration (such as aberrant methylation) underlying a specific disorder (genotyping analysis and mutational screening of disease-causing genes).

Table 4.1 Salivary DNA markers identified for several oral and systemic diseases

Pathophysiological condition	Type of sample	Methodology	Major findings	Refs.
Dental caries	Unstimulated WS	DNA extraction kit + real-time PCR	Increased *Streptococcus mutans* genomic DNA	[37]
Oral squamous cell carcinoma (OSCC)	Unstimulated WS	DNA extraction kit + PCR + DNA sequencing	Mutation of p53 codon 63	[38]
Pityriasis rosea	Unstimulated WS	DNA extraction kit + nested PCR	Presence of HHV-6 and HHV-7 viral DNA	[39]
Head and neck squamous cell carcinoma (HNSCC)	Unstimulated WS	Cloned p53 sequences amplified by PCR + radiolabeled oligonucleotide probes	Mutations in p53 gene; promoter hypermethylation patterns: p16; MGMT; DAP-K; increased mtDNA content	[40–42]
		DNA extraction kit + PCR Real-time qPCR		
Pancreatic cancer	Unstimulated WS	DNA extraction kit + microarray + qPCR	*Atopobium parvulum*; *Granulicatella adiacens*; *Neisseria elongata*; *Prevotella nigrescens*; *Streptococcus australis*; *Streptococcus mitis* bacterial DNA specific variation	[13]

MGMT O^6-methylguanine-DNA-methyltransferase, *DAP-K* dead-associated protein kinase, *mtDNA* mitochondrial DNA, *HHV-6* human herpesvirus type 6, *HHV-7* human herpesvirus type 7, *PCR* polymerase chain reaction

On the other hand, salivary DNA can be used to identify specific bacterial species that triggers an inflammatory response [36]. Thus, DNA tests can identify the bacterial targets for therapy and assist in monitoring the concentration of these pathogens during therapy. For instance, the possibility of quantification of bacteria through salivary DNA (Table 4.1) without cultivation of samples, which is laborious and lengthy, represents a useful and practical diagnosis approach of infectious diseases. Nevertheless, salivary DNA is mainly applied in pharmacogenomic and epidemiologic studies and for forensics [16].

The search for genetic determinants underlying common diseases such as cardiovascular diseases, cancer, osteoporosis, and diabetes can also be revolutionized through large population-based epidemiologic studies utilizing salivary DNA instead of blood DNA [43]. Salivary DNA markers have become appealing since the presence of tumor markers in saliva has been reported (Table 4.1), such as aberrant methylation of tumor suppressor genes in cancer cells [31].

Biomedical Applications of Salivary Transcriptomics

Alongside DNA, RNA can also be found in saliva because salivary RNAs are protected by specific mechanisms against the saliva nucleases including association with macromolecules (such as mucins and salivary chaperone Hsp70) and exosomes [20, 44, 45]. Even more interestingly, saliva contains not only transcripts of genes related to immune defense, digestion, and electrolyte and water metabolism as expected but also transcripts of most metabolic processes in the body [26]. Therefore, the transcriptomic signature holds valuable information to discover novel biomarkers for oral and systemic diseases. In 2004, the human salivary transcriptome in CFS was discovered by applying microarray technology [26].

It was discovered that RNA in saliva exists from partial to full-length forms and it is of vital importance to understand the characteristics of salivary RNA network in order to use RNA markers in clinical diagnosis and surveillance. Furthermore, different types of RNA coexist in

Table 4.2 Salivary RNA markers identified for several oral and systemic diseases

Pathophysiological condition	Type of sample	Methodology	Major findings	Refs.
Breast cancer	Unstimulated CFS	RNA extraction and amplification kits + microarray + RT-qPCR	Upregulated: CSTA; TPT1; IGF2BP1; GRM1; GRIK1; H6PD; MDM4; S100A8	[47]
Esophageal cancer	Unstimulated CFS	RNA extraction and amplification kits + microarray + RT-qPCR	Upregulated: miRNA-10b; miRNA-144; miRNA-21; miRNA-451	[48]
Malignant parotid gland tumors	Unstimulated CFS	RNA extraction and amplification kits + microarray + RT-qPCR	Upregulated: hsa-miRNA-132; hsa-miRNA-15b; mmu-miRNA-140; hsa-miRNA-223	[49]
Oral squamous cell carcinoma (OSCC)	Unstimulated CFS	RNA extraction and amplification kits + microarray + qPCR	Upregulated: DUSP1; H3F3A; IL1B; IL8; OAZ1, S100P; SAT	[50]
Resective pancreatic cancer	Unstimulated CFS	RNA extraction and amplification kits + microarray + qPCR	Upregulated: KRAS, MBD3L2, ACRV1 Downregulated: DPM1	[51]
Sjögren's syndrome (SS)	Stimulated CFS	RNA extraction and amplification kits + microarray + real-time qPCR	Upregulated: G1P2; proteasome subunit β(beta) type 9; guanylate-binding protein 2, IFN-induced protein 44; β(beta)2-microglobulin	[52]
Sleep deprivation	Unstimulated CFS	RNA extraction and amplification kits + microarray + qPCR	Upregulated: salivary amylase	[53]

ACRV1 acrosomal vesicle protein 1, *CSTA* cystatin A, *DPM1* dolichyl-phosphate mannosyltransferase polypeptide 1, *DUSP1* dual-specificity phosphatase 1, *G1P2* ISG15 ubiquitin-like modifier, *GRIK1* glutamate receptor, ionotropic, kainate 1, *GRM1* glutamate receptor, metabotropic 1, *H3F3A* H3 histone, family 3A, *H6PD* hexose-6-phosphate dehydrogenase, *IFN* interferon, *IGF2BP1* insulin-like growth factor 2 mRNA-binding protein 1, *IL1B* interleukin-1 β(beta), *IL8* interleukin-8, *KRAS* V-Ki-ras2 Kirsten rat sarcoma viral oncogene homologue, *MBD3L2* methyl-CpG-binding domain protein 3-like 2, *MDM4* Mdm4 p53-binding protein homologue (mouse), *OAZ1* ornithine decarboxylase antizyme 1, *S100A8* S100 calcium-binding protein A8, *S100P* S100 calcium-binding protein P, *SAT* serine acetyltransferase, *TPT1* tumor protein, translationally controlled 1

saliva leading to the saliva RNA interactome concept. They all have implicated roles in gene regulation, and therefore, a complete characterization of mRNAs, microRNAs (miRNAs), small nucleolar RNAs (snoRNAs), and other RNA species found in saliva should be made in order to understand their impact and interplay in biological and pathological processes [16, 26]. The salivary mRNAs are of extreme importance because viral mRNA can be detected in saliva, which indicates viral infections [46]. miRNAs have gained increased attention in the salivary diagnostics field due to their roles in cell growth, differentiation, apoptosis, host-pathogen interactions, stress responses, and immune function. These short RNA transcripts are differentially expressed in several cancer cell types compared with normal cells and may accurately distinguish poorly differentiated tumors [31]. Consequently, miRNA cancer biomarkers are potentially very powerful in cancer diagnoses using salivary tests. The utility of salivary RNAs in biomedical applications is being explored, and candidate markers for several diseases have been found (Table 4.2).

In the near future, focus should be given to specific salivary RNA types, such as miRNAs and snoRNAs, to achieve more specificity and sensitivity in clinical diagnostics and to ensure a complete profile of the transcriptomic signature in certain pathophysiological conditions. For instance, salivary miRNAs found in exosomes seem to hold great interest as biomarkers for autoimmune disorders in order to reduce the probability of false-negative results [54].

The future of salivary genomics and transcriptomics relies not only in the optimization and standardization of methodological protocols but also in the enlargement of studied populations in cross-sectional longitudinal studies to validate and translate DNA and RNA markers for routine clinical analysis.

Salivary Proteomics

The term "proteomics" concerns the study of the entire protein asset of a specific biofluid, cell type, or tissue. It represents a tool for a better understanding of protein function and how it interacts with other proteins, envisioning the assessment of health or disease states [55]. Saliva proteome holds several essential roles, such as digestive processes, antimicrobial activity, ion storage, microorganism aggregation, tooth surface protection, lubrication, and buffering actions [56]. A life cycle of a salivary protein comprises the basic cellular process of protein biosynthesis and posttranslational modifications—PTMs (comprehending glycosylation, phosphorylation, proteolysis, and sulfation)—prior to and after secretion of the protein into the oral cavity. Therefore, the salivary proteome is highly dynamic and variable depending on time, nature, and number of agents capable of inducing protein modifications [57].

Proteomic studies allow the analysis of salivary composition, investigating the major families of salivary proteins, the different contributions of salivary glands, and the physiological and pathological modifications of saliva. Currently, the salivary proteome is essentially characterized with more than 3,000 different proteins already identified [55]. The major salivary protein families involve salivary proline-rich proteins (PRPs), histatins, statherin, cystatins, and α(alpha)-amylases. Whereas these protein classes can be considered specific of saliva, there are many other proteins present in whole saliva that are common to other organs and biofluids such as mucins; lysozyme; lactoferrin; agglutinin; peroxidase; carbonic anhydrase; serum proteins like salivary IgA, IgG, and albumin; proteins of the S100 class and other calcium-binding proteins; defensins; and thymosin β(beta)4 [57, 58]. Remarkably, approximately 20 % of total salivary proteins are also seen in plasma and show comparable functional diversity and disease linkage [59]. This fact abets the potential of salivary proteomics in the diagnosis and monitoring not only of oral diseases but also of systemic conditions.

Salivary proteomics aims to discriminate between healthy and pathological states through the identification of proteins that are uniquely correlated to a specific state [60]. The understanding of each protein's role in the oral cavity will contribute to improving the scientific knowledge of several oral and systemic diseases' pathogenesis.

Methodologies Used in Salivary Proteomics

The application of salivary proteins in the biomedical field as disease markers has only been possible due to the combination of conceptual innovations and technical breakthroughs in separation techniques, mass spectrometry, and bioinformatics for data analysis and integration. Proteomic approaches can be divided into four main classes: structural, expression, functional, and targeted proteomics [61]. All these types of proteomics can be applied to saliva in order to find patterns of salivary proteins that can be used for diagnosis, prognosis, monitoring, and therapeutic targets of human diseases. On one hand, the structural characterization (structural proteomics) of proteins and their interactions and assemblies may be important for drug targets [62]. On the other hand, the quantification (expression proteomics) and functional characterization (functional proteomics) of salivary proteins can assist in a specific and reliable diagnosis. Targeted proteomics is a more recent approach and focuses on the study of only one or a preselected group of proteins in order to evaluate its importance in a certain physiological or pathological event. Regarding salivary proteomics, all these approaches can be employed to enhance the knowledge of disease pathogenesis and to find salivary biomarkers.

Overall, proteome characterization is achieved through different tools classified in top-down or bottom-up proteomics. In top-down proteomics approach, proteins are analyzed without proteolytic digestion. Hence, intact proteins are introduced into the mass spectrometer (MS), and after ionization the ions generated are subjected to separation, fragmentation, and automated interpretation of MS data, yielding both the molecular weight of the intact protein and the protein fragmentation ladders [63]. In contrast, the bottom-up proteomics approach involves enzymatic and/or chemical cleavage of protein-originating peptides. The peptide analysis requires chromatographic or electrophoretic strategies to decrease the complexity of peptide mixtures before MS analysis [64]. In order to characterize the salivary proteome, both approaches have been widely applied to saliva, contributing toward demystifying its complexity.

The salivary proteomics workflow is divided in sample preparation, protein separation, characterization, and functional validation. The first step in the salivary proteome characterization is sample preparation that encompasses all the experimental steps performed to obtain a protein extract. Secondly, the separation of proteins is required, and the major approaches utilized can be divided into gel-based approaches (e.g., 2-dimensional gel electrophoresis (2-DE)) and gel-free-based approaches (e.g., liquid chromatography). After the separation step, the proteins are analyzed by mass spectrometry, commonly matrix-assisted laser desorption/ionization time-of-flight with tandem mass spectrometry (MALDI-TOF-MS/MS) or electrospray ionization with tandem mass spectrometry (ESI-MS/MS) [55]. The main strategies for protein identification by MS comprise database searching, de

novo sequencing, and peptide sequence tag [65]. Database searching with MASCOT [66] and SEQUEST [67] is the most popular. Protein quantification in gel-free-based approaches is based on labeling methods, the most common being the isobaric tagging for relative and absolute quantitation (iTRAQs) or label-free methods based on the comparison of related peak areas between MS runs [68, 69]. The last step of a proteomic workflow stands in functional validation through standard methods as western blot and enzyme-linked immunosorbent assay (ELISA). With the plethora of technologies available for proteomic studies, the choice of the methodological strategy is based on sample amount and on the goal of the study. If the aim is the characterization of salivary glycoproteome or phosphoproteome in a certain pathological condition, such as periodontitis, enrichment strategies should be employed.

Biomedical Applications of Salivary Proteomics

The comprehensive analysis of human saliva proteome, through the application of the different methodologies described previously, will contribute to the understanding of disease pathogenesis and might provide a foundation for the recognition of potential disease biomarkers. Indeed, clinical proteomics tries to highlight the relationships between proteins and defined physiological conditions connecting these biomolecules to disease diagnosis, monitoring of therapies, therapeutic outcomes, and disease progression [59]. Indeed, several protein candidate markers have been described in several oral and systemic diseases as dental caries, periodontitis, Sjögren's syndrome (SS), oral squamous cell carcinoma (OSCC), head and neck squamous cell carcinoma (HNSCC), oral lichen planus (OLP), autism spectrum disorders, diabetes, breast cancer, and lung cancer (Table 4.3).

Analyzing the biomarkers highlighted in Table 4.3, it is observed that certain biomarkers are present in more than one disease (e.g., annexin A1 in HNSCC and lung cancer).

Table 4.3 Salivary protein markers identified for several oral and systemic diseases

Pathophysiological condition	Type of sample	Methodology	Major findings	Refs.
Aggressive periodontitis	Unstimulated WS	2DE-ESI-MS/MS	Increased: albumin; Ig γ(gamma)2 chain C region; Ig α(alpha)2 chain C region; vitamin D-binding protein; amylase; zinc α(alpha)2 glycoprotein Decreased: lactotransferrin; elongation factor 2; 14-3-3 sigma; SPLUNC-2; carbonic anhydrase VI	[70]
Autism spectrum disorders	Unstimulated WS	RP-HPLC-ESI-MS	Hypophosphorylation: histatin 1; statherin; entire and truncated isoforms of aPRPs	[71]
Breast cancer	Unstimulated WS	Enzyme-linked immunosorbent assay 2DE-MALDI-MS/MS	Increased: c-erbB-2; carbonic anhydrase VI	[47, 72]
Chronic periodontitis	Unstimulated WS	2DE-MALDI-MS/MS and LC-ESI-MS/MS	Increased: albumin; hemoglobin; Ig proteolysis Decreased: cystatin	[73]
Cystic fibrosis	Unstimulated WS	RIA and RRA assays	Present a less efficient form of salivary EGF	[74]
Dental caries	Unstimulated WS	2DE-MALDI-MS/MS IEF-SDS-PAGE-MALDI-TOF/TOF	Increased: amylase, Ig A, lactoferrin Decreased: lipocalin, cystatins S; cystatins SN; statherin; truncated cystatin S	[75, 76]
Gingivitis	Unstimulated WS	2DE-MALDI-MS/MS and LC-ESI-MS/MS	Increased: albumin; amylase	[77]
Head and neck squamous cell carcinoma (HNSCC)	Unstimulated WS	SDS-PAGE-MALDI-MS/MS	Increased: annexin A1; β(beta)- and γ(gamma)-actin; cytokeratins 4 and 13; zinc finger proteins; P53 pathway proteins; β(beta)-fibrin; S100A9; transferrin; Ig heavy chain constant region γ(gamma); cofilin-1; α(alpha)-1B-glycoprotein; complement factor B	[78–80]
	Stimulated WS	2DE-MALDI-TOF-MS SDS-PAGE-LC-MS/MS	Decreased: cystatin S; parotid secretory protein; poly-4-hydrolase β(beta)-subunit	
Lung cancer	Unstimulated WS	2DE-(DIGE)-MALDI-MS/MS	Increased: annexin A1; HBA2; cystatins D and S; zinc α(alpha)2 glycoprotein; human calprotectin Decreased: carbonic anhydrase VI; lipocalin; S100A9; S100A8	[81]
Oral lichen planus (OLP)	Unstimulated WS	2DE-MALDI-TOF-MS	Increased: urinary prekallikrein Decreased: PLUNC	[82]

(continued)

Table 4.3 (continued)

Pathophysiological condition	Type of sample	Methodology	Major findings	Refs.
Oral squamous cell carcinoma (OSCC)	Unstimulated WS Stimulated WS	2DE-MALDI-TOF-MS SELDI RP-LC-MS/MS ELISA (sandwich type) Multiplex bead-based flow cytometric assay Real-time qPCR + ELISA	Increased: transferrin; truncated cystatin SA-1; S100A9, profiling, CD59, catalase; M2BP; soluble CD44; IL-8; IL-8; IL-1β	[83–88]
Periodontitis	Unstimulated WS	2DE-MALDI-MS/MS 2DE-ESI-MS/MS Enzyme-linked immunosorbent assay	Increased: S100A8; S100A9; S100A6; albumin; Ig γ(gamma)2 chain C region; Ig α(alpha)2 chain C region; vitamin D-binding protein; amylase; zinc α(alpha)2 glycoprotein; MMP-8; IL-1β(beta) Decreased: lactotransferrin, elongation factor 2, 14-3-3 sigma, SPLUNC-2; carbonic anhydrase VI	[70, 89, 90]
Rheumatoid arthritis	Unstimulated WS	2DE-MALDI-MS/MS	Increased: GRP78/BiP	[91]
Sjögren's syndrome (SS)	*Unstimulated WS* Parotid saliva Unstimulated WS	*2DE-MALDI-TOF-MS* SELDI + 2DE-MALDI-TOF-MS 2DE-LC-ESI-MS/MS	Increased: *β(beta)2-microglobulin*; lactoferrin; *Ig kappa light chain*; polymeric Ig receptor; lysozyme C; cystatin C; *α(alpha)-enolase; E-FABP;* amylase; α(alpha)-enolase; actin; carbonic anhydrases I and II Decreased: *carbonic anhydrase VI; amylase precursor*; carbonic anhydrase VI; *G3PDH; SPLUNC-2*; cystatins (S, SA, C, SN, D); carbonic anhydrase VI	[52, 92–94]
Type 1 diabetes	Unstimulated WS	RP-HPLC-ESI-MS	Increased: α(alpha)-defensins 1, 2, and 4; S100A9 Decreased: statherin, histatins 1 and 5	[95]
Type 2 diabetes	Unstimulated WS	2DE-LC-MS/MS	Increased: A1AT, cystatin C, α(alpha)2-macroglobulin; transthyretin	[96, 97]

2DE two-dimensional electrophoresis, *A1AT* α(alpha)1-antitrypsin, *aPRPs* acidic proline-rich proteins, *DIGE* difference gel electrophoresis, *E-FABP* epidermal fatty acid-binding protein, *EGF* epidermal growth factor, *ESI* electrospray ionization, *G3PDH* glyceraldehyde-3-phosphate dehydrogenase, *HBA2* hemoglobin α(alpha)2, *HPLC* high-performance liquid chromatography, *Ig* immunoglobulin, *IL* interleukin, *LC* liquid chromatography, *M2BP* mac-2-binding protein, *MALDI* matrix-assisted laser desorption/ionization, *MMP* matrix metalloproteinase MS/MS tandem mass spectrometry, *PLUNC* palate, lung, and nasal epithelium carcinoma-associated protein, *qPCR* quantitative polymerase chain reaction, *RIA* radioimmunoassays, *RP* reverse phase, *RRA* radioreceptor assays, *SDS-PAGE* Sodium dodecyl sulfate polyacrylamide gel electrophoresis, *SELDI* Surface-enhanced laser desorption/ionization, *SPLUNC-2* short palate, lung, and nasal epithelium clone 2, *TOF* time of flight, *WS* whole saliva

Moreover, accordingly with the proteomic methodology used, the biomarkers found for one particular disease can be different. The first issue can be overcome through the reliance in a panel of proteins as a signature of a certain disease instead of only one protein marker. If valuable data obtained from salivary genomics and transcriptomics come attached with that panel of protein markers found for a specific disease, a reliable, specific, and sensitive diagnostic will be achieved. The second problem is more challenging because it requires a standardization of saliva proteome analysis methodology in order to get more robust and consistent results. Efforts through this standardization are already being made through several studies that were designed to discover the best methods for saliva collection, handling, processing, storage, and further protein identification and quantification [98–100]. Notwithstanding these difficulties, in SS there are common biomarkers between different studies (increased β[beta]2-microglobulin, Ig kappa light chain, α[alpha]-enolase, and E-FABP and decreased carbonic anhydrase VI, G3PDH, and SPLUNC-2) giving consistency and foundation for further studies of validation. The ultimate goal will be the translation of this biomarker panel into clinics as a diagnostic tool for SS [101].

Additionally, the dissimilar biomarker profile obtained for a particular disease may be explained by distinct variables such as gender, age, diet, circadian rhythm, interindividual variability, and sample stability that influence protein composition of saliva. In order to manage these variables, appropriate controls and inclusion and exclusion criteria should be taken into account to diminish the heterogeneity between different studies [59].

After standardization of the proteomic methodology, the future of salivary proteomics relies in long-term longitudinal and cohort studies in large-scale population and development of predictive models to evaluate and translate the potential protein markers previously identified to clinical medicine [99].

Methodologies Used in Salivary Peptidomics

Nowadays, it seems evident that many proteins hide within their superior structures, videlicet peptide substructures, which may exert relevant biological activities after their release of these substructures, according to precise temporal events [102] other than those of the parent protein. One relevant example is represented by salivary proteins. Indeed, one of the main PTMs faced by salivary proteins is proteolysis, by which they are cleaved into smaller fragments before, during, and after secretion in the oral cavity [103–105].

The action of a complex mix of endo- and exo-proteases leads to the production of a huge number of naturally occurring peptides, which represent approximately 40–50 % of the total secreted proteins in the whole saliva. In consideration of the very likely pathophysiological significance of salivary peptides, the interest in their characterization is growing, and several groups have investigated the techniques of extraction, enrichment, and detection of salivary peptides [98], as reported in several reviews [55, 100]. One important point to be considered in view of the application of salivary peptidomics to biomarker discovery is the influence of sample handling on salivary peptide composition. Indeed, several papers have shown that sample-handling factors may affect peptide abundance and composition [58, 106].

Schipper et al. demonstrated by SELDI-TOF-MS that delayed processing time resulted in both increase and decrease of peak numbers consistent with proteolysis and that profiles also changed, depending on storage temperature—although sample processing by centrifugation and numbers of freeze-thaw cycles had a minimal impact [107].

The naturally occurring cleavage events cannot be obviously investigated by bottom-up platforms, because this information is definitively lost during the trypsin digestion carried out before the separation [100]. Conversely, top-down platforms for the analysis of salivary peptide-rich extracts, obtained by ultrafiltration or using TFA, provide the possibility to detect naturally occurring fragments of proteins, as well as to achieve their structural characterization by high-resolution MS/MS fragmentation, and their quantification by labeling or by label-free methods [108, 109].

Gel-free MS methods for peptidomics investigations included surface-enhanced laser desorption/ionization time-of-flight (SELDI-TOF) MS [110], matrix-assisted laser desorption/ionization time-of-flight (MALDI-TOF) MS [111], and MS approach using electrospray ionization [112]. Both LC-MS/MS and MALDI-TOF MS require minimal sample preparation and allow detecting low-molecular-weight peptides with adequate resolution and sensitivity, making it a useful tool for peptide pattern profiling. Functionalized beads with peptide library, weak cation-exchanger magnetic beads, and mesoporous silica particles have been also used for selective enrichment of salivary peptides before MS analysis [113, 114].

A thorough overview of the multiple highly homologous peptides generated by pre-secretory and post-secretory cleavages from many salivary proteins has been obtained by using "in solution" top-down platforms. A comprehensive example is represented by the characterization of the proteolytic events occurring to the proproteins expressed by *PRB1*, *PRB2*, and *PRB4* polyallelic loci before secretion that lead to the generation of a lot of bPRP peptides with dimensions ranging from about 30 to 70 aa residues [115, 116]. Moreover, salivary peptidomics allowed evidencing the activity of an oral glutamine endoproteinase from *Rhodia* species localized in the dental plaque [117, 118] that cleaves bPRPs into smaller fragments (7–20 aa residues) at a XPQ consensus sequence, where X is prominently K. Similar fragmentations were observed with a lesser extent for P-C peptide and statherin [105, 119].

Also histatins are submitted to extensive pre- and post-secretory cleavage. Twenty-four naturally occurring fragments of histatin 3 have been identified in whole saliva by LC-MS/MS, and their structural characterization has permitted to postulate a sequential fragmentation process before secretion during granule maturation [103]. The same fragmentation pattern was observed in

another study by using a top-down approach on an ultrafiltered low molecular fraction from parotid saliva [120].

C-terminal residue removal also occurs in salivary glands by the action of carboxypeptidases active toward substrates with C-terminal basic amino acids, i.e., in the formation of histatin 5 from histatin 6 [103] as well as in the generation of the C-truncated forms of IB-1, II-2, and P-E bPRPs missing the C-terminal Arg [121] The exopeptidase can remove other C-terminal residues in statherin generating SV-1 (statherin Des-Phe-43) and statherin Des-Thr-42 Phe-43 and Pro and Gln in the P-C peptide and in the aPRP Pa-dimer [121, 122].

Recently, a specific chymotrypsin-like activity has been evidenced in saliva of human preterm newborns generating two fragments of cystatin B, a salivary protein of nonglandular origin [123]. Fragments were abundant in preterm newborns and decreased as a function of the post-conceptional age, disappearing in at-term newborns and adults. Proteolytic products of other nonsecretory proteins were observed in preterm newborns' saliva by top-down approaches, such as those deriving from peroxiredoxin 6, polymeric Ig receptor, and glyceraldehyde-3-phosphate dehydrogenase [112]. These fragments, detected and quantified by HPLC-ESI-MS top-down platform, highlighted the presence of still unknown fetal oral proteolytic activities. Recent studies are indicating that some variations of the concentration of these peptides, of their PTMs, and/or of naturally occurring fragments could be utilized as biomarkers or clues of multifactorial diseases. Anomalous fragment levels from different peptides (P-C, P-B, statherin, histatins) were established in type 1 (insulin-dependent) diabetic patients [95, 124, 125].

A minor contribution to whole saliva is ensured by gingival crevicular fluid, as transudate arising in minute quantities from the gingival plexus of gingival corium. Top-down platforms have evidenced that this fluid contains high concentrations of interesting peptides, such as α(alpha)-defensins [126] and thymosins β(beta)$_4$ and β(beta)$_{10}$ [127]. The high amount of α(alpha)-defensins probably originates from different leukocyte families transmigrating in high number in the gingival pocket, while the origin of the high levels of β(beta)-thymosins is currently unknown.

An Outlook of Salivary Findings

Salivary diagnostics is quickly augmenting its range of biomedical applications due to the identification and quantification of several molecules (biomarkers) in saliva that can be used for health and disease surveillance. Currently, it is crucial to define reference ranges for these biomarkers in order to clearly define physiological and pathological conditions. Thus, disease diagnosis can be done through the analysis of saliva in a standardized manner and salivary diagnosis can move toward clinicians worldwide. In this regard, next-generation salivary diagnostic platforms (POC devices), such as the oral fluid nanosensor test device (OFNASET), are being developed with encouraging outcomes. OFNASET detects salivary constituents within minutes and holds the potential of providing a highly sensitive medical diagnostic infrastructure to the general public or even the most deprived regions in the world. Furthermore, it is the first platform that allows parallel multiple detections of RNA and protein markers and has been optimized for salivary biomarker detection [128].

Accordingly with the literature, among all the salivary candidate biomarkers found using genomic, transcriptomic, and proteomic approaches, transcriptomic analysis is the one that achieved the most progress in terms of sensitivity and specificity progressing toward clinical implementation [31]. Nonetheless, unraveling the salivary genomics, transcriptomics, and proteomics signature in oral and systemic diseases will revolutionize the diagnostic and monitoring tools since an upright specificity and sensitivity can be achieved, in a noninvasive and cost-effective manner, combining all information set by the genes, transcripts, and proteins present in the oral environment. For example, using only the proteomic markers found in OSCC (Table 4.3), a specific diagnostic is not obtained since some of the markers are also found altered in other diseases (e.g., HNSCC and periodontitis). However, by adding DNA and RNA characteristic markers found in OSCC (Tables 4.1 and 4.2) to the equation, salivary biomarkers can be used to diagnose OSCC with a reliable confidence. Gathering all the putative salivary biomarkers found in Tables 4.1, 4.2, and 4.3, a network was made to evaluate the biomarkers' overlap between the various pathological conditions (Fig. 4.2). This network highlights the requirement of combining different types of biomarkers to accurately diagnose a specific disease. A comprehensive analysis of the biological processes behind the upregulated and downregulated markers from Fig. 4.2 uncovered that same specific pathways and processes are activated in different pathological conditions (Fig. 4.3). Acute inflammatory response, platelet degranulation, response to oxidative stress, killing of cells of other organisms, and regulation of signaling cascades are the main processes that are upregulated in saliva in response to certain pathologies as infections, cancers, and autoimmune diseases. The upcoming studies should focus in these particular affected pathways in a certain pathological condition and attempt to find precise therapeutic targets. By this approach, saliva components may be useful not only for prognosis, diagnosis, and monitoring but also to assess, in fact, therapeutic efficacy of certain drugs.

Taking this in consideration, a good initiative toward salivary diagnostics was the creation of a "Salivaomics Knowledge Base" (SKB). SKB is a Web-based data management system that contains valuable information of genomic, transcriptomic, proteomic, and metabolomic profiling of human saliva that can be used to identify disease-specific salivary biomarkers for human diseases [129]. Ideally, in the future of salivary diagnostics, a drop of saliva will be used for the concurrent detection of multiple disease-specific salivary biomarkers in real time and in a cost-effective manner. For that, saliva-based biosensor technologies—"lab-on-a-chip"—will be established and translated into the real world through an industrial partner. This technology will also provide the possibility for POC diagnostics that can revolutionize our

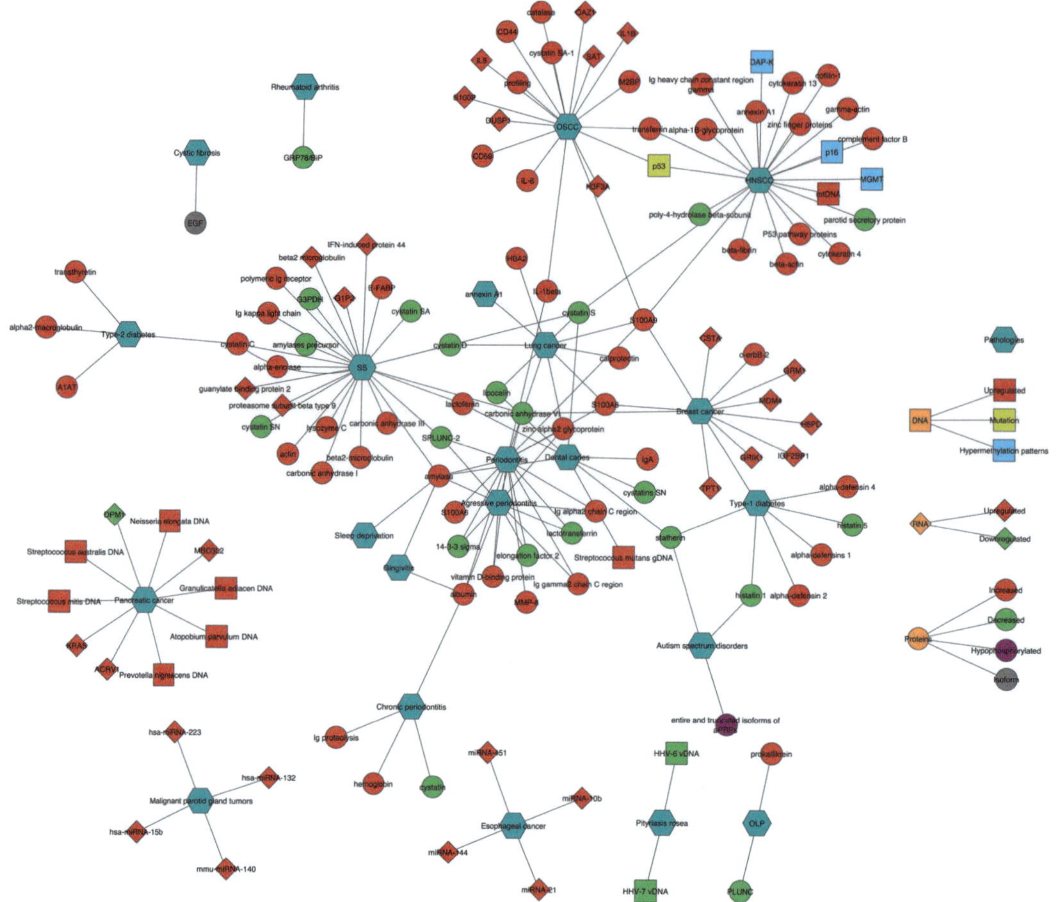

Fig. 4.2 A network visualizing the overlap between diseases of the salivary candidate biomarkers

approach to screening, risk assessment, and therapeutic management for a range of health conditions [130]. The design and development of saliva-based POC devices will transform the use of a minute amount of saliva suitable for population-based screening programs, confirmatory diagnosis, risk stratification, prognosis determination, and therapy response monitoring [131]. The "lab-on-a-chip" conjugates components and achievements from nanotechnology, clinical chemistry, bioinformatics, microfluidics, optics, image analysis, and pattern recognition to create a powerful new integrated measurement approach in a small device footprint. Therefore, this technology allows for personal and private diagnosis outside of a laboratory, and applying it to saliva will enhance healthcare delivery, reduce health disparities, and improve access to care [2].

Conclusion

A global analysis of all salivary components will enrich the oral and systemic disease pathogenesis knowledge (Fig. 4.4) and shape a solid foundation for the characterization of salivary biomarkers for noninvasive diagnosis of the most common and life-threatening diseases.

Acknowledgments The authors would like to thank Fundação para a Ciência e a Tecnologia (FCT) grants PTDC/EXPL/BBB-BEP/0317/2012; QREN (FCOMP-01-0124-FEDER-027554), QOPNA research unit (project PEst-C/QUI/UI0062/2013).

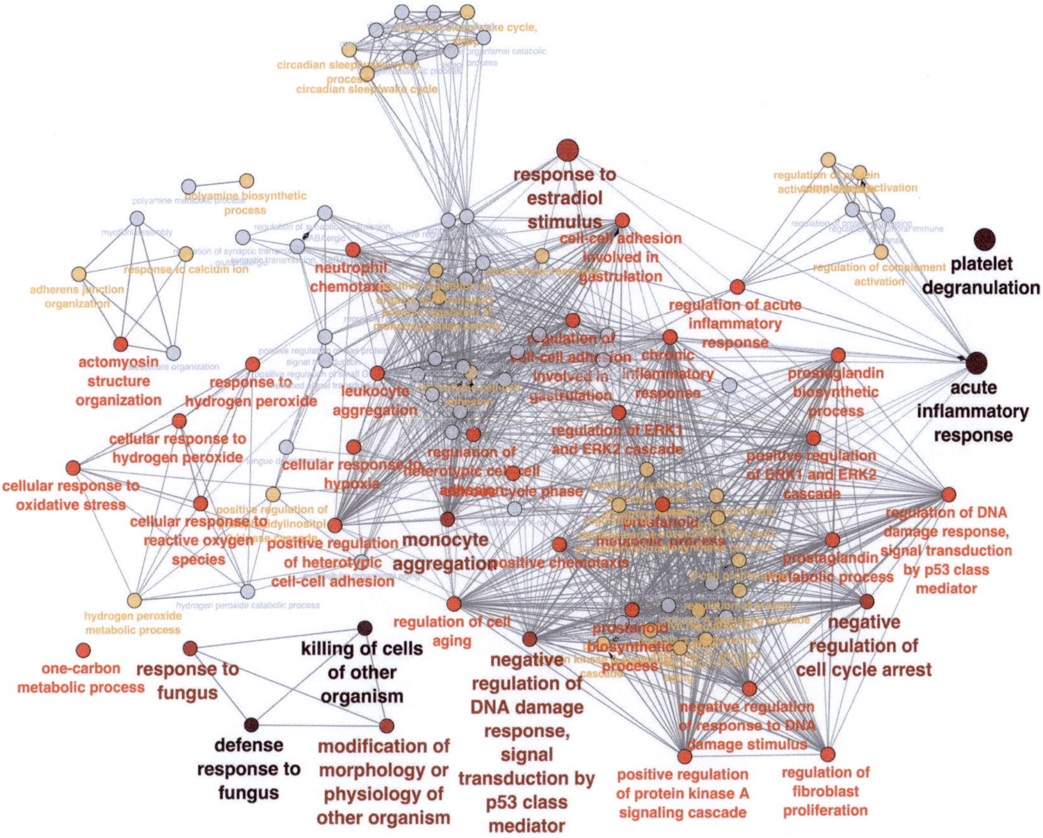

Fig. 4.3 Biological process analysis of the salivary candidate biomarkers for the diseases mentioned in biomedical applications of saliva. The main biological processes (represented by *red* intensity) are the ones that hold more saliva biomarkers associated. Regardless of the saliva biomarkers found for each disease, there are common pathways that are activated in response to disease state being responsible for organism defense or exacerbation of the pathological condition

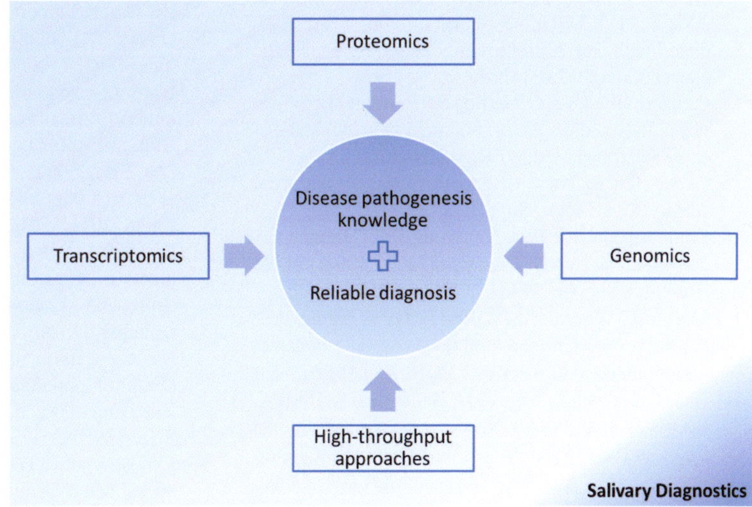

Fig. 4.4 The future of salivary diagnostics to improve scientific knowledge about human diseases and to become a valuable diagnostic tool

References

1. Lee Y-H, Wong DT. Saliva: an emerging biofluid for early detection of diseases. Am J Dent. 2009;22(4): 241–8.

2. Liu J, Duan Y. Saliva: a potential media for disease diagnostics and monitoring. Oral Oncol. 2012;48(7): 569–77.

3. Lima DP, Diniz DG, Moimaz SAS, Sumida DH, Okamoto AC. Saliva: reflection of the body. Int J Infect Dis. 2010;14(3):e184–8.

4. Siqueira WL, Dawes C. The salivary proteome: challenges and perspectives. Proteomics Clin Appl. 2011;5(11–12):575–9 [Research Support, Non-U.S. Gov't Review].

5. Michael P. Saliva as an aid in the detection of diathetic diseases. Dent Dig. 1901;7:105–10.

6. Kirk EC. Saliva as an index of faulty metabolism. Dent Dig. 1903;9:1126–38.

7. Mandel ID. Salivary studies in cystic fibrosis. Arch Pediatr Adolesc Med. 1967;113(4):431.

8. Oppenheim FG. Preliminary observations on the presence and origin of serum albumin in human saliva. Helv Odontol Acta. 1970;14(1):10–7.

9. Yeh C-K, Christodoulides NJ, Floriano PN, Miller CS, Ebersole JL, Weigum SE, et al. Current development of saliva/oral fluid-based diagnostics. Tex Dent J. 2010;127(7):651–61.

10. Malamud D. Saliva as a diagnostic fluid. Dent Clin N Am. 2011;55(1):159–78.

11. Wong DTW. Salivaomics. J Am Dent Assoc. 2012; 143(10 Suppl):19S–24.

12. Sugimoto M, Wong DT, Hirayama A, Soga T, Tomita M. Capillary electrophoresis mass spectrometry-based saliva metabolomics identified oral, breast and pancreatic cancer-specific profiles. Metabolomics. 2010;6(1):78–95.

13. Farrell JJ, Zhang L, Zhou H, Chia D, Elashoff D, Akin D, et al. Variations of oral microbiota are associated with pancreatic diseases including pancreatic cancer. Gut. 2012;61(4):582–8.

14. Farnaud SJC, Kosti O, Getting SJ, Renshaw D. Saliva: physiology and diagnostic potential in health and disease. Sci Transl Med. 2010;10:434–56.

15. Genco RJ. Salivary diagnostic tests. J Am Dent Assoc. 2012;143(10 Suppl):3S–5.

16. Zimmermann BG, Park NJ, Wong DT. Genomic targets in saliva. Ann N Y Acad Sci. 2007;1098:184–91 [Research Support, N.I.H., Extramural Review].

17. Martin KJ, Fournier MV, Reddy GPV, Pardee AB. A need for basic research on fluid-based early detection biomarkers. Cancer Res. 2010;70(13):5203–6.

18. Haas C, Hanson E, Anjos MJ, Banemann R, Berti A, Borges E, et al. RNA/DNA co-analysis from human saliva and semen stains – results of a third collaborative EDNAP exercise. Forensic Sci Int Genet. 2013;7(2):230–9.

19. Bowden A, Fleming R, Harbison S. A method for DNA and RNA co-extraction for use on forensic samples using the Promega DNA IQ system. Forensic Sci Int Genet. 2011;5(1):64–8 [Comparative Study Research Support, Non-U.S. Gov't].

20. Park NJ, Li Y, Yu T, Brinkman BMN, Wong DT. Characterization of RNA in saliva. Clin Chem. 2006;52(6):988–94.

21. Rylander-Rudqvist T, Hakansson N, Tybring G, Wolk A. Quality and quantity of saliva DNA obtained from the self-administered oragene method – a pilot study on the cohort of Swedish men. Cancer Epidemiol Biomarkers Prev. 2006;15(9):1742–5 [Research Support, Non-U.S. Gov't].

22. Hu Z, Zimmermann BG, Zhou H, Wang J, Henson BS, Yu W, et al. Exon-level expression profiling: a comprehensive transcriptome analysis of oral fluids. Clin Chem. 2008;54(5):824–32.

23. Li Y, Zhou X, St John MAR, Wong DTW. RNA profiling of cell-free saliva using microarray technology. J Dent Res. 2004;83(3):199–203.

24. Bahlo M, Stankovich J, Danoy P, Hickey PF, Taylor BV, Browning SR, et al. Saliva-derived DNA performs well in large-scale, high-density single-nucleotide polymorphism microarray studies. Cancer Epidemiol Biomarkers Prev. 2010;19(3):794–8.

25. Yano A, Kaneko N, Ida H, Yamaguchi T, Hanada N. Real-time PCR for quantification of streptococcus mutans. FEMS Microbiol Lett. 2002;217(1):23–30.

26. Spielmann N, Ilsley D, Gu J, Lea K, Brockman J, Heater S, et al. The human salivary RNA transcriptome revealed by massively parallel sequencing. Clin Chem. 2012;58(9):1314–21.

27. Maron JL, Johnson KL, Rocke DM, Cohen MG, Liley AJ, Bianchi DW. Neonatal salivary analysis reveals global developmental gene expression changes in the premature infant. Clin Chem. 2010; 56(3):409–16.

28. Kumar SV, Hurteau GJ, Spivack SD. Validity of messenger RNA expression analyses of human saliva. Clin Cancer Res. 2006;12(17):5033–9 [Research Support, N.I.H., Extramural].

29. Ogawa Y, Taketomi Y, Murakami M, Tsujimoto M, Yanoshita R. Small RNA transcriptomes of two types of exosomes in human whole saliva determined by next generation sequencing. Biol Pharm Bull. 2013;36(1):66–75.

30. Lee Y-H, Zhou H, Reiss JK, Yan X, Zhang L, Chia D, et al. Direct saliva transcriptome analysis. Clin Chem. 2011;57(9):1295–302.

31. Bonne NJ, Wong DT. Salivary biomarker development using genomic, proteomic and metabolomic approaches. Genome Med. 2012;4(10):82.

32. Quinque D, Kittler R, Kayser M, Stoneking M, Nasidze I. Evaluation of saliva as a source of human DNA for population and association studies. Anal Biochem. 2006;353(2):272–7.

33. Rogers NL, Cole SA, Lan H-C, Crossa A, Demerath EW. New saliva DNA collection method compared to buccal cell collection techniques for epidemiological studies. Am J Hum Biol. 2007;19(3):319–26.

34. Rylander-Rudqvist T, Håkansson N, Tybring G, Wolk A. Quality and quantity of saliva DNA obtained from the self-administered oragene method – a pilot

study on the cohort of Swedish men. Cancer Epidemiol Biomark Prev. 2006;15(9):1742–5.

35. Segal A, Wong DT. Salivary diagnostics: enhancing disease detection and making medicine better. Eur J Dent Educ. 2008;12 Suppl 1:22–9 [Research Support, Non-U.S. Gov't Research Support, U.S. Gov't, Non-P.H.S. Review].

36. Oblath EA, Henley WH, Alarie JP, Ramsey JM. A microfluidic chip integrating DNA extraction and real-time pcr for the detection of bacteria in saliva. Lab Chip. 2013;13(7):1325–32 [Research Support, N.I.H., Extramural Research Support, Non-U.S. Gov't].

37. Vieira AR, Deeley KB, Callahan NF, Noel JB, Anjomshoaa I, Carricato WM, et al. Detection of streptococcus mutans genomic DNA in human DNA samples extracted from saliva and blood. ISRN Dent. 2011;2011:543561.

38. Liao PH, Chang YC, Huang MF, Tai KW, Chou MY. Mutation of p53 gene codon 63 in saliva as a molecular marker for oral squamous cell carcinomas. Oral Oncol. 2000;36(3):272–6 [Research Support, Non-U.S. Gov't].

39. Watanabe T, Kawamura T, Jacob SE, Aquilino EA, Orenstein JM, Black JB, et al. Pityriasis rosea is associated with systemic active infection with both human herpesvirus-7 and human herpesvirus-6. J Invest Dermatol. 2002;119(4):793–7.

40. Boyle JO, Mao L, Brennan JA, Koch WM, Eisele DW, Saunders JR, et al. Gene mutations in saliva as molecular markers for head and neck squamous cell carcinomas. Am J Surg. 1994;168(5):429–32.

41. Rosas SL, Koch W, da Costa Carvalho MG, Wu L, Califano J, Westra W, et al. Promoter hypermethylation patterns of p16, o6-methylguanine-DNA-methyltransferase, and death-associated protein kinase in tumors and saliva of head and neck cancer patients. Cancer Res. 2001;61(3):939–42 [Research Support, U.S. Gov't, P.H.S].

42. Jiang WW, Masayesva B, Zahurak M, Carvalho AL, Rosenbaum E, Mambo E, et al. Increased mitochondrial DNA content in saliva associated with head and neck cancer. Clin Cancer Res. 2005;11(7):2486–91 [Comparative Study Research Support, N.I.H., Extramural Research Support, Non-U.S. Gov't Research Support, U.S. Gov't, P.H.S].

43. Hansen TV, Simonsen MK, Nielsen FC, Hundrup YA. Collection of blood, saliva, and buccal cell samples in a pilot study on the Danish nurse cohort: comparison of the response rate and quality of genomic DNA. Cancer Epidemiol Biomarkers Prev. 2007;16(10):2072–6.

44. Fabian TK, Fejerdy P, Nguyen MT, Soti C, Csermely P. Potential immunological functions of salivary hsp70 in mucosal and periodontal defense mechanisms. Arch Immunol Ther Exp (Warsz). 2007;55(2):91–8 [Research Support, Non-U.S. Gov't Review].

45. Lasser C, Alikhani VS, Ekstrom K, Eldh M, Paredes PT, Bossios A, et al. Human saliva, plasma and breast milk exosomes contain RNA: uptake by macrophages. J Transl Med. 2011;9:9 [Research Support, Non-U.S. Gov't].

46. Fabian TK, Fejerdy P, Csermely P. Salivary genomics, transcriptomics and proteomics: the emerging concept of the oral ecosystem and their use in the early diagnosis of cancer and other diseases. Curr Genomics. 2008;9(1):11–21.

47. Zhang L, Xiao H, Karlan S, Zhou H, Gross J, Elashoff D, et al. Discovery and preclinical validation of salivary transcriptomic and proteomic biomarkers for the non-invasive detection of breast cancer. PLoS One. 2010;5(12):e15573 [Research Support, N.I.H., Extramural Research Support, Non-U.S. Gov't].

48. Xie Z, Chen G, Zhang X, Li D, Huang J, Yang C, et al. Salivary microRNAs as promising biomarkers for detection of esophageal cancer. PLoS One. 2013;8(4):e57502.

49. Matse JH, Yoshizawa J, Wang X, Elashoff D, Bolscher JG, Veerman EC, et al. Discovery and pre-validation of salivary extracellular microRNA biomarkers panel for the noninvasive detection of benign and malignant parotid gland tumors. Clin Cancer Res. 2013;19(11):3032–8 [Research Support, N.I.H., Extramural].

50. Li Y, St John MA, Zhou X, Kim Y, Sinha U, Jordan RC, et al. Salivary transcriptome diagnostics for oral cancer detection. Clin Cancer Res. 2004;10(24):8442–50 [Comparative Study Research Support, N.I.H., Extramural Research Support, Non-U.S. Gov't Research Support, U.S. Gov't, P.H.S].

51. Zhang L, Farrell JJ, Zhou H, Elashoff D, Akin D, Park N-H, et al. Salivary transcriptomic biomarkers for detection of resectable pancreatic cancer. Gastroenterology. 2010;138(3):949–57, e941–7.

52. Hu S, Wang J, Meijer J, Ieong S, Xie Y, Yu T, et al. Salivary proteomic and genomic biomarkers for primary Sjögren's syndrome. Arthritis Rheum. 2007;56(11):3588–600 [Research Support, N.I.H., Extramural].

53. Seugnet L, Boero J, Gottschalk L, Duntley SP, Shaw PJ. Identification of a biomarker for sleep drive in flies and humans. Proc Natl Acad Sci U S A. 2006;103(52):19913–8.

54. Gallo A, Tandon M, Alevizos I, Illei GG. The majority of microRNAs detectable in serum and saliva is concentrated in exosomes. PLoS One. 2012;7(3):e30679.

55. Amado FM, Ferreira RP, Vitorino R. One decade of salivary proteomics: current approaches and outstanding challenges. Clin Biochem. 2013;46(6):506–17 [Research Support, Non-U.S. Gov't Review].

56. Yamada N, Yuji R, Suzuki E. The current status and future prospects of the salivary proteome. J Health Sci. 2009;55(5):682–8.

57. Helmerhorst EJ, Oppenheim FG. Saliva: a dynamic proteome. J Dent Res. 2007;86(8):680–93 [Research Support, N.I.H., Extramural Review].

58. Messana I, Inzitari R, Fanali C, Cabras T, Castagnola M. Facts and artifacts in proteomics of body fluids. What proteomics of saliva is telling us? J Sep Sci. 2008;31(11):1948–63 [Research Support, Non--U.S. Gov't Review].

59. Zhang A, Sun H, Wang P, Wang X. Salivary proteomics in biomedical research. Clin Chim Acta. 2013;415:261–5 [Research Support, Non-U.S. Gov't Review].

60. Ruhl S. The scientific exploration of saliva in the post-proteomic era: from database back to basic function. Expert Rev Proteomics. 2012;9(1):85–96 [Research Support, N.I.H., Extramural Review].

61. Graves PR, Haystead TA. Molecular biologist's guide to proteomics. Microbiol Mol Biol Rev. 2002;66(1):39–63, table of contents.

62. Serpa JJ, Parker CE, Petrotchenko EV, Han J, Pan J, Borchers CH. Mass spectrometry-based structural proteomics. Eur J Mass Spectrom (Chichester, Eng). 2012;18(2):251–67 [Research Support, Non-U.S. Gov't Review].

63. Capriotti AL, Cavaliere C, Foglia P, Samperi R, Lagana A. Intact protein separation by chromatographic and/or electrophoretic techniques for top-down proteomics. J Chromatogr A. 2011;1218(49):8760–76. Review.

64. Manadas B, Mendes VM, English J, Dunn MJ. Peptide fractionation in proteomics approaches. Expert Rev Proteomics. 2010;7(5):655–63 [Research Support, Non-U.S. Gov't].

65. Zhang W, Zhao X. Method for rapid protein identification in a large database. Biomed Res Int. 2013; 2013:414069.

66. Perkins DN, Pappin DJ, Creasy DM, Cottrell JS. Probability-based protein identification by searching sequence databases using mass spectrometry data. Electrophoresis. 1999;20(18):3551–67 [Research Support, Non-U.S. Gov't].

67. Eng JK, McCormack AL, Yates JR. An approach to correlate tandem mass spectral data of peptides with amino acid sequences in a protein database. J Am Soc Mass Spectrom. 1994;5(11):976–89.

68. Al Kawas S, Rahim ZH, Ferguson DB. Potential uses of human salivary protein and peptide analysis in the diagnosis of disease. Arch Oral Biol. 2012;57(1):1–9. Review.

69. Zhao Y, Lee WN, Xiao GG. Quantitative proteomics and biomarker discovery in human cancer. Expert Rev Proteomics. 2009;6(2):115–8 [Editorial Research Support, N.I.H., Extramural Research Support, Non-U.S. Gov't Review].

70. Wu Y, Shu R, Luo LJ, Ge LH, Xie YF. Initial comparison of proteomic profiles of whole unstimulated saliva obtained from generalized aggressive periodontitis patients and healthy control subjects. J Periodontal Res. 2009;44(5):636–44 [Comparative Study].

71. Castagnola M, Messana I, Inzitari R, Fanali C, Cabras T, Morelli A, et al. Hypo-phosphorylation of salivary peptidome as a clue to the molecular pathogenesis of autism spectrum disorders. J Proteome Res. 2008;7(12):5327–32 [Research Support, Non-U.S. Gov't].

72. Streckfus C, Bigler L. The use of soluble, salivary c-erbB-2 for the detection and post-operative follow-up of breast cancer in women: the results of a five-year translational research study. Adv Dent Res. 2005;18(1):17–24 [Research Support, N.I.H., Extramural Review].

73. Goncalves Lda R, Soares MR, Nogueira FC, Garcia C, Camisasca DR, Domont G, et al. Comparative proteomic analysis of whole saliva from chronic periodontitis patients. J Proteomics. 2010;73(7): 1334–41 [Comparative Study Research Support, Non-U.S. Gov't].

74. Aubert B, Cochet C, Souvignet C, Chambaz EM. Saliva from cystic fibrosis patients contains an unusual form of epidermal growth factor. Biochem Biophys Res Commun. 1990;170(3):1144–50 [Research Support, Non-U.S. Gov't].

75. Vitorino R, de Morais Guedes S, Ferreira R, Lobo MJ, Duarte J, Ferrer-Correia AJ, et al. Two-dimensional electrophoresis study of in vitro pellicle formation and dental caries susceptibility. Eur J Oral Sci. 2006;114(2):147–53 [Research Support, N.I.H., Intramural].

76. Rudney JD, Staikov RK, Johnson JD. Potential biomarkers of human salivary function: a modified proteomic approach. Arch Oral Biol. 2009;54(1):91–100 [Research Support, N.I.H., Extramural].

77. Goncalves Lda R, Soares MR, Nogueira FC, Garcia CH, Camisasca DR, Domont G, et al. Analysis of the salivary proteome in gingivitis patients. J Periodontal Res. 2011;46(5):599–606 [Research Support, Non-U.S. Gov't].

78. Jarai T, Maasz G, Burian A, Bona A, Jambor E, Gerlinger I, et al. Mass spectrometry-based salivary proteomics for the discovery of head and neck squamous cell carcinoma. Pathol Oncol Res. 2012;18(3):623–8 [Comparative Study Research Support, Non-U.S. Gov't].

79. Dowling P, Wormald R, Meleady P, Henry M, Curran A, Clynes M. Analysis of the saliva proteome from patients with head and neck squamous cell carcinoma reveals differences in abundance levels of proteins associated with tumour progression and metastasis. J Proteomics. 2008;71(2):168–75 [Research Support, Non-U.S. Gov't].

80. Ohshiro K, Rosenthal DI, Koomen JM, Streckfus CF, Chambers M, Kobayashi R, et al. Pre-analytic saliva processing affect proteomic results and biomarker screening of head and neck squamous carcinoma. Int J Oncol. 2007;30(3):743–9.

81. Xiao H, Zhang L, Zhou H, Lee JM, Garon EB, Wong DT. Proteomic analysis of human saliva from lung cancer patients using two-dimensional difference gel electrophoresis and mass spectrometry. Mol Cell Proteomics. 2012;11(2):M111 012112 [Comparative Study Research Support, N.I.H., Extramural Research Support, Non-U.S. Gov't].

82. Yang LL, Liu XQ, Liu W, Cheng B, Li MT. Comparative analysis of whole saliva proteomes for the screening of biomarkers for oral lichen planus. Inflamm Res. 2006;55(10):405–7.

83. Jou YJ, Lin CD, Lai CH, Chen CH, Kao JY, Chen SY, et al. Proteomic identification of salivary transferrin as a biomarker for early detection of oral cancer. Anal Chim Acta. 2010;681(1–2):41–8 [Research Support, Non-U.S. Gov't].

84. Shintani S, Hamakawa H, Ueyama Y, Hatori M, Toyoshima T. Identification of a truncated cystatin

SA-I as a saliva biomarker for oral squamous cell carcinoma using the SELDI ProteinChip platform. Int J Oral Maxillofac Surg. 2010;39(1):68–74 [Comparative Study].

85. Hu S, Arellano M, Boontheung P, Wang J, Zhou H, Jiang J, et al. Salivary proteomics for oral cancer biomarker discovery. Clin Cancer Res. 2008;14(19):6246–52 [Research Support, N.I.H., Extramural].

86. Franzmann EJ, Reategui EP, Pedroso F, Pernas FG, Karakullukcu BM, Carraway KL, et al. Soluble CD44 is a potential marker for the early detection of head and neck cancer. Cancer Epidemiol Biomarkers Prev. 2007;16(7):1348–55 [Comparative Study Multicenter Study Research Support, N.I.H., Extramural Research Support, Non-U.S. Gov't].

87. St John MA, Li Y, Zhou X, Denny P, Ho CM, Montemagno C, et al. Interleukin 6 and interleukin 8 as potential biomarkers for oral cavity and oropharyngeal squamous cell carcinoma. Arch Otolaryngol Head Neck Surg. 2004;130(8):929–35 [Comparative Study Evaluation Studies Research Support, Non-U.S. Gov't Research Support, U.S. Gov't, P.H.S].

88. Arellano-Garcia ME, Hu S, Wang J, Henson B, Zhou H, Chia D, et al. Multiplexed immunobead-based assay for detection of oral cancer protein biomarkers in saliva. Oral Dis. 2008;14(8):705–12 [Comparative Study Research Support, N.I.H., Extramural Research Support, Non-U.S. Gov't].

89. Haigh BJ, Stewart KW, Whelan JR, Barnett MP, Smolenski GA, Wheeler TT. Alterations in the salivary proteome associated with periodontitis. J Clin Periodontol. 2010;37(3):241–7 [Research Support, Non-U.S. Gov't].

90. Miller CS, King Jr CP, Langub MC, Kryscio RJ, Thomas MV. Salivary biomarkers of existing periodontal disease: a cross-sectional study. J Am Dent Assoc. 2006;137(3):322–9 [Research Support, N.I.H., Extramural Research Support, Non-U.S. Gov't].

91. Giusti L, Baldini C, Ciregia F, Giannaccini G, Giacomelli C, De Feo F, et al. Is grp78/bip a potential salivary biomarker in patients with rheumatoid arthritis? Proteomics Clin Appl. 2010;4(3):315–24.

92. Giusti L, Baldini C, Bazzichi L, Ciregia F, Tonazzini I, Mascia G, et al. Proteome analysis of whole saliva: a new tool for rheumatic diseases–the example of Sjogren's syndrome. Proteomics. 2007;7(10):1634–43.

93. Ryu OH, Atkinson JC, Hoehn GT, Illei GG, Hart TC. Identification of parotid salivary biomarkers in Sjogren's syndrome by surface-enhanced laser desorption/ionization time-of-flight mass spectrometry and two-dimensional difference gel electrophoresis. Rheumatology. 2006;45(9):1077–86.

94. Baldini C, Giusti L, Ciregia F, Da Valle Y, Giacomelli C, Donadio E, et al. Proteomic analysis of saliva: a unique tool to distinguish primary Sjogren's syndrome from secondary Sjogren's syndrome and other sicca syndromes. Arthritis Res Ther. 2011;13(6):R194.

95. Cabras T, Pisano E, Mastinu A, Denotti G, Pusceddu PP, Inzitari R, et al. Alterations of the salivary secretory peptidome profile in children affected by type 1 diabetes. Mol Cell Proteomics. 2010;9(10):2099–108 [Research Support, Non-U.S. Gov't].

96. Rao PV, Reddy AP, Lu X, Dasari S, Krishnaprasad A, Biggs E, et al. Proteomic identification of salivary biomarkers of type-2 diabetes. J Proteome Res. 2009;8(1):239–45.

97. Prathibha KM, Johnson P, Ganesh M, Subhashini AS. Evaluation of salivary profile among Type 2 diabetes mellitus patients in South India. J Clin Diagn Res. 2013;7(8):1592–5.

98. Vitorino R, Guedes S, Manadas B, Ferreira R, Amado F. Toward a standardized saliva proteome analysis methodology. J Proteomics. 2012;75(17):5140–65 [Evaluation Studies Research Support, Non-U.S. Gov't].

99. Hu S, Loo JA, Wong DT. Human saliva proteome analysis and disease biomarker discovery. Expert Rev Proteomics. 2007;4(4):531–8 [Research Support, N.I.H., Extramural Review].

100. Castagnola M, Cabras T, Iavarone F, Fanali C, Nemolato S, Peluso G, et al. The human salivary proteome: a critical overview of the results obtained by different proteomic platforms. Expert Rev Proteomics. 2012;9(1):33–46 [Research Support, Non-U.S. Gov't Review].

101. Al-Tarawneh SK, Border MB, Dibble CF, Bencharit S. Defining salivary biomarkers using mass spectrometry-based proteomics: a systematic review. OMICS. 2011;15(6):353–61 [Research Support, N.I.H., Extramural Research Support, Non-U.S. Gov't Review].

102. Giardina B, Messana I, Scatena R, Castagnola M. The multiple function of haemoglobin. Crit Rev Biochem Mol Biol. 1995;30(3):165–96 [Research Support, Non-U.S. Gov't Review].

103. Castagnola M, Inzitari R, Rossetti DV, Olmi C, Cabras T, Piras V, et al. A cascade of 24 histatins (histatin 3 fragments) in human saliva. Suggestions for a pre-secretory sequential cleavage pathway. J Biol Chem. 2004;279(40):41436–43 [Research Support, Non-U.S. Gov't].

104. Thomadaki K, Helmerhorst EJ, Tian N, Sun X, Siqueira WL, Walt DR, et al. Whole-saliva proteolysis and its impact on salivary diagnostics. J Dent Res. 2011;90(11):1325–30.

105. Vitorino R, Calheiros-Lobo MJ, Williams J, Ferrer-Correia AJ, Torner KB, Duarte JA, et al. Peptidomic analysis of human acquired enamel pellicle. Biomed Chromatogr. 2007;21(11):1107–17.

106. de Jong EP, van Riper SK, Koopmeiners JS, Carlis JV, Griffin TJ. Sample collection and handling considerations for peptidomic studies in whole saliva; implications for biomarker discovery. Clin Chim Acta. 2011;412(23–24):2284–8.

107. Schipper R, Loof A, de Groot J, Harthoorn L, van Heerde W, Dransfield E. Salivary protein/peptide profiling with SELDI-TOF-MS. Ann N Y Acad Sci. 2007;1098:498–503.

108. Vitorino R, Barros A, Caseiro A, Domingues P, Duarte J, Amado FM. Towards defining the whole salivary peptidome. Proteomics Clin Appl. 2009;3(5):528–40.

109. Messana I, Cabras T, Iavarone F, Vincenzoni F, Urbani A, Castagnola M. Unraveling the different proteomic platforms. J Sep Sci. 2013;36(1):128–39 [Research Support, Non-U.S. Gov't Review].

110. Schipper R, Loof A, de Groot J, Harthoorn L, Dransfield E, van Heerde W. SELDI-TOF-MS of saliva: methodology and pre-treatment effects. J Chromatogr B Analyt Technol Biomed Life Sci. 2007;847(1):45–53.

111. Huang CM, Zhu W. Profiling human saliva endogenous peptidome via a high throughput MALDI-TOF-TOF mass spectrometry. Comb Chem High Throughput Screen. 2009;12(5):521–31.

112. Castagnola M, Cabras T, Iavarone F, Vincenzoni F, Vitali A, Pisano E, et al. Top-down platform for deciphering the human salivary proteome. J Matern Fetal Neonatal Med. 2012;25 Suppl 5:27–43 [Research Support, Non-U.S. Gov't].

113. Terracciano R, Preianò M, Palladino GP, Carpagnano GE, Barbaro MP, Pelaia G, et al. Peptidome profiling of induced sputum by mesoporous silica beads and MALDI-TOF MS for non-invasive biomarker discovery of chronic inflammatory lung diseases. Proteomics. 2011;11(16):3402–14.

114. Jou YJ, Lin CD, Lai CH, Tang CH, Huang SH, Tsai MH, et al. Salivary zinc finger protein 510 peptide as a novel biomarker for detection of oral squamous cell carcinoma in early stages. Clin Chim Acta. 2011;412(15–16):1357–65.

115. Vitorino R, Alves R, Barros A, Caseiro A, Ferreira R, Lobo MC, et al. Finding new posttranslational modifications in salivary proline-rich proteins. Proteomics. 2010;10(20):3732–42.

116. Messana I, Cabras T, Inzitari R, Lupi A, Zuppi C, Olmi C, et al. Characterization of the human salivary basic proline-rich protein complex by a proteomic approach. J Proteome Res. 2004;3(4):792–800 [Research Support, Non-U.S. Gov't].

117. Helmerhorst EJ, Zamakhchari M, Schuppan D, Oppenheim FG. Discovery of a novel and rich source of gluten-degrading microbial enzymes in the oral cavity. PLoS One. 2010;5(10):e13264.

118. Fernandez-Feo M, Wei G, Blumenkranz G, Dewhirst FE, Schuppan D, Oppenheim FG, et al. The cultivable human oral gluten-degrading microbiome and its potential implications in coeliac disease and gluten sensitivity. Clin Microbiol Infect. 2013;19(9):E386–94.

119. Helmerorst EJ, Sun X, Salih E, Oppenheim FG. Identification of Lys-Prof-Gln as a novel cleavage site specificity of saliva-associated proteases. J Biol Chem. 2008;283(29):19957–66.

120. Hardt M, Thomas LR, Dixon SE, Newport G, Agabian N, Prakobphol A, et al. Toward defining the human parotid gland salivary proteome and peptidome: identification and characterization using 2D SDS-PAGE, ultrafiltration, HPLC, and mass spectrometry. Biochemistry. 2005;44(8):2885–99.

121. Messana I, Cabras T, Pisano E, Sanna MT, Olianas A, Manconi B, et al. Trafficking and postsecretory events responsible for the formation of secreted human salivary peptides: a proteomics approach. Mol Cell Proteomics. 2008;7(5):911–26 [Research Support, Non-U.S. Gov't].

122. Inzitari R, Cabras T, Rossetti DV, Fanali C, Vitali A, Pellegrini M, et al. Detection in human saliva of different statherin and P-B fragments and derivatives. Proteomics. 2006;6(23):6370–9 [Research Support, Non-U.S. Gov't].

123. Iavarone F, Cabras T, Pisano E, Sanna MT, Nemolato S, Vento G, et al. Top-down HPLC-ESI-MS detection of S-glutathionylated and S-cysteinylated derivatives of cystatin B and its 1–53 and 54–98 fragments in whole saliva of human preterm newborns. J Proteome Res. 2013;12(2):917–26 [Research Support, Non-U.S. Gov't].

124. Caseiro A, Vitorino R, Barros AS, Ferreira R, Calheiros-Lobo MJ, Carvalho D, et al. Salivary peptidome in type 1 diabetes mellitus. Biomed Chromatogr. 2012;26(5):571–82.

125. Caseiro A, Ferreira R, Padrão A, Quintaneiro C, Pereira A, Marinheiro R, et al. Salivary proteome and peptidome profiling in type 1 diabetes mellitus using a quantitative approach. J Proteome Res. 2013;12(4):1700–9.

126. Pisano E, Cabras T, Montaldo C, Piras V, Inzitari R, Olmi C, et al. Peptides of human gingival crevicular fluid determined by HPLC-ESI-MS. Eur J Oral Sci. 2005;113(6):462–8 [Research Support, Non-U.S. Gov't].

127. Inzitari R, Cabras T, Pisano E, Fanali C, Manconi B, Scarano E, et al. HPLC-ESI-MS analysis of oral human fluids reveals that gingival crevicular fluid is the main source of oral thymosins beta(4) and beta(10). J Sep Sci. 2009;32(1):57–63 [Research Support, Non-U.S. Gov't].

128. Gau V, Wong D. Oral fluid nanosensor test (OFNASET) with advanced electrochemical-based molecular analysis platform. Ann N Y Acad Sci. 2007;1098:401–10 [Research Support, N.I.H.,Extramural].

129. Ai J, Smith B, Wong DT. Saliva ontology: an ontology-based framework for a salivaomics knowledge base. BMC Bioinformatics. 2010;11:302 [Research Support, N.I.H.,Extramural].

130. Miller CS, Foley JD, Bailey AL, Campell CL, Humphries RL, Christodoulides N, et al. Current developments in salivary diagnostics. Biomark Med. 2010;4(1):171–89.

131. Pfaffe T, Cooper-White J, Beyerlein P, Kostner K, Punyadeera C. Diagnostic potential of saliva: current state and future applications. Clin Chem. 2011; 57(5):675–87.

Salivary Diagnostics and the Oral Microbiome

5

Jennifer E. Kerr and Gena D. Tribble

Abstract

Our oral cavity hosts an extraordinary variety of microorganisms. Recent work has started to look at the composition of the oral microbiome in both healthy and disease states. Various stages of caries, gingivitis, and periodontitis, plus novel work understanding the role of bacteria in other diseases/conditions and carcinogenesis, reveal that our oral microbiome has an intriguing link to our global health. Together, these studies have combined a number of techniques, including human oral microbe identification microarray (HOMIM) and high-throughput sequencing, to survey the oral flora composition. Microorganisms' sensitivity to small changes in the environment including pH, nutrients and metabolites, oxygen and water levels, and host immune factors has been broadly studied. Ideally, the high sensitivity of oral microorganisms should forecast subtle changes in the health status and potentially serve as a biomarker for early detection of disease. Paired with other host saliva biomarkers, the oral microbiome presents a novel noninvasive diagnostic tool for monitoring changes in human physiology and a potential shift toward disease.

Introduction

The number of bacteria in the human microbiome is estimated to outnumber human cells by a factor of more than 10 [1]. These microorganisms (bacteria, fungi, and viruses) form diverse communities in different body locations (the skin, the respiratory system, the intestinal and vaginal mucosa, and the oral cavity) as the normal "flora" with distinct compositions and vital functions. The distribution and ratios of these microorganisms at specific body sites have been found to be more similar between humans (e.g., comparing two salivary microbiomes) than comparing different body sites within the same person (e.g., intestine versus saliva) [2–4]. This suggests that the various microbiome communities have coevolved with their body sites, leading to separate functional

J.E. Kerr, PhD (✉)
Department of Biology – Oral Microbiology, Notre Dame of Maryland University, Baltimore, MD, USA
e-mail: jkerr@ndm.edu

G.D. Tribble, PhD
Department of Periodontics, University of Texas Health Science Center, School of Dentistry, Houston, TX, USA

C.F. Streckfus (ed.), *Advances in Salivary Diagnostics,*
DOI 10.1007/978-3-662-45399-5_5, © Springer-Verlag Berlin Heidelberg 2015

repertoires. Novel work in recent years is starting to reveal that our microbiome functions as a unit and thus is more comparable to an essential organ than just a set of random hitchhikers [5–11]. Overall, these microbial communities are thought to maintain a healthy homeostatic balance with the host as a functional community, but environmental perturbations can allow for significant changes within these sites.

Given the opportunity, members of the microbial flora can also act as pathogens and can cause life-threatening problems. There have been numerous studies showing a direct link between specific combinations of bacteria, fungi, or viruses that are associated with specific disease states. As part of the disease process, the microbial community may undergo a shift in composition, and bacteria associated with disease may transition from a minority to a majority of the community [12–14]. This shift in composition may happen for a variety of reasons but at least in part as a response to changes in the host environment. This change in proportions of microorganisms not only may allow certain opportunistic pathogens to become dominant but also acts as an indicator of a systemic problem.

In order to understand how these microbial communities might undergo shifts in response to various changes in the body, we must first identify what microorganisms commonly inhabit healthy individuals. Extensive work has started to determine these healthy compositions of the human microbiome at different locations throughout the body, including the oral cavity. Work analyzing the human microbiome has shown clear overlap among individuals, especially between oral samples [3, 4, 15, 16]. This overlap allows for the establishment of a "core microbiome" profile of healthy individuals, and the noninvasive sampling of the mouth makes it an ideal candidate for comparing microbiome profiles among different populations. The oral environment presents a variety of niches for harboring a wide variety of microorganisms (bacterial, fungal, and viral). These microbes often subvert and survive attack from the host immune system and persist even during significant changes in pH, nutrient availability, temperature, and moisture throughout the course of a day. The

ideal healthy oral environment provides a neutral pH and a constant supply of host molecules and nutrients (e.g., saliva, diet). A prolonged change in the oral microenvironment over time will lead to a shift in the predominant microbial organisms. While many diseases often go undiagnosed until primary or secondary symptoms are recognized by the patient, our microbiome may be "detecting" these changes well before the host does. Microorganisms' sensitivity to small changes in the environment has been studied extensively [17–20]. The hope is these changes within the microbiome can be a predictor of disease *before* prominent symptoms associated with disease progression become apparent.

Researchers have recently started to look at the overall differences observed in healthy versus disease states. This work has oftentimes taken advantage of the recently developed human oral microbe identification microarray (HOMIM) profiling technology to assess changes in oral microflora [21–26]. This technology simultaneously detects more than 300 of the most prevalent oral bacterial species, including bacteria that have not been successfully cultured. HOMIM and high-throughput sequencing has the potential to allow scientists to discover microbial biomarkers that can be paired with host biomarkers, leading to the increased likelihood of early disease detection. With more than 700 identified bacterial phylotypes, the oral microbiome provides a complex, quantifiable signal capable of responding to minute changes in the environment and likely mirroring changes in the body.

The establishment of the core microbiome serves as a baseline comparison for altered states of the human body. These states might include healthy changes such as pregnancy, healthy weight loss, or cancer remission as well as unhealthy changes such as diabetes, infection, obesity, or cancer. All of these changes have the potential to alter the host environment in dramatic ways. For instance, altering circulating levels of hormones or immune cells, changes in local oxygen levels within tissue, shifts in pH, and even marked difference in salivary flow represent possible differences. These changes may be prolonged or temporary given the host's situation. Disease states often will set off a domino effect that will eventually lead to dramatic changes in overall physiology. Being able to identify minute changes in the body that suggest disease before they lead to more severe, potentially life-altering symptoms is paramount to improving patient outcomes. Due to the highly responsive nature of microorganisms, monitoring the microbiome has the potential to provide this early indicator that something may be wrong, even before primary disease symptoms are noticed. Ideally, a wellness checkup could include traditional testing such as heart rate and blood pressure monitoring but would also include a microbiome sample for analysis. This noninvasive test would allow for a simple and quick way to screen large populations for overall health.

Oral sampling presents one of the easiest locations for obtaining a microbiome profile as well as other host biomarkers. Work with saliva microbial or host biomarkers individually may sometimes yield unclear results when predicting disease states [27–30]. A single sample with dual testing capability provides the opportunity for increased testing sensitivity and specificity. While fungi and viruses do form a part of our microbiome, most of the work surveying the human microbiome has primarily focused on the bacterial communities present at different sites within and on the human body. Therefore, this chapter will mainly focus on the core oral bacterial microbiome and how the bacterial composition shifts in response to various diseases/conditions, briefly outline the new emerging research in the human mycobiome and virome, and finally present future directions in using the oral microbiome as part of salivary diagnostics. Designing a dual biomarker salivary test approach presents a novel future on the horizon as we come to better understand how we as hosts are linked to our microbial residents.

Oral Microbiome Composition

The human oral microbiome presents an intriguing and varied composition of thousands of different species of bacteria. New molecular techniques have greatly improved our ability to monitor the composition of this diverse group of organisms, since many of these bacteria are not able to be cultured in the laboratory. In fact, experts are now finding more evidence to support the hypothesis that bacteria must be treated as a community versus singling out an individual bacterium as being responsible for causing incidents of disease or heath. This community involves not only communication and dealings between multiple types of bacteria but also complex interactions with the environment. In the case of humans, we are that environment, and researchers are finding that humans have a much closer relationship to their microbiome than was ever imagined.

Here we will focus on the oral microbiome relationship. Multiple studies, including the Human Microbiome Project and HOMIM, have worked to identify the normal flora present in the oral cavity. The commensal oral microbiota serves in a protective capacity for the host by occupying the space that would otherwise be colonized by microbial pathogens. The oral cavity supports a number of niche environments that maintain a relatively diverse microbial profile. Studies have shown that while there is a "core oral microbiome," the relative composition of these species varies somewhat within the oral cavity. Both solid (e.g., teeth) and shedding (e.g., mucosal) surfaces are available for microbial colonization in the mouth. The microbiome has been analyzed in various locations in the mouth including the tongue, cheek, palate, teeth, tonsils, gingiva, and saliva. The oral microbial composition will be discussed in total and relative to some of these oral micro-niches to better understand a typical profile.

Healthy Oral "Core Microbiome"

Numerous studies have looked at the oral composition of healthy humans (Table 5.1) [31–34, 36–39]. Several species are commonly found in healthy individuals. For example, *Streptococcus* spp. and *Veillonella* spp. (Gram-positive cocci) are prevalent in healthy individuals and on average comprise greater than 20 % of the oral microbiome [16, 23, 31, 32, 35, 37, 38, 40]. These microbes are considered "pioneers" and are able to

Table 5.1 Healthy oral microbiome profile studies

References	[31]	[32]	[2]	[33]	[34]	[35]	[16]	[36]	[37]	[38]	[3]
Number of subjects	5	71; 98	7	3	120	12	3	10	5	1	242
Locations analyzed	Multiple sites	Saliva; Sp-ging	Two sites	Two sites	Saliva	Saliva	Multiple sites	Un-saliva	Un-saliva	Multiple sites	Multiple sites
Specific sites	Buccal H-palate Sb-ging Teeth tongue Tonsils	–	Saliva tongue	Saliva O-P	–	–	Buccal H-palate St-saliva Sp-ging Teeth Tongue	–	–	St-saliva Sp-ging Teeth Tongue Un-saliva	Buccal H-Palate Saliva Sb-ging Sp-ging Throat Tongue Tonsils
Notes	–	–	4 time points	–	12 worldwide locations	–	–	3 time points	–	–	–

H-palate hard palate, *O-P* oropharyngeal, *Sb-ging* subgingival, *Sp-ging* supragingival, *St-Saliva* stimulated saliva, *Un-saliva* unstimulated saliva

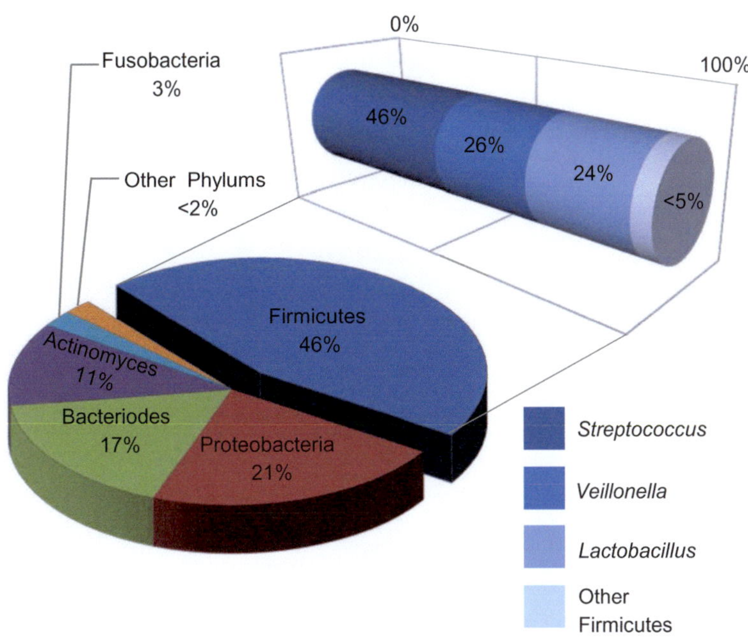

Fig. 5.1 Shared oral microbiome. Average phylum- and genus-level classification of common bacteria colonizing the oral cavity (Data compiled from studies highlighted in Table 5.1)

rapidly attach and colonize bacteria-free surfaces in the mouth (i.e., the salivary pellicle) [41]. Microscopic counts from healthy oral sites showed that 62–79 % are cocci, 10–20 % are nonmotile rods, 1–6 % are motile rods, and spirochetes represent 1–3 % [42–44]. The shared oral microbiome shows that Firmicutes represent the largest phylum followed closely by Proteobacteria, Bacteroidetes, Actinobacteria, and finally Fusobacteria (Fig. 5.1). The rest of the phyla represented less than 2 % in total of the oral microbiome [16, 45]. Altogether, there are predicted to be approximately 150–500 common "species-level" phylotypes present when testing combined oral samples from a single healthy person [40, 45, 46], but there are estimates of more than 19,000 "species-level" phylotypes contributing to the total oral species diversity when considering the entire human population [32].

Pooled sample studies are working toward identifying a global oral microbiome profile for healthy individuals. One study found 72 % of the genus level or above, which accounted for 99.8 % of all the organisms present in the mouth, was the same among unrelated healthy volunteers [16]. Another group found that 15 genera were found to overlap between 10 unrelated healthy individuals [40]. Of these genera, 13 were found to be in

common between both studies: *Streptococcus, Corynebacterium, Neisseria, Rothia, Veillonella, Actinomyces, Granulicatella, Fusobacterium, Haemophilus, Prevotella, Campylobacter, Capnocytophaga,* and *Cardiobacterium* [16, 40]. This overlap creates an outline of the typical organisms and their relative amounts present within healthy individuals, defining the so-called oral "core" microbiome.

Thorough evaluation of oral micro-niches has recently become possible thanks to the culture-independent methods of high-throughput sequencing. Multiple studies have been published outlining the normal microorganisms found in various locations in the mouth. Analysis in one study revealed that at each oral site tested, there was an average of 200–300 different "species-level" phylotypes [16]. Interestingly, comparison between these unrelated healthy volunteers showed a significant overlap in the typical organisms present in each location. When samples were compared across various sampling sites in the mouth, saliva showed the closest relationship to the tongue first, then palate, mucosa and gingiva, and finally plaque [3, 15, 16, 32, 38, 47] (Fig. 5.2). Firmicutes were the dominant species in saliva followed by Bacteroidetes, Proteobacteria, and Actinobacteria [16, 32, 34, 36]. Together, these

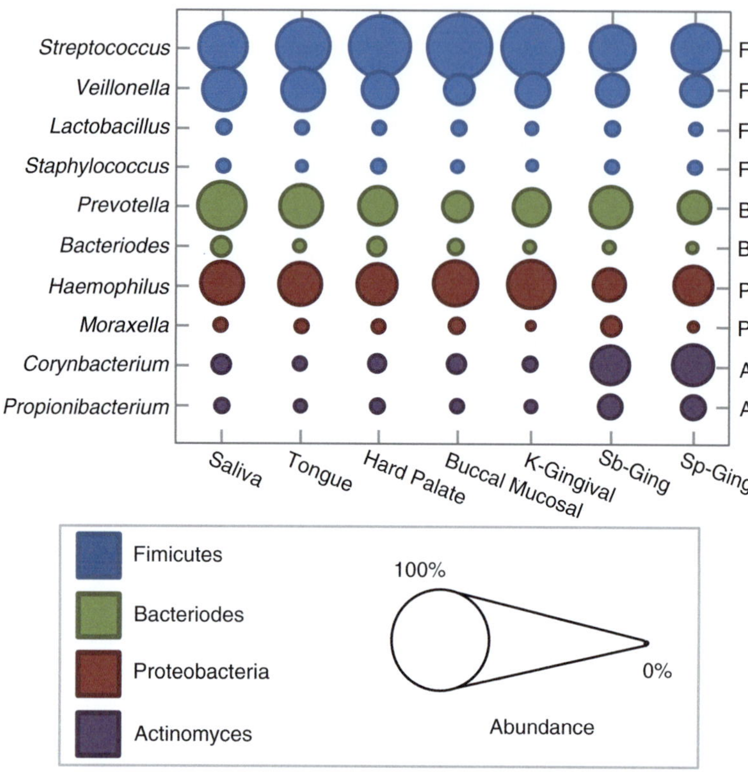

Fig. 5.2 Comparison between bacterial abundance from typical sites in the oral cavity. Relative prevalence of selected oral bacteria shown for a healthy population. *K-Gingival* keratinized gingiva, *Sb-ging* subgingival plaque, *Sp-Ging* supragingival plaque, *F* Firmicutes, *P* Proteobacteria, *B* Bacteroides, *A* Actinomyces (Based on data from [3, 15])

four phyla made up >96 % of the total bacterial composition. Salivary samples were also found to be relatively stable in composition over time among healthy individuals [2, 36, 48, 49]. Samples taken at three separate time points over a period of 29 days showed consistent results in their overall salivary microbiome profile [36]. Overall, these studies revealed that each oral location tested resulted in a relatively unique profile or relative number of microorganisms and these healthy communities are stably maintained over time.

This persistent maintenance of the "normal" flora appears to be a key feature not only in the oral cavity but also in the gut, skin, and vaginal locations [2–4, 11, 15, 16, 31, 48, 50]. Strikingly, the oral environment was found to have the most consistent "core" microbiome maintained between unrelated people in comparison to other microbial sites such as the gut [2, 36, 40]. The other microbiome sites in the body showed a diverse population of bacteria, but there was considerable variation between unrelated individuals [2, 40]. Defining

this "core" microbiome is one of the primary steps that allow for future comparison studies to define profiles that shift away minimally or aggressively from the normal profile.

Shaping the Normal Oral Microbiome

Oral bacteria have preferences for specific sites in the mouth including the teeth, tongue, hard and soft pallet, buccal mucosa, tonsils, gingival tissue, and saliva. Several factors influence the formation and maintenance of the oral ecosystem including the host (host tissues, fluids and signals, diet, genetics), the local environment (pH, temperature, oxygen, amount of nutrients), and the microorganisms themselves (adherence, coaggregation, inter-/intraspecies interactions, virulence mechanisms). The particular community of microorganisms is normally maintained in a state of symbiosis with the host. Yet this diversity can be shifted with changes in the local host condition along with the influence from beneficial and/or antagonistic microbial interactions. In fact, many oral pathogens are opportunist. These pathogens only show virulence when presented with a susceptible host or when a normal host undergoes a number of changes within their oral physiology. Multiple studies have shown that microbial species show distinct properties when part of a multispecies community versus growing in isolation [51–59]. Specifically, work by Foster and Kolenbrander [54] showed that the adherence of certain oral species to an artificial tooth surface was dependent on specific microbial binding partners. These multispecies communities generally respond to changes as a group. The microbial population is continuously undergoing a process of turnover. New microorganisms colonize and persist at the expense of others and based on complex interactions will then influence subsequent population compositions [57].

The foundation of these oral communities starts with the deposit of the salivary pellicle on surfaces. The pellicle is primarily composed of glycoproteins derived from saliva that are recognized by bacterial adhesions, allowing selective binding of mainly Gram-positive cocci to the pellicle surface. In addition to providing a binding surface for bacteria, saliva also provides nutrients for bacterial growth from both endogenous (glycoproteins) and exogenous (carbohydrates and peptides) sources. The saliva also shapes the composition by introducing antimicrobial elements and clearance of bacterial species (see later). Bacteria that have attached to the pellicle generate bacterial products as they grow and multiply that influences the subsequent colonizers. A number of organisms are dependent on coaggregation in order to form part of the microbial community [57]. Once the initial microbial population is established, there is a shift observed in composition as more organisms attach and also based on growth rate differences. The majority of these bacterial communities must be constantly rebuilt in response to the mouth's natural cleansing activities such as saliva production, abrasion, and swallowing.

The Role of Saliva in Forming the Oral Microbial Environment

Saliva is a complex mixture of salivary gland secretions, gingival crevicular fluid, microorganisms, microbial by-products, epithelial cells, and other chemical components. Saliva is secreted by three primary glands, the sublingual, the parotid, and the submandibular, as well as by many minor glands [60]. The amount and type of components present in saliva are known to affect many aspects of oral health and influence bacterial growth [19, 54, 57, 61–66]. The bicarbonates, phosphates, and urea within saliva act to modulate the pH and buffer the oral cavity. Salivary proteins contribute to oral microbial metabolism, aggregation, and attachment as well as bacterial cleansing. Immunoglobulins, enzymes, and proteins in saliva manage bacterial growth through antimicrobial action. Finally, saliva is primarily composed of water and therefore provides the necessary moisture for bacterial survival.

The normal pH of saliva is slightly acidic from 6 to 7; however, the range varies based on salivary flow, with values near 7.8 during high flow, and the pH can approach 5.3 at low flows [60]. Bacteria are able to survive in a wide range of pH conditions, but the healthy microbiome composition is primarily supported by a neutral pH range [19]. Circulating bicarbonate and phosphate systems work together to buffer saliva and maintain pH levels [60]. Bacteria also help to buffer saliva by breaking down urea to ammonia and CO_2, resulting in an increase in pH [67, 68]. The buffering action of saliva is greatly dependent on high flow rate, allowing regulation of the pH in regions such as the oral plaque environment on and around the teeth [69]. The amount of saliva produced in the mouth displays regional variation, with different areas of the mouth producing various volumes. This variation in saliva volume has been directly linked to the regional clearance rate of acid produced by oral bacteria, generating pH micro-niches within the oral cavity [60]. This variation explains some of the regional differences in bacterial composition seen in the oral cavity (Fig. 5.2). A shift toward acidic pH is known to support the growth of acid-producing and acid-tolerant organisms while killing off acid-susceptible bacteria.

There is a large variability in individual flow rates of saliva [70]. Salivary flow is commonly triggered by mechanical chewing and the taste or smell of food. Other factors that influence salivary flow rates are pain, certain medications, and various local and systemic diseases [71–76]. The salivary glands are linked to the sympathetic and parasympathetic nervous system [77]. There are also a number of neurotransmitters and hormones that can influence the rate of salivary flow. Insufficient salivary flow has been clearly associated with a significantly increased risk of oral disease [64, 72, 74, 78, 79] coinciding with a shift in the oral flora [55, 61, 72, 80, 81] (see later). Nutritional changes and deficiencies have also been shown to affect salivary function [19, 82–84] (see later). Salivary flow rates correlate with clearance of fermentable carbohydrates and buffering around high-dental-plaque zones.

Colonization of oral surfaces by bacteria depends on binding to the salivary pellicle (Fig. 5.3). The acquired salivary pellicle is a proteinaceous layer that covers all exposed surfaces in the oral cavity. This complex layer is composed of approximately 90–130 different proteins derived from saliva and crevicular fluid serum [60]. These proteins have been grouped based on various roles including binding calcium and/or phosphate, interaction with other proteins, antimicrobial activity, inflammatory response, immune defense, lubrication, and/or buffering and remineralization. Pellicle formation depends in part on the presence of intact mucins and proline-rich proteins (PRPs). Mucins are glycoproteins mainly secreted by sublingual, submandibular, and palatal glands [87–89]. PRPs constitute the majority of the human parotid saliva [90]. Mucins and PRPs help initiate colonization by healthy oral flora and are incorporated into the bacterial biofilm structure [87, 88, 91, 92]. Healthy bacteria and the mucin pellicle component provide a protective layer that shields

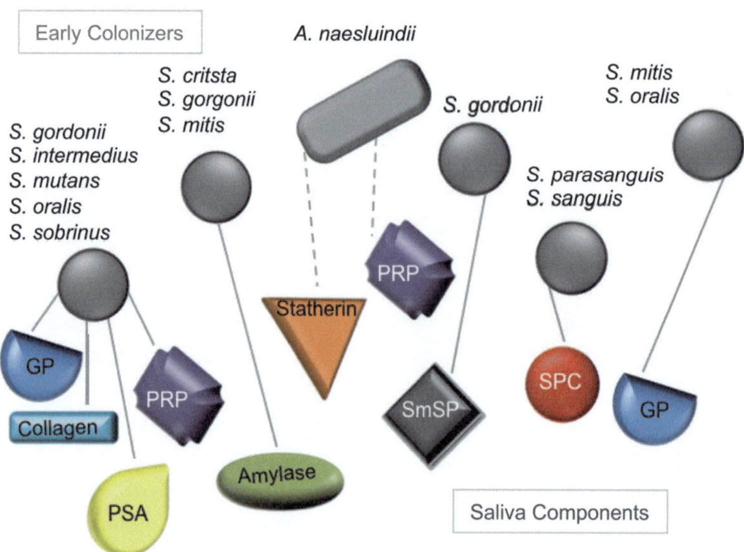

Fig. 5.3 Oral bacteria mediate initial attachment to salivary pellicle. Early colonizers bind to various salivary molecules to initiate attachment to oral surfaces. These connections are mediated by surface adhesions (*solid lines*) or fibrillar appendages (*dashed lines*). These early colonizers provide the main binding capability of the biofilm. Few late colonizers are known to interact with salivary molecules, but one example is *Fusobacterium nucleatum* interacting with statherin [85]. Saliva component abbreviations shown *GP* glycoprotein, *PSA* parotid salivary agglutinin, *PRP* proline-rich protein, *SmSP* submandibular salivary protein, *SCP* salivary component in pellicle, *Streptococcus* genus, except for *Actinomyces naeslundii* (Based on compiled information in [41, 86])

against acids and excessive wear of oral surfaces [88, 93]. If excess colonization takes place, mucins are able to aggregate oral bacteria and clear them from oral surface [93]. Mucins are also critical in hydration and lubrication in the oral cavity and thought to play a role in binding toxins [93–95].

The antimicrobial activity of saliva is primarily maintained by production of immunoglobulins and enzymes. Salivary glands secrete immunologic agents to protect the teeth and mucosal surfaces. IgA, IgG, and IgM are common immunological salivary components. Secretory IgA is the dominant immunoglobulin on all mucosal surfaces, and it works to neutralize viruses and to aggregate bacteria and functions as an antibody to bacterial antigens [96, 97]. Mucin had been shown to work with secretory IgA and bind bacterial pathogens with greater affinity than either molecule working alone [98]. IgM is thought to work in a similar way to IgA but is more susceptible to proteolytic degradation [99]. IgG is primarily added to saliva via crevicular fluid and has been found to inhibit colonization of the oral pathogen *Streptococcus mutans* [100]. Saliva-based enzymes (lactoferrin, lysozyme, peroxidase, amylase) protect the teeth from microbial insults [19, 60]. Nutritional immunity is enacted when lactoferrin binds salivary ferric iron, a necessary nutrient for some oral bacterial species [101, 102]. Lysozyme destroys bacterial cell walls and also promotes clearance through bacterial aggregation [19, 103]. Peroxidase catalyzes the production of bactericidal by-products such as thiocyanate [104]. Amylase is a well-known digestive enzyme secreted by the parotid gland [105]. It functions to modulate the adhesion of certain oral species (e.g., *Streptococcus gordonii* and *Streptococcus mitis*) while forming part of the salivary pellicle and as a component in free saliva [19]. Finally, amylase has been specifically found to inhibit the growth of bacterial pathogens *Legionella pneumophila*, *Neisseria gonorrhoeae*, and *Neisseria meningitidis* [106–109].

Different salivary glands produce saliva with various levels of key salivary components [87, 110]. Differences are seen in the growth of oral bacteria on saliva from different glands [111]. This alone demonstrates that variations in saliva components are able to influence the microbiome of a healthy adult. At the outset, studies have looked at the direct effect on saliva composition and flow rates based on medication, radiation treatment, diet, or disease/trauma directly linked to the salivary gland functionality [73, 76, 79, 101, 112, 113]. A classic example is seen with the autoimmune disease Sjögren's syndrome. Patients with Sjögren's have chronic inflammation that affects their salivary glands leading to reduced salivary flow [76, 113]. Radiation has also been shown to decrease not only the salivary flow rate but also buffering capacity and pH [79, 114]. Together, altering the buffering capacity, salivary flow, and/or protein levels can all lead to major changes in the oral environment.

Mechanisms of Oral Bacterial Colonization

Bacterial Adherence and Coaggregation

Coaggregation is a process whereby two or more species of bacteria adhere to each other via specific adhesin-receptor interactions. Coaggregation is highly selective and dependent on interaction of multiple binding receptors in order to build the structured and complex multispecies community that resides in the oral cavity. Coaggregation allows for colonization of microbial species that lack pellicle receptor sites. This colonization is based on cell-cell interactions that were found to be mediated by existing surface molecules from both viable and dead cells attached to the salivary pellicle or floating in free saliva [54, 57, 58]. These interactions are dependent on multiple factors, including physical proximity, nutrient sources, bacterial factors, and host factors. The spatial location of adhesins and their receptors has been identified using antibodies and microscopy [115]. Confocal microscopy revealed that bacterial cells with complimentarily binder/receptors were found to be adjacent to each other within the biofilm structures [86, 116]. Further studies with electron microscopy demonstrated that there appears to be a competition for binding sites between common partners when using the same binding mechanisms. A classic example of this is seen when coccoid cells (streptococci) bind to long rods such as *Fusobacterium nucleatum* or *Corynebacterium matruchotii* forming a "corncob structure" [117].

If different mechanisms are used in coaggregation, then some organisms may serve as a bridge to connect other species. Indeed, *Prevotella loescheii* was found to link *Streptococcus oralis* to *Actinomyces israelii* [118–120]. The presence of simple sugars in the local environment is also able to change the coaggregation dynamic of several interspecies pairs [63, 119, 121–124]. Dextrans are produced by streptococci, encouraging coaggregation and forming part of the intracellular matrix in the biofilms [121]. The enhanced binding of multiple bacterial partners also has the potential to prevent colonization of pathogenic species as the binding sites are blocked [124]. Collectively, the ability of multiple species to coaggregate with each other plays a key role in the spatial architecture and volume of oral biofilms (Fig. 5.4).

Bacterial Metabolic Products, Food Webs, and Nutrient Sharing

Bacterial metabolic products and food sharing also have the ability to shape the biofilm, encouraging the growth of some species while deterring others. For example, lactic acid is produced by a number of microorganisms in the mouth as a result of carbohydrate fermentation. Some of the most notable acid producers are from *Streptococcus* and *Actinomyces*. This lactic acid can then be used by *Veillonella* allowing for the production of menadione that enriches for growth of *Porphyromonas* and *Prevotella*. *Fusobacterium* creates fatty acids that are used by *Treponema*. *Porphyromonas gingivalis* then works together with *Treponema* to generate products used by *Mogibacterium timidum* [169].

Cooperative nutritional behaviors have also been studied for bacteria growing in saliva as its sole nutrient source [54, 57]. Some species are able to be grown individually with saliva as the sole food source, but many common oral bacteria are not. *Veillonella parvula*, *Aggregatibacter actinomycetemcomitans*, and *Fusobacterium nucleatum* are unable to grow in saliva by themselves. However, pairwise and all together, these three species are able to thrive in saliva. *Actinomyces oris* paired with *Porphyromonas gingivalis*, *V. parvula* paired with *A. oris*, and *V. parvula* paired with *P. gingivalis* all show increased growth in saliva; yet, together the three-species group refuses to grow. *Streptococcus oralis*, *P. gingivalis*, and *V. parvula* grow together, while *S. oralis* paired with *P. gingivalis* does not. This dependency on the presence of certain species before others can survive leads to a defined spatial architecture within the oral biofilms. This spatial dependence is thought to influence the survival of certain microorganisms within these dynamic oral biofilms, and coaggregation used in conjunction with saliva represents a key mechanism of group bacterial clearance [88, 170] and facilitates symbiotic relationships [58].

In contrast to coaggregation and food webs, oral bacteria may also have antagonistic relationships. Thus, production of certain by-products by established microbiota may act to exclude or inhibit growth of other incompatible microbes. A classic example is the production of acid by *S. mutans*, which eliminates competitors that are less tolerant of low pH [171–174]. Streptococcal species may also compete by production of hydrogen peroxide or bacteriocins in an effort to establish certain bacterial species as dominant in a particular host.

The Dynamic Oral Microbiome: Shifting Bacterial Compositions in Response to Change

Changes in salivary flow can greatly influence the microbial composition present in the oral cavity [54, 55, 60, 72, 80, 114]; pH buffering, bacterial nutrient access, and components of the host response all shape the oral environment [19, 60]. While bacterial populations are able to remain relatively stable throughout the day with multiple shifts in saliva production levels and access to

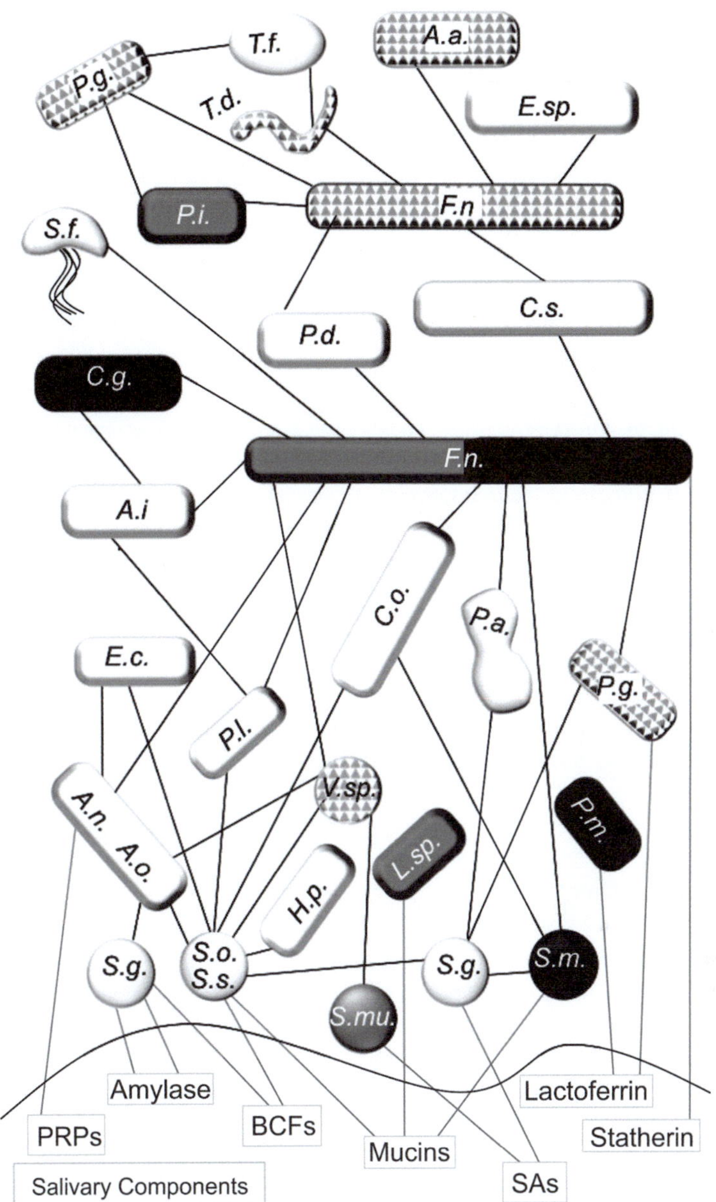

Fig. 5.4 Spatial model of oral bacterial colonization. These bacteria present some common relationships seen in the oral cavity. The salivary component recognition and coaggregation between bacterial binding partners is shown. Bacteria used as part of biomarker studies in cancer diagnosis are indicated in black (see Table 5.4), and biomarkers for oral health diseases are shown in gray (see Table 5.2). The diamond pattern denotes bacterial shifts associated with oral health diseases and selected systemic disease states (see Tables 5.2 and 5.3). *Fusobacterium nucleatum*, in particular, was found to be associated with several different diseases. The saliva component abbreviations shown are proline-rich proteins (*PRPs*), bacterial cell fragments (*BCFs*), and salivary agglutinin (*SAs*). The bacterial species shown are *Aggregatibacter actinomycetemcomitans* (*A.a.*), *Actinomyces israelii* (*A.i.*), *Actinomyces naeslundii* (*A. n.*), *Actinomyces oris* (*A.o.*), *Capnocytophaga gingivalis* (*C.g.*), *Capnocytophaga ochracea* (*C. o.*), *Capnocytophaga sputigena* (*C. s.*), *Eikenella corrodens* (*E. c*), *Eubacterium* spp. (*E. sp.*), *Fusobacterium nucleatum* (*F.n.*), *Haemophilus parainfluenzae* (*H.p.*), *Lactobacillus* spp. (*L.sp.*), *Porphyromonas gingivalis* (*P.g.*), *Prevotella denticola* (*P. d.*), *Prevotella intermedia* (*P.i*), *Prevotella loescheii* (*P.l.*), *Prevotella melaninogenica* (*P.m.*), *Propionibacterium acnes* (*P.a.*), *Selenomonas flueggei* (*S.f.*), *Streptococcus gordonii* (*S.g.*), *Streptococcus mitis* (*S.m.*), *Streptococcus mutans* (*S.mu.*), *Streptococcus oralis* (*S.o.*), *Streptococcus sanguinis* (*S.s.*), *Treponema denticola* (*T.d.*), *Veillonella* spp (*V.sp.*) (This image was adapted from [86] with data added from [166–168] and Tables 5.2, 5.3, and 5.4)

fermentable substrates, prolonged difference in the salivary composition or flow rate can result in a dramatic shift in the oral population. Bacterial mechanisms to tolerate external stress have been well documented [172, 175–177]. Cell-cell communication and biofilm formation oftentimes allow these microbial communities to quickly adapt and survive short-term extreme changes in the environment (e.g., lack or food, host antimicrobial factors). Yet, these complex communities inevitably demonstrate changes in species composition after persistent changes occur in the host environment. On the microbial scale, even minute changes that are not readily perceivable by the host, if consistent, will impact the microbial composition. These shifts in host-microbial homeostasis demonstrate that, instead of considering our microbiome as something peripheral, we need to recognize our flora as an integral part of our body systems.

Next, we will discuss how the oral microbiome shifts away from the oral core microbiome in response to oral-specific diseases and systemic diseases/conditions.

Diseases of the Oral Cavity

Some of the most well-documented relationships between health, disease, and the oral flora can be observed with the common dental ailments of tooth decay (caries) and periodontitis, including gingivitis. These diseases represent two of the most common chronic diseases seen worldwide [178–180]. Several decades of research by dental scientists have clearly illustrated that dental caries and periodontitis are caused by ecological changes in the homeostatic balance between host and bacterial flora (Table 5.2). While initial work assumed that the presence or absence of a single species would be linked to cause and effect for these diseases, it was quickly discovered that these diseases develop along a more complex story line. These oral diseases involve regulation by many sources such as multispecies bacterial connections, host-bacterial interactions, and behavioral or environmental shifts. This body of work begins to demonstrate that changes in the microbial balance can both lead to and result from active oral disease profiles in humans. Oral biofilms have been studied extensively in oral diseases. There is a general progression seen in the buildup of the oral composition as early/primary colonizers attach to the salivary pellicle, additional bacteria bind to the primary colonizers, and finally late colonizers join the group only after a complex community is present. These later colonizers include a number of key oral disease-linked bacteria.

Caries

Dental caries lesions are localized demineralization of tooth enamel as a result of acid

Table 5.2 Bacteria connected to oral health conditions

Oral health condition	Caries	Periodontitis/gingivitis	Healthy
Bacteria	*Actinomyces* spp.	Aggregatibacter actinomycetemcomitans	*Actinomyces* spp.
	Lactobacillus spp.	**Campylobacter rectus**	Capnocytophaga sputigena
	Propionibacterium acidifaciens	**Fusobacterium nucleatum**	Cardiobacterium hominis
	Streptococcus mutans*/*sobrinus	Porphyromonas gingivalis	Haemophilus parainfluenzae
	Veillonella spp.	**Prevotella intermedia/ nigrescens**	Rothia dentocariosa/mucilaginosa
	–	Treponema denticola/ forsythensis	Streptococcus sanguinis
References	[46, 134–145]	[27, 146–151]	[2, 3, 16, 31–38]

Bold indicates organism was used as disease biomarker

production by dental plaque biofilms. Caries progression has been well documented from superficial white spot lesion to deep-dentin cavitations [56]. This decay is due to chronic acid production from bacterial fermentation of carbohydrates in the vicinity of the tooth enamel [56]. Previous work looking for the causative agent of dental caries showed that mutans streptococci (*Streptococcus mutans* and *Streptococcus sobrinus*) appeared to be the primary acid producers associated with enamel caries [56, 134–136, 171, 181]. These bacteria were consistently shown to create the extreme acidic environment necessary for caries conditions, a pH <5.5 [182–184]. More recent research has shown that *Lactobacillus* spp. are also prevalent at active caries site and appear to create the necessary cariogenic conditions in the absence of the *S. mutans* or *S. sobrinus* [137, 138, 185]. These species are all aciduric, meaning that they thrive in low pH environments, while other members of the oral flora do not survive long exposures to acid conditions. The loss of competing species during low pH events creates a feedback loop that ultimately yields more acid production, due to the enrichment of aciduric species in the population, leading to the progressive destruction of enamel and dentin, if left untreated. Thus, caries patients display an increasing accumulation of these cariogenic bacteria. Modern techniques using sequencing technology have allowed for further characterization of not just a few select species but analysis of the entire microbiome at the disease sites. More detailed microbiome sequencing reveals an apparent distinct overall microbial shift as the tooth deterioration progresses from mild white spot lesion to caries dentin involvement and finally to severe disease with deep-dentin lesions [21, 46]. The attachment of specific oral flora to the salivary pellicle was directly tied to the particular binding partners that were present or absent during multispecies biofilm formation [51, 116]. Organisms that would normally be able to bind to the pellicle may be outcompeted for binding sites by other common oral species, while others are completely dependent on "helper" bacteria to mediate any active binding to the pellicle surface. These multispecies interactions appear to significantly influence the makeup of the biofilm composition as well as the circulating bacteria in saliva. These interactions must be constantly reestablished following removal from common oral practices such as swallowing, mechanical abrasion from mastication, and toothbrushing.

Lapses in oral hygiene and increased access to fermentable carbohydrates correlate with increased acid production from certain oral species leading to a localized drop in pH at sites with high levels of dental plaque [83, 186, 187]. This drop in pH then starts an environmental feedback cycle shifting some of the oral flora in the mouth. The decrease in pH starts to kill off susceptible oral bacterial species and selects for acid-tolerant organisms while simultaneously dissolving mineral from the tooth enamel. As the caries disease progresses, the environment has been shown to enrich growth of acid-producing and acid-tolerant bacteria including *S. mutans*, *S. sobrinus*, *Propionibacterium acidifaciens*, *Lactobacillus* spp., *Veillonella* spp., and *Actinomyces* spp. [138, 188]. Allowed to persist, this localized loss of mineral from of tooth enamel can lead to significant structural deterioration and pain.

While these acid-tolerant species increase in numbers, it should be emphasized that the remaining oral species do not completely disappear, but instead are less prevalent at the disease site. It was mentioned earlier that the oral environment normally undergoes a number of environmental shifts throughout the day; nonetheless, the overall composition of the oral flora remains constant in healthy individuals [177, 189]. Thus, bacterial and host biomarker profiles can then be used to infer the risk of developing dental disease as well as monitor dental treatment effectiveness. For example, caries risk has been assessed by the amount of lactobacilli, mutans streptococci, and *Actinomyces* spp. in the patient's saliva [46, 135, 137, 139, 140, 185]. Young children with high levels of *S. mutans* and *S. sobrinus* were more than five times as likely to develop dental caries than individuals with lower levels [135, 136, 141, 190]. Sweden has used salivary levels of lactobacilli (>100,000/ml saliva) and mutans streptococci (>1 million/ml saliva) to determine caries risk for more than 30 years [142–144]. The progression of dental caries was also studied by looking at the microbial composition in white spot lesions, dentin lesions, and deep-dentin lesions [46]. They saw a continuous shift in the bacterial composition as the caries sites progress through the stages of disease. Together, these works indicate that while the presence of key bacterial species is necessary for caries development, a microbial community is crucial to supporting the persistence of those pathogenic species in the oral cavity. This change appears to be driven by changes in the local environmental conditions, such as a lower pH and changes in the host response. Therefore, monitoring known caries pathogens as well as the rest of the microbial community should provide a global picture of the oral disease state and can act as a tool to predict caries risk and treatment outcomes.

Periodontology

Periodontal diseases range from basic inflammation of the gum tissue to major damage of oral connective tissue and bone. Gingivitis is mild to moderate inflammation of the gum tissue, and diseased tissue can normally be reversed to a healthy state with a proper oral hygiene regimen [191, 192]. In contrast, periodontitis is diagnosed when inflammation begins to cause permanent damage to the connective tissue surrounding a tooth or the teeth. As the body tries to respond to the presence of bacterial biofilms on the tooth, the host's immune system actually starts to damage oral tissue. Left untreated, this host-pathogen interaction can lead to loss of gum tissue, loss of attachment of connective tissue to the tooth and bone, and can potentially lead to the loss of teeth [193]. Extensive research has linked the pathology of gingivitis and periodontitis to certain microbial species such as *Porphyromonas gingivalis*, *Treponema denticola*, *Tannerella forsythia*, *Aggregatibacter actinomycetemcomitans*, *Prevotella intermedia/nigrescens*, and *Campylobacter rectus* [146, 147, 194, 195]. These etiological agents are dependent on other members

of the oral flora to allow for colonization, and many times there is also an increase in salivary viral load (see later). These bacteria are late colonizers of the biofilm and are not often allowed access to gum tissue when excellent oral hygiene standards are followed.

Reminiscent of dental caries, periodontitis progression is underpinned by a global shift in microbial species [13, 23, 196]. Extensive work has looked at outlining the composition of the periodontal microbiota in order to help develop more effective treatments and diagnostic testing [12, 13, 193]. The predicted periodontitis microbiome shift was analyzed using the microarray technology HOMIM to discover the major differences between healthy control patients and those patients that responded well to treatment versus those that suffered from refractory periodontitis [23]. More species of bacteria in total were detected in diseased patients in comparison to healthy subjects, where 28 % of the 300 species were not detected in healthy individuals. The putative periodontal pathogens were found in much higher numbers than those with healthy periodontium. Those patients with treatable periodontitis were also distinguishable from those with refractory periodontitis based on their unique bacterial profiles. Significantly higher accumulations of common perio-pathogens such as *T. forsythia*, *P. gingivalis*, and *Prevotella* spp. were found within patients with refractory periodontitis compared to treatable but also more "unusual" species that were present, such as *Brevundimonas diminuta*, *Mycoplasma salivarium*, and *Filifactor alocis* [23]. The microbial profile of the healthy individuals revealed that certain bacterial species were more prevalent in subgingival plaque samples and have been found consistently associated with oral health in other studies, including *Actinomyces* spp. [16, 23], *Capnocytophaga sputigena* [23, 46, 138], *Cardiobacterium hominis* [16, 23], *Haemophilus parainfluenzae* [16, 23], *Rothia dentocariosa/mucilaginosa* [16, 23], *and Streptococcus sanguinis* [23, 46, 138].

Periodontal pathogens have been found to colonize the tongue and other non-periodontal sites [38, 197, 198]. The whole saliva provides the immediate source of bacteria for oral biofilm formation and is therefore predicted to have bacterial profiles that are coupled to the biofilm composition. *P. gingivalis*, *P. nigrescens T. denticola*, and *P. intermedia* were found to have a statistical relationship when comparing saliva and periodontal pocket samples [199]. Additional research has shown both genetic and environmental factors influence bacterial colonization in saliva and the periodontal pocket [200–202]. Several groups have assessed the severity of periodontal disease by using levels of both pathogenic bacteria and host-response biomarkers in saliva [199, 203–206]. Interestingly, investigations have started to show that the bacterial composition shift paired with host biomarkers is correlated with detecting disease stability or periodontitis disease progression [27, 204]. Those patients who showed low bacterial and host biomarker levels fared better than those with high bacterial and host biomarker amounts. Kinney et al. [27] showed that the elevated presence of *Fusobacterium nucleatum*, *C. rectus*, and *P. intermedia* predicted disease progression in 82 % of patients. Low levels of host biomarkers, matrix metalloproteinases 8 and 9 (host-derived enzymes involved with tissue and bone degradation), osteoprotegerin (inhibitor of differentiation and activation of osteoclasts involved in bone resorption), and IL-1 (inflammatory cytokine) predicted periodontal site stability 78 % of the time. These studies present some of the novel work that is starting to link microbiome composition to disease progression and treatment outcomes [13, 193]. Overall, patients who were successfully treated for periodontitis showed a shift back toward a healthy oral microbiome [13].

Defining the oral microbiome has allowed researchers to start to understand the normal commensal organisms that are consistent with health. Key work looking at oral-specific disease supported the hypothesis that the oral microbiome usually harbors a core microbiome, and changes in the core composition are directly related to oral disease progression due to dysbiosis. However, it was still unclear if other disease states were linked to the oral microbiome. This shift from homeostasis to dysbiosis reflects a common theme seen across many microbiome profiles that a disease state may not show complete removal and/or enrichment of certain species but instead results in a dramatic shift in the overall proportions of the total microbiome. The microbiome acts like a community that is influenced by the overall presence of key players that may aid in attachment, acquiring nutrients, surviving fluctuations in the environment, etc. Work outlined in the next section will focus on how the oral microbiome has ties to other systemic diseases such as diabetes, autoimmune disorders, hematologic diseases, vitamin deficiencies, and cancer.

The Oral Microbiome and Systemic Conditions

Saliva contains a number of components that could be used for disease risk assessment. Saliva microbial components are already commonly used for the diagnosis of many dental diseases including caries risk, periodontal disease, saliva gland dysfunction and disease, and oral-based fungal infections [13, 138, 145, 160, 161, 207]. Additional recent work has used microbial and/or host markers in saliva to identify tuberculosis, cancers, gastric ulcers, liver malfunction, and Sjögren's syndrome [60, 80, 81, 133, 208–210].

Based on the relatively new fields of microbiomics and metabolomics, research is just starting to test these predicted shifts in microbial profiles in a number of systemic diseases. Mapping these alternate oral microbiomes may help us better understand what happens as the body challenges these microorganisms with a new environment in response to disease (Tables 5.3 and 5.4).

Diabetes

Numerous studies have started to uncover the link between oral health and type 2 diabetes [211]. High, uncontrolled blood sugar levels are associated with excess bleeding and poor healing overall [212–214]. Diabetic patients have been

Table 5.3 Oral manifestations and associated oral flora shift in selected disease states

Disease or condition	Diabetes	Autoimmune: Crohn's disease	Autoimmune: Sjögren's disease	Nutrition/vitamin deficiency
Oral manifestation	↑Risk caries, gingivitis, periodontitis	Oral lesions	Chronic inflammation of salivary glands	↓Salivary flow
		Oral swelling	↓Saliva production	↑ Caries
		↑ Caries	Xerostomia (dry mouth)	↑Periodontitis
			↑Caries	Oral lesions
				Enamel defects
				Inflammation
				Delayed dental eruption
Bacteria	↑*P. gingivalis*	↓*Fusobacteria* spp.	↑*S. mutans*	–
	↑*A. actinomycetemcomitans*	↓Firmicutes	↑*Lactobacillus* spp.	
	↑*F. nucleatum*	↑*Prevotella melaninogenica*	↑*Staphylococcus aureus*	
	↑*Veillonella parvula/dispar*	↑*Neisseria mucosa*	↓*Fusobacterium nucleatum*	
	↑*Eikenella corrodens*		↓*P. intermedia/nigrescens*	
	↑*C. rectus*			
Fungi			↑*Candida albicans*	↑*C. albicans*
References	[152–157]	[158, 159]	[80, 81, 160–163]	[112, 164, 165]

found to have a significantly higher risk for gingivitis and periodontitis [211, 212, 215]. One large-scale study that looked at 4,343 adults revealed that diabetics have an odds ratio of 2.9 for periodontitis compared to those not suffering from diabetes [216]. Diabetic patients who better controlled their glycemic levels saw their odds ratio fall to approximately 1.56 [216]. When patients are failing to control their diabetes, they show a consistent flare in oral diseases [215, 216]. Systemic problems with increased blood glucose levels lead to chronic inflammatory immune response leading to excess production of inflammatory proteins, which may help to keep the microbiome in check [12, 211, 217]. While the subgingival bacterial profile showed the same type of species in periodontal patients with diabetes in comparison to those periodontal patients without diabetes, the relative abundance was different between diabetic and nondiabetic [152, 153]. The diabetic patients show higher numbers overall of assessed perio-pathogens (Table 5.3). Diabetic patients appear to show an exaggerated inflammatory response to the same oral periodontal pathogens and in some cases

increased apoptosis (programmed cell death). This enhanced inflammation and apoptosis is thought to be involved with delayed wound healing and likely explains some of the excess periodontal tissue damage seen in diabetic patients [218]. Interestingly, a key relationship was found between one particular oral pathogen, *P. gingivalis*, and insulin. Lipopolysaccharide released from *P. gingivalis* has been shown to be toxic to some cytokine proteins that regulate insulin levels in the body [219, 220]. Proinflammatory cytokines, including interleukins 1 and 6 along with tumor necrosis factor-alpha, are produced in inflamed periodontal tissue [221–223]. These factors gain access to the body's general circulation via the periodontal microcirculation [224, 225], which then allows them to systemically antagonize insulin [226]. Whole-body insulin resistance was also found to be triggered by bacterial infection [154].

Research has demonstrated that treatment for periodontitis, which also shifts the microbial microbiome, improves the overall health outcomes for these patients [12, 211, 222]. However, diabetes can also lead to additional oral disorders

Table 5.4 Oral bacterial shifts observed in cancer patients

Disease	OSCC	Head and neck cancer	Upper GI tract cancer	Colorectal cancer	Gastric precancerous lesions	Pancreatic diseases (cancer)
Bacteria	*Fusobacterium naviforme* *S. aureus* **Streptococcus mitis** **Prevotella melaninogenica** **Capnocytophaga gingivalis**	*Streptococcus anginosus*	*S. anginosus* *T. denticola*	*F. nucleatum*	*A. actinomycetemcomitans*	***Neisseria elongata*** ***S. mitis***
References	[47, 125, 126]	[45, 47, 127]	[128]	[129, 130]	[131, 132]	[133]

OSCC oral squamous cell carcinoma, *Bold* indicates organism was used as disease biomarker

including fungal infections, salivary functional disorders, dental caries, and burning mouth syndrome [154, 227, 228]. Together, this systemic disorder leads to major changes in the body and importantly the oral environment. Diabetes and oral infections have a bidirectional relationship where the presence of one seems to further provoke the other and leads to a global increase in symptoms and decrease in quality of life. Here we see that a systemic disorder can significantly advance the periodontitis infection resulting in a shift in the microbial profiles with increased frequency of perio-pathogens consistent with diabetes plus periodontitis.

Autoimmune Disorders

Autoimmune disorders represent a wide-ranging group of diseases that can impact the human body with varied severity. Oftentimes, autoimmune disorder patients suffer cyclical disease presentation where "flares" coincide with severe disease symptoms and times when symptoms are manageable to nonexistent [162, 229, 230]. There are some autoimmune diseases that show consistent oral presentations in addition to other symptoms [230]. In some cases, the oral symptoms have been known to precede more classic symptoms [230]. This is sometimes seen with Crohn's disease oral lesions. Crohn's disease is an autoimmune disorder that primarily impacts the intestines, but secondary symptoms are seen with the joints, skin, and liver [229]. Oral manifestations have been used for Crohn's diagnosis [78, 231, 232]. These symptoms include mucosal tags; gingival, labial, or mucosal swelling; and ulcers. The patterns of oral symptoms and histology mimic those seen in the intestine with inflammation, ulcers, and swelling. The severity of the oral lesions has been shown to predict the extent of disease in the intestine [230]. In some cases, the oral presentation will precede the systemic symptoms and could be used as an indicator for further confirmatory testing [230, 231, 233]. Microbial shifts were seen in Crohn's disease patients including an overall decrease in Firmicutes and increases in *Prevotella melaninogenica* and

Neisseria mucosa [158, 159]. Patients with Crohn's disease show an increased risk for caries development [159]. In addition, inflammation in the intestine has been shown to lead to malabsorption [234, 235]. This nutritional deficiency can lead to significant changes in the oral environment (see later).

Sjögren's syndrome is an autoimmune disease that attacks the endocrine glands, including the salivary glands that lead to a significant decrease in the production of saliva [113, 162]. The dry mouth conditions means there is considerable risk for severe dental diseases [62, 162]. Predictably, patients with primary Sjögren's syndrome were found to have increased levels of *S. mutans*, *Lactobacillus* spp., and *Candida albicans* within their supragingival plaque samples [81]. The smooth mucosa and tongue samples also showed increased prevalence of *Staphylococcus aureus* and *Candida albicans* [80, 81, 160, 163]. The greatest shift in microbial differences was observed by patients who had a stimulated saliva secretion rate of <0.5 ml/min [81]. The primary risk factor that seems to be associated with this shift in the bacterial profile is the reduced saliva production. There is, however, a change seen in the protein levels of Sjögren's syndrome patients as well [114, 236]. This suggests that reduced salivary flow combined with changes in the salivary composition shapes the microbial accumulation in the mouth. These shifts may therefore be used to predict "flares" along with assessing treatment progress.

Nutrition and Vitamin Deficiencies

Changes in the diet are known to alter the overall composition of some species within the oral flora [177, 237–239]. Malnutrition has been linked to reduced salivary flow rates, changes in bacterial numbers, and shifts in salivary composition [82, 164, 239–241]. There has been a documented increase in the prevalence of oral pathogens that are involved with caries development as our modern human diets have increased in refined sugar consumption [83, 242]. Scarcity of certain foods and nutrients can dramatically alter the oral environment. The mucous membranes in the mouth show a high cell turnover rate (3–7 days) versus the skin (up to 28 days) [243, 244]. The oral cavity may, therefore, exhibit signs and symptoms more quickly from direct nutritional deficiencies or systemic diseases that lead to nutritional/vitamin depletion. Vitamin deficiencies can lead to generalized issues in the oral cavity [164]. Many deficiencies are associated with oral-specific symptoms including caries, delayed dental eruption, enamel defects, and oral lesions [164, 235, 239, 241]. Dentists may be involved with diagnosis of vitamin deficiencies based on presenting oral symptoms when no other obvious cause is present. For example, megaloblastic anemia, due to a lack of the vitamin B12, displays oral mucosal membrane change in approximately 50–60 % of the patients [195, 245, 246]. In general, low iron levels are known to contribute to diminished bactericidal activity from leukocytes, impaired cellular immunity, epithelial abnormality, and inadequate antibody response. These changes in the host lead to generalized oral problems including inflammation, higher prevalence of oral candidiasis, and predicted shifts in oral flora that are sensitive to low iron levels [239, 247–252]. Vitamin A deficiency leads to dry mouth, impaired tooth growth, and increased susceptibility to infection [164, 253, 254]. Vitamin C is important for healthy collagen formation and serves to enhance iron absorption [164, 255–257]. Vitamin C deficiency has been shown to contribute to the severity of periodontal disease [165, 241]. Patients that were suffering from vitamin C deficiency displayed more attachment loss than those with normal vitamin C levels. Together, these missing nutrients and many others may indicate the start of systemic disease that impacts the oral cavity early on and left untreated can result in severe damage [112, 164, 214, 235, 239].

Cancer

There is a new and novel work that is following potential links between the oral microbiome and various cancers (Table 5.4). This field is just starting to highlight microbiome differences observed in cancer patients versus healthy individuals. A majority of the work, so far, has looked at the oral flora composition and its link to oral and other head-/neck-associated cancers (e.g., esophagus, pharyngeal, etc.). Oral, head, and neck cancers are the sixth most common cancer seen worldwide [258]. Despite many advances in cancer diagnosis and treatment, in general, the overall prognosis for oral cancer patients has not improved much in recent years [259–261]. Improving early detection of many different types of cancers remains a key objective of salivary diagnostics, and here we will emphasize some of the promising research in that field.

A few groups have started to survey the bacteria that colonize different regions in the mouth, focusing on both malignant and healthy sites in oral and upper gastrointestinal locations [47, 127, 128, 133, 262, 263]. These groups found that the microbial composition differed significantly for at least some of the bacterial species when comparing normal, healthy tissue to malignant sites. For example, Hooper et al. [125, 126] conducted two studies that looked at the bacterial composition of oral squamous cell carcinoma tissue samples. The oral cancer tissues showed a distinct profile of several oral species including *Fusobacterium naviforme* and *Staphylococcus aureus*. In contrast, analysis of various upper gastrointestinal tract carcinomas found a distinct link with one particular species, *Streptococcus anginosus* [128]. *S. anginosus* DNA was also found in carcinoma tissue from head and neck squamous cell biopsies but not in those from other cancer types, including oral cancer [127, 264, 265]. One potential explanation given for these observed differences in bacterial composition between cancer and cancer-free sites is that certain oral bacterial cells may actually be influencing signals that initiate and advance oral and head-/neck-associated cancers [266], as well as other cancers [267, 268]. There are several cases where microorganisms are considered the primary source of cancer, including the classic bacterial example of *Helicobacter pylori* infection leading to gastric cancer formation [269, 270] plus numerous viral-associated cancers [271–276]. In these cases, the microorganisms were directly involved with influencing the development of specific cancers. Intriguingly, preliminary studies have found a link between *H. pylori* infection and oral cancer diagnosis [263, 277, 278]. In addition, several normal oral bacterial residents have been shown to have a direct influence on stimulating an inflammatory response in the mouth [153, 211, 279]. Although many of the exact mechanisms leading from bacterial infection to carcinogenesis remain largely unclear, there is a general link between upregulation of cytokines and other inflammatory mediators that leads to an increased risk of carcinogenesis [280–282].

Because the aforementioned studies imply that the presence of certain bacterial species may actually increase the likelihood of developing certain cancers, these and other bacterial species can potentially be used as a portent for diagnosing cancer early. One particular study looked at comparing the bacterial salivary composition from 229 healthy controls versus 45 patients with oral cancer [47]. This work found principal increases in *Streptococcus mitis*, *Prevotella melaninogenica*, and *Capnocytophaga gingivalis* among patients with oral squamous cell carcinoma in comparison to the controls. Further analyses showed that these species could be used as a diagnostic biomarker for oral cancer. The three-species diagnostic marker predicted 80 % of the cancer cases correctly while excluding the controls approximately 82 % of the time. Importantly, this research group found that the soft tissue bacterial composition was similar to that of the saliva composition. As mentioned earlier, different locations in the mouth may have large differences in the oral microbiome structure. This represents a key feature of testing since the cancerous or precancerous oral lesions may not be obvious in patients and will have to be diagnosed from a shift in saliva alone.

Several groups have also found an interesting link between the oral microbial composition and other cancers [47, 262, 263, 268, 283, 284]. Gastric precancerous lesion risk was found to positively correlate with high levels of periodontal bacterial pathogens [131, 132]. Gastric cancer has the second highest mortality rate worldwide and is the fourth most common cancer [285]. Patients with periodontitis that showed an increased colonization

by *Actinobacillus actinomycetemcomitans* were more likely to have precancerous gastric lesions. Of interest, *A. actinomycetemcomitans* is associated with systemic infections along with being a general cause of periodontitis; therefore, its association with the oral flora may have been directly influenced by additional signals from the host resulting in favorable colonization. *Fusobacterium nucleatum* was recently shown to have a link to colorectal cancer [129, 130]. Colorectal adenomas, colorectal cancer tissue, and feces from colorectal cancer patients all showed significantly higher rates of *Fusobacterium* spp. in comparison to healthy controls. A mouse model of intestinal tumorigenesis demonstrated a rise in proinflammatory markers and increased infiltration of myeloid immune cells in *F. nucleatum* treated animals [129]. Human colon tissue samples also showed a strong correlation between the *F. nucleatum* levels and the expression of proinflammatory markers (COX-2, IL-1β[beta], IL-6, IL-8, and TNF-α[alpha]) [129, 286, 287]. A proposed mechanism for *Fusobacterium* involvement in colorectal cancer is based on the cell-surface *Fusobacterium* adhesion molecule (FadA) binding to E-cadherin on the surface of host epithelial cells [288]. Binding activates β(beta)-catenin signaling, *F. nucleatum* invasion, and inhibition of tumor suppressor activity promoting colorectal cancer formation. FadA levels are presented as a proposed marker for early diagnosis of colorectal cancer. However, it is still unclear whether *Fusobacterium* is acting as a commensal to modify the forming tumor microenvironment or instead it is an opportunistic pathogen and directly responsible for the promotion of colorectal cancer.

Finally, HOMIM was used to look at the oral microbiota in patients with various pancreatic diseases. The salivary microbiome was observed to be significantly different in patients with pancreatic disease, including cancer, in comparison to the healthy controls [133]. Pancreatic cancer patients had an increase in 31 bacterial clusters/species and decrease in 21 bacterial clusters/species. Further analysis, testing 16 species/clusters as a pancreatic disease biomarker, showed that combining *Neisseria elongata* and *Streptococcus mitis* were the most valid biomarkers. The combination biomarker resulted in a 96.4 %

sensitivity and 82.1 % specificity in determining pancreatic cancer patients from healthy individuals. Novel recent work from the same lab has presented evidence for a mechanism connecting systemic disease with salivary changes. Lau et al. [210] found that pancreatic cancer-derived exosomes, "cell-specific lipid vesicles," provide a link between the primary cancer site and saliva biomarker production in mice. These exosomes that are able to travel through the vascular systems are involved with intercellular communication and are thought to be associated with a number of functions including immune response regulation and tumor invasion promoters [289, 290]. A number of host factors were shown to be upregulated based on saliva comparison from healthy and diseased mice using microarray analysis. Some of these host factors have the potential to influence the bacterial compositions observed in the cancer patients versus cancer-free individuals (Table 5.5). The presence of human serum was also shown to influence the adhesion and coaggregation phenotypes in a number of oral species [55]. This leads to a tempting mechanism that exosomes have the potential to travel from newly forming cancer sites to deliver disease-specific products directly to saliva, which can then shape the oral microbial environment through direct messages or trigger secondary messages such as hormones and cytokines (Fig. 5.5). These oral changes can, therefore, presumably be used to monitor distant body sites throughout disease progression.

Table 5.5 Upregulated saliva gene products in response to pancreatic cancer and the predicted bacterial association

Gene product	Predicted function	Bacterial association
sema6d	Immune response (CD4+ T cell regulation) and gastric cancer [291, 292]	Commensal gut bacteria displays CD4+ T cells response [293]
daf2	Associated with insulin receptor [294]	*Caenorhabditis elegans daf2* mutants are resistant to bacterial pathogens [295–297]
aspn	Binds collagen and calcium [298]	Divalent cation concentrations influence bacterial adhesion [299–302]

The Other Microbiomes: Mycobiome and Virome

The majority of work looking at the human microbiome has focused on bacteria composition. In reality the microbiome contains fungal and viral components as well. While this is still an emerging area of study, there are some intriguing research efforts coming to light related to fungal and viral shifts in response to systemic disease.

Mycobiome

Candida albicans has been consistently seen as an indicator of oral microbiome imbalance and other oral diseases [303, 304]. This overgrowth of *Candida albicans* is commonly known as oral thrush. Thrush is seen in the immunocompromised and immunosuppressed patients, including patients with human immunodeficiency virus (HIV), cancer patients, infants, elderly, etc. As many as 90 % of HIV patients will present with reoccurring oral candidiasis [305–308]. Diabetic patients with high blood sugar and patients with Sjögren's are also more prone to candidiasis infections [160, 163, 309]. The generalized presentation of candidiasis is a good visual indictor that something is systemically wrong with the patient, though infant oral thrush does not indicate a problem unless the infection continues for several weeks. Unfortunately, because a variety of conditions can lead to candidiasis, it is not specific and thus provides limited information about the potential systemic issue without further testing. Just like the bacterial composition, a defined oral mycobiome will need to be established to determine differences between conditions of health and disease. One group has started this work by looking at the oral mycobiome of 20 healthy individuals [207]. They were able to detect 74 culturable and 11 unculturable fungal genera in the oral cavity. As few as 3 and as many as 39 genera were found in these healthy volunteers. *Candida* spp. were present in more than 75 % of the individuals, followed by *Cladosporium* at 65 % and Saccharomycetales and *Aureobasidium* at 50 % each. Intriguingly, a

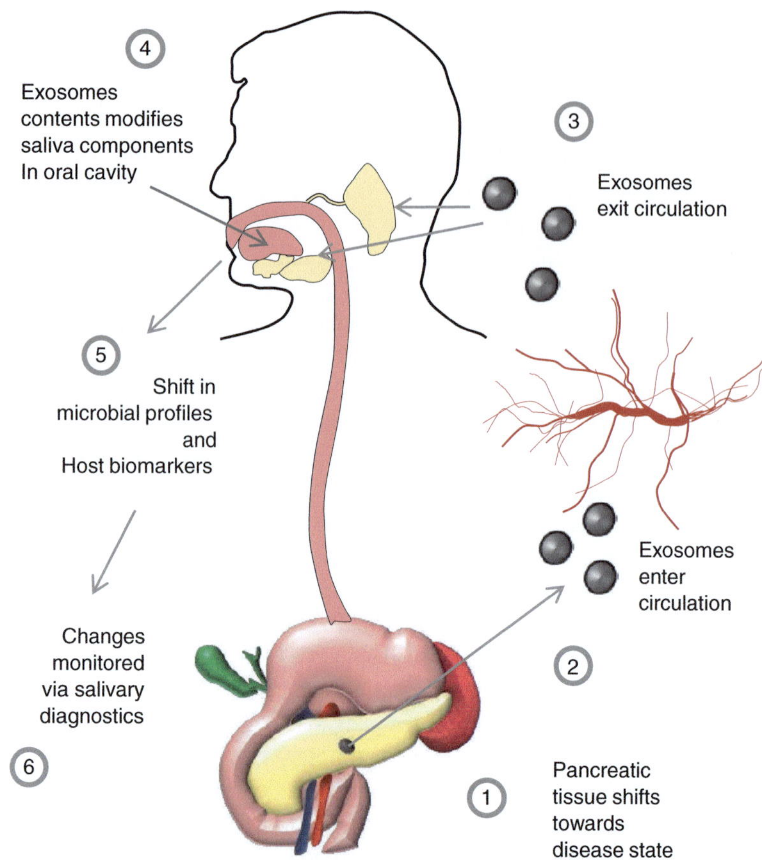

Fig. 5.5 Model for pancreatic disease detection using salivary diagnostics. (*1*) Pancreas tissue transitions toward a disease state. (*2*) Exosomes from the pancreas enter the circulatory system. (*3*) Exosomes deliver disease-specific products directly to the salivary glands. (*4*) The oral microbiome is changed through direct signaling or secondary message effects within the saliva. (*5, 6*) Saliva samples can be used to detect changes in host biomarkers and the oral microbiome providing noninvasive feedback of disease progression and/or treatment outcomes

cluster analysis showed that mycobiome profiles of males and females were separate from one another. This study represents the first survey of the fungal species present in the oral cavity and only surveyed a small number of people. Similar to the bacterial microbiome surveys, the oral mycobiome is predicted to reveal a core set of fungal organisms present within healthy populations along with unique species specific to each individual. In fact, efforts have shown that the total composition of an individual's human microbiome is just as unique as a fingerprint with no two people alike [310].

Virome

The persistent presence of viruses in saliva can be observed for a number of reasons. Viruses can be transferred by direct contact with infected individuals, a blood-borne viral infection can allow for salivary gland involvement, or the oral cavity itself may be infected in the mucosa or diseased periodontal sites [148]. Like with candidiasis patients, those with compromised or suppressed immune systems will also likely display a viral load increase in saliva. The presence of viruses in saliva presents another noninvasive disease diagnosis opportunity. In light of this, a number of groups have developed saliva-based viral detection tests for common human viruses including HIV [311], hepatitis viruses [312], herpes viruses [312, 313], and measles virus [314]. Researchers are starting to characterize the human virome; however, this field is still emerging. One key problem lies in detecting the presence of unknown viruses. Unlike bacteria that have a conserved 16s ribosomal region within their DNA, viruses have little DNA sequence in common. Plus, the majority of viruses in the human body are specific for bacteria hosts (bacteriophage) and not humans [315, 316]. Those bacteriophages are able to indirectly impact humans by changing the abundance or function of our resident bacteria. With the advent of shotgun sequencing, we can now look at all the DNA whether it is human, bacterial, fungal, or viral. Studies using this approach on the gut virome found that mothers and children, and identical twins have similar viromes [317, 318]. Another study looked at the viral composition present inside the lungs of cystic fibrosis (CF) patients in comparison to non-CF patients [319]. They found some differences in the viral composition but significant changes in metabolic functions as a result of these viruses in the lung. These variations are thought to influence the severity of cystic fibrosis; however, this was a small-scale study with five CF and five non-CF patients. A larger analysis used nasal swabs from 176 children, some healthy and some with unexplained fevers. The children with unexplained fevers had more viruses on average than those that were healthy, suggesting the fevers may have been viral in nature and not bacterial [320].

New human viruses and bacteriophages are discovered every day; nonetheless, new viruses that posses DNA or RNA that is unlike any other known sequence will likely be missed in these large-scale sequence surveys until a more universal method of identifying viruses becomes available. Much of the work to date has, therefore, focused on quantifying the viral load of known human viruses, mainly those belonging to the herpes-type viruses.

Herpes Viruses

Herpes viruses are the most common viral type found in human saliva [321–323]. There are eight known herpes viruses that infect humans: herpes simplex types 1 and 2, cytomegalovirus, Epstein-Barr virus, varicella zoster virus, herpes virus 6, herpes virus 7, and herpes virus 8 (Kaposi's sarcoma) [324]. Herpes viral infections can lead to diseases of the periodontium and oral mucosa or may present asymptomatically but still with active viral shedding into saliva [322, 324]. Herpes viruses exist in either the lytic (active) or latent (dormant) phase [324] and persist as a

permanent infection of the host. The change from dormant to active replication in healthy adults can happen spontaneously or more likely is caused by environmental changes (e.g., physical or emotional stress) [325–332]. Those suffering from systemic diseases (e.g., HIV, cancer) or immunosuppression (e.g., elderly) often display a reactivation of herpes viruses that may exacerbate or create new symptoms.

Thorough work looking at astronauts has shown that in space otherwise healthy adults shift into a state of immuno-dampening [326, 333]. Viruses that are normally kept in check by the body's immune system start to flourish and result in oral shedding. Epstein-Barr virus and varicella zoster are found in enormous quantities while the astronauts are in space for several weeks after returning to earth [326, 328, 329]. A similar herpes zoster viral shedding is also seen in some pregnant women [334]. Cold sores caused by herpes simplex 1 virus tend to come back during times of stress [334, 335]. This allows the normally latent virus to take hold and cause an active disease again. Aging adults often fail to control reactivation of Epstein-Barr virus, cytomegalovirus, and/or varicella zoster viruses [336]. The latter virus results in the development of painful shingles disease that can last for several weeks or months. All of the patients mentioned above exhibited some type of change or challenge to their immune system leading to increased viral load in their saliva. Yet, healthy adults can also continually shed various herpes viruses. These healthy adults are often asymptomatic and may easily spread the viruses [333, 335, 337].

Interesting research has shown that herpes virus infection is associated with periodontitis. A dual infection of both oral pathogenic bacteria and a herpes virus leads to immune signaling impairment, enhanced proinflammatory cytokine release, and more severe periodontitis [223, 313, 338, 339]. A distinct correlation has been found with Epstein-Barr and cytomegalovirus between both gingivitis and periodontitis. The prevalence of Epstein-Barr genome copies in dental patients was evaluated in separate studies and showed an average of 8 % in healthy individuals and 20 % in those suffering from gingivitis [149, 150, 323,

340–343] along with 46 % for chronic periodontitis and 58 % for aggressive periodontitis [149, 150, 340, 343–347]. Studies focused on cytomegalovirus showed similar results with a positive correlation between gingivitis/periodontitis and viral infection (average 8 % healthy, 33 % gingivitis, 52 % chronic periodontitis, and 42 % aggressive periodontitis) [149, 150, 221, 323, 341, 343, 344, 346, 348]. Periodontal lesions have been implicated as the main salivary source of the cytomegalovirus [341]. Together these studies suggest that herpes virus infection may contribute to gingivitis and periodontitis infection in at least a subset of patients. Not surprisingly, periodontal treatment leads to a significant decrease in salivary viral load [344, 349]. These herpes virus infections are hypothesized by some to actually contribute to the inconsistent infections seen with periodontitis. Many patients will have healthy tissue right next to chronic or aggressive periodontitis infections. The presence of active periodontitis infection means that periodontal pathogens are circulating in the saliva; yet, they do not infect all tissue sites. These viruses are therefore predicted to create an initial infection site and then create a gateway for bacterial pathogens.

Other diseases/conditions have also been linked to the presence of herpes viruses [323, 343, 347]. High levels of herpes simplex 1 viral DNA were found in 31 % of the patients (parotid and submandibular saliva samples) with Bell's palsy (peripheral facial paralysis) on their affected side versus the unaffected side [350]. The presence of oropharyngeal herpes zoster lesions resulted in an increased viral load in saliva versus herpes zoster skin lesions, and these saliva levels correlated with reactivation of the virus within the facial nerve seen in the Ramsay Hunt syndrome [351, 352]. HIV infection has a clear relationship with herpes simplex virus (HSV) reactivation; as CD4 cell counts decrease, the herpes viral loads increase [271, 321, 353–357]. Herpes simplex regulatory proteins were also shown to increase HIV replication when HIV-infected CD4 cells are recruited to HSV-infected lesions [321, 358]. Down syndrome is associated with a systemic shift in the immune system. Neutrophil and monocyte chemotaxis reduction, phagocytosis impairment, and decline in T-lymphocyte counts are all seen as complications of Down syndrome [359]. Down syndrome children have a higher frequency of herpes simplex viruses, cytomegalovirus, and Epstein-Barr virus than children without Down syndrome [348, 360]. Finally, patients receiving bone marrow and stem cell transplants showed reactivation of cytomegalovirus in their saliva [361].

Bacterial-Viral Interactions

Considerable work indicates that human viruses and bacteria have distinct synergistic interactions that aid in pathogenic behavior. Herpes virus infections are typically associated with a rise in the amount of oral pathogenic bacteria [313]. Hormonal changes during puberty have been shown to reactivate oral cytomegalovirus infection sites, leading to a localized change in the immune system allowing for enrichment of perio-pathogens such as *A. actinomycetemcomitans* [149, 313, 362]. Copy numbers of cytomegalovirus and Epstein-Barr virus of severe periodontitis sites were linked to abundance of *P. gingivalis* and/or *T. forsythia* [149, 363]. Cytomegalovirus was shown to enhance the binding of *A. actinomycetemcomitans* to primary periodontal epithelial cells [364]. These bacterial-viral interactions likely work bidirectionally. Oral bacterial pathogens can take advantage of immune dysregulation by active herpes-type virus infection, and the established bacteria have the potential to reactivate latent viruses in oral tissues [313, 365].

Based on these aforementioned close connections, viral saliva load may be used as a risk indicator for developing certain diseases, as well as provide further testing for patients to modify their current treatment regimen to specifically inhibit herpes viral replication. The ease of testing saliva for viruses has already been used commercially for a number of viruses, including in-home testing kits for HIV. Currently, these kits rely on testing for a specific virus. Having access to the core human virome will prove crucial to developing a more comprehensive test. Many viral and host factors are known to cause universal reactivation of dormant viruses [366]. Furthermore, conditions of stress, disease, and general immunosuppression can influence the viral load numbers in saliva [148]. Consequently, the human virome relative composition can work together with other microbiome data and salivary host biomarkers to provide a comprehensive look at the health status of patients.

Conclusion

To the Future

We have seen that systemic disease states have the potential to shift our resident microbiome toward imbalance. Several studies have found a progressive shift in the composition of bacteria associated with various oral diseases, and new analysis with systemic diseases shows they may also result in a significant change. Ideally, taking a sample from the mouth could prove to be the key to diagnosing oral and systemic diseases. As multispecies bacterial identification techniques become less costly, these methods could potentially be offered by a medical care provider or paired with a dental office visit. Several groups have started creating fully automated diagnostic units that can be used to help identify viral and bacterial levels in saliva [236, 312, 367, 368]. In fact, both saliva and tongue swabs could easily be used to screen for human biomarkers and the microbial profile in a single test. Together, these results should allow for an "early alert system" for patients to follow up with their physician. With these diagnostic tools in place, early detection should increase treatment options, decrease potential hospitalizations, and has the potential to improve quality of life overall.

In looking toward the future, the microbiome composition of bacteria, fungi, and/or viruses may actually be used routinely as markers of host physiological changes and preferably diagnostic tools that would allow for earlier recognition before global symptoms are present in patients.

Using host biomarkers together with the oral microbiome profile should provide a stronger specificity for these diagnostic tests. Important primary research is currently underway to understand what are the normal microorganisms present in healthy humans. These microbial surveys will determine the baseline, and more work will need to continue to identify predicted shifts in these normal profiles under different disease states.

Right now, these microbial surveys have the potential to diagnose malignancies and disease states and provide surveillance for reoccurrence; however, more extensive work with host salivary biomarkers has shown that these tests are not necessarily definitive across large populations. In the future, a single saliva sample could be used to evaluate not only host biomarkers but microbial biomarkers as well. Together, these two indicators should dramatically increase the validity across the population, yielding specific and sensitive testing for a variety of diseases before any key symptoms start to show up. Patients can get further testing to confirm the presumptive diagnosis and start treatment well before traditional timelines. This early detection using noninvasive diagnostic biomarkers has the potential to be lifesaving for particularly aggressive diseases, such as pancreatic cancer, yielding a new age in clinical medicine.

References

1. Gill SR, Pop M, Deboy RT, Eckburg PB, Turnbaugh PJ, Samuel BS, et al. Metagenomic analysis of the human distal gut microbiome. Science. 2006; 312(5778):1355–9.
2. Costello EK, Lauber CL, Hamady M, Fierer N, Gordon JI, Knight R. Bacterial community variation in human body habitats across space and time. Science. 2009;326(5960):1694–7.
3. Gevers D, Knight R, Petrosino JF, Huang K, McGuire AL, Birren BW, et al. The human microbiome project: a community resource for the healthy human microbiome. PLoS Biol. 2012;10(8):e1001377.
4. Grice EA, Segre JA. The human microbiome: our second genome. Annu Rev Genomics Hum Genet. 2012;13:151–70.
5. Baquero F, Nombela C. The microbiome as a human organ. Clin Microbiol Infect. 2012;18 Suppl 4:2–4.

6. Saei AA, Barzegari A. The microbiome: the forgotten organ of the astronaut's body–probiotics beyond terrestrial limits. Future Microbiol. 2012;7(9):1037–46.

7. Possemiers S, Bolca S, Verstraete W, Heyerick A. The intestinal microbiome: a separate organ inside the body with the metabolic potential to influence the bioactivity of botanicals. Fitoterapia. 2011;82(1):53–66.

8. O'Hara AM, Shanahan F. The gut flora as a forgotten organ. EMBO Rep. 2006;7(7):688–93.

9. Kutikhin AG, Yuzhalin AE, Brusina EB, Kutikhin AG, Yuzhalin AE, Brusina EB. Infectious agents and cancer. Dordrecht: Springer; 2012.

10. Foxman B, Goldberg D, Murdock C, Xi C, Gilsdorf JR. Conceptualizing human microbiota: from multicelled organ to ecological community. Interdiscip Perspect Infect Dis. 2008;2008:613979.

11. Evans JM, Morris LS, Marchesi JR. The gut microbiome: the role of a virtual organ in the endocrinology of the host. J Endocrinol. 2013;218(3):R37–47.

12. Zarco MF, Vess TJ, Ginsburg GS. The oral microbiome in health and disease and the potential impact on personalized dental medicine. Oral Dis. 2012;18(2):109–20.

13. Jünemann S, Prior K, Szczepanowski R, Harks I, Ehmke B, Goesmann A, et al. Bacterial community shift in treated periodontitis patients revealed by ion torrent 16S rRNA gene amplicon sequencing. PLoS ONE. 2012;7(8):e41606.

14. Pflughoeft KJ, Versalovic J. Human microbiome in health and disease. Annu Rev Pathol Mech Dis. 2012;7(1):99–122.

15. Methé BA, Nelson KE, Pop M, Creasy HH, Giglio MG, Huttenhower C, et al. A framework for human microbiome research. Nature. 2012;486(7402):215–21.

16. Zaura E, Keijser BJF, Huse SM, Crielaard W. Defining the healthy "core microbiome" of oral microbial communities. BMC Microbiol. 2009;9:259.

17. Bowden GHW, Hamilton IR. Survival of oral bacteria. Crit Rev Oral Biol Med. 1998;9(1):54–85.

18. Donoghue HD, Perrons CJ. Effect of nutrients on defined bacterial plaques and streptococcus mutans C67-1 implantation in a model mouth. Caries Res. 1991;25(2):108–15.

19. Scannapieco FA. Saliva-bacterium interactions in oral microbial ecology. Crit Rev Oral Biol Med. 1994;5(3–4):203–48.

20. Gibbons RJ, Houte JV. Bacterial adherence in oral microbial ecology. Annu Rev Microbiol. 1975;29(1):19–42.

21. Torlakovic L, Klepac-Ceraj V, Ogaard B, Cotton SL, Paster BJ, Olsen I. Microbial community succession on developing lesions on human enamel. J Oral Microbiol. 2012;4:16125. doi:10.3402/jom.v4i0.16125.

22. Docktor MJ, Paster BJ, Abramowicz S, Ingram J, Wang YE, Correll M, et al. Alterations in diversity of the oral microbiome in pediatric inflammatory bowel disease. Inflamm Bowel Dis. 2012;18(5):935–42.

23. Colombo APV, Boches SK, Cotton SL, Goodson JM, Kent R, Haffajee AD, et al. Comparisons of subgingival microbial profiles of refractory periodontitis, severe periodontitis, and periodontal health using the human oral microbe identification microarray. J Periodontol. 2009;80(9):1421–32.

24. Belstrøm D, Fiehn N, Nielsen CH, Kirkby N, Twetman S, Klepac-Ceraj V, et al. Differences in bacterial saliva profile between periodontitis patients and a control cohort. J Clin Periodontol. 2014;41(2):104–12.

25. Colombo APV, Bennet S, Cotton SL, Goodson JM, Kent R, Haffajee AD, et al. Impact of periodontal therapy on the subgingival microbiota of severe periodontitis: comparison between good responders and individuals with refractory periodontitis using the human oral microbe identification microarray. J Periodontol. 2012;83(10):1279–87.

26. Albandar JM, Khattab R, Monem F, Barbuto SM, Paster BJ. The subgingival microbiota of Papillon-Lefèvre syndrome. J Periodontol. 2012;83(7):902–8.

27. Kinney JS, Morelli T, Braun T, Ramseier CA, Herr AE, Sugai JV, et al. Saliva/pathogen biomarker signatures and periodontal disease progression. J Dent Res. 2011;90(6):752–8.

28. Al-Tarawneh SK, Border MB, Dibble CF, Bencharit S. Defining salivary biomarkers using mass spectrometry-based proteomics: a systematic review. OMICS. 2011;15(6):353–61.

29. Siqueira WL, Dawes C. The salivary proteome: challenges and perspectives. Proteomics Clin Appl. 2011;5(11–12):575–9.

30. Giannobile WV. Salivary diagnostics for periodontal diseases. J Am Dent Assoc. 2012;143(10 Suppl):6S–11.

31. Aas JA, Paster BJ, Stokes LN, Olsen I, Dewhirst FE. Defining the normal bacterial flora of the oral cavity. J Clin Microbiol. 2005;43(11):5721–32.

32. Keijser BJF, Zaura E, Huse SM, van der Vossen JMBM, Schuren FHJ, Montijn RC, et al. Pyrosequencing analysis of the oral microflora of healthy adults. J Dent Res. 2008;87(11):1016–20.

33. Lazarevic V, Whiteson K, Huse S, Hernandez D, Farinelli L, Osterås M, et al. Metagenomic study of the oral microbiota by illumina high-throughput sequencing. J Microbiol Methods. 2009;79(3):266–71.

34. Nasidze I, Li J, Quinque D, Tang K, Stoneking M. Global diversity in the human salivary microbiome. Genome Res. 2009;19:636–43.

35. Nasidze I, Quinque D, Li J, Li M, Tang K, Stoneking M. Comparative analysis of human saliva microbiome diversity by barcoded pyrosequencing and cloning approaches. Anal Biochem. 2009;391(1):64–8.

36. Lazarevic V, Whiteson K, Hernandez D, François P, Schrenzel J. Study of inter- and intra-individual variations in the salivary microbiota. BMC Genomics. 2010;11:523.

37. Lazarevic V, Whiteson K, Gaïa N, Gizard Y, Hernandez D, Farinelli L, et al. Analysis of the salivary microbiome using culture-independent techniques. J Clin Bioinforma. 2012;2:4.

38. Simón-Soro A, Tomás I, Cabrera-Rubio R, Catalan MD, Nyvad B, Mira A. Microbial geography of the oral cavity. J Dent Res. 2013;92(7):616–21.

39. Zaura E. Next-generation sequencing approaches to understanding the oral microbiome. Adv Dent Res. 2012;24(2):81–5.

40. Bik EM, Long CD, Armitage GC, Loomer P, Emerson J, Mongodin EF, et al. Bacterial diversity in the oral cavity of 10 healthy individuals. ISME J. 2010; 4(8):962–74.

41. Rosan B, Lamont RJ. Dental plaque formation. Microbes Infect. 2000;2(13):1599–607.

42. Bimstein E, Ram D, Naor R, Sela MN. The composition of subgingival microflora in two groups of children with and without primary dentition alveolar bone loss. Pediatr Dent. 1996;18(1):42–7.

43. Africa CW, Parker JR, Reddy J. Darkfield microscopy of the flora of subgingival plaque of patients with severe periodontitis and its use in therapeutic assessment. J Dent Assoc S Afr. 1985;40(1):5–9.

44. Addy M, Newman H, Langeroudi M, Gho JG. Dark-field microscopy of the microflora of plaque. Br Dent J. 1983;155(8):269–73.

45. Pushalkar S, Mane SP, Ji X, Li Y, Evans C, Crasta OR, et al. Microbial diversity in saliva of oral squamous cell carcinoma. FEMS Immunol Med Microbiol. 2011;61(3):269–77.

46. Aas JA, Griffen AL, Dardis SR, Lee AM, Olsen I, Dewhirst FE, et al. Bacteria of dental caries in primary and permanent teeth in children and young adults. J Clin Microbiol. 2008;46(4):1407–17.

47. Mager D, Haffajee A, Devlin P, Norris C, Posner M, Goodson J. The salivary microbiota as a diagnostic indicator of oral cancer: a descriptive, non-randomized study of cancer-free and oral squamous cell carcinoma subjects. J Transl Med. 2005;3(1):27.

48. Ley RE, Lozupone CA, Hamady M, Knight R, Gordon JI. Worlds within worlds: evolution of the vertebrate gut microbiota. Nat Rev Microbiol. 2008; 6(10):776–88.

49. Stahringer SS, Clemente JC, Corley RP, Hewitt J, Knights D, Walters WA, et al. Nurture trumps nature in a longitudinal survey of salivary bacterial communities in twins from early adolescence to early adulthood. Genome Res. 2012;22(11):2146–52.

50. Human Microbiome Project Consortium. Structure, function and diversity of the healthy human microbiome. Nature. 2012;486(7402):207–14.

51. Kolenbrander PE. Oral microbial communities: biofilms, interactions, and genetic systems. Annu Rev Microbiol. 2000;54:413–37.

52. Falsetta ML, Klein MI, Colonne PM, Scott-Anne K, Gregoire S, Pai C, et al. Symbiotic relationship between Streptococcus mutans and Candida albicans synergizes the virulence of plaque-biofilms in vivo. Infect Immun. 2014;82:1968–81.

53. Wessel SW, Chen Y, Maitra A, van den Heuvel ER, Slomp AM, Busscher HJ, et al. Adhesion forces and composition of planktonic and adhering oral microbiomes. J Dent Res. 2014;93(1):84–8.

54. Foster JS, Kolenbrander PE. Development of a multi-species oral bacterial community in a saliva-conditioned flow cell. Appl Environ Microbiol. 2004;70(7):4340–8.

55. Biyikoğlu B, Ricker A, Diaz PI. Strain-specific colonization patterns and serum modulation of multi-species oral biofilm development. Anaerobe. 2012; 18(4):459–70.

56. Selwitz RH, Ismail AI, Pitts NB. Dental caries. Lancet. 2007;369(9555):51–9.

57. Kolenbrander PE. Multispecies communities: inter-species interactions influence growth on saliva as sole nutritional source. Int J Oral Sci. 2011;3(2):49–54.

58. Kolenbrander PE, Andersen RN, Blehert DS, Egland PG, Foster JS, Palmer RJ. Communication among oral bacteria. Microbiol Mol Biol Rev. 2002; 66(3):486–505, table of contents.

59. Periasamy S, Kolenbrander PE. Mutualistic biofilm communities develop with Porphyromonas gingivalis and initial, early, and late colonizers of enamel. J Bacteriol. 2009;191(22):6804–11.

60. Humphrey SP, Williamson RT. A review of saliva: normal composition, flow, and function. J Prosthet Dent. 2001;85(2):162–9.

61. Culp DJ, Robinson B, Parkkila S, Pan P, Cash MN, Truong HN, et al. Oral colonization by Streptococcus mutans and caries development is reduced upon deletion of carbonic anhydrase VI expression in saliva. Biochim Biophys Acta. 2011;1812(12):1567–76.

62. Melvin JE. Saliva and dental diseases. Curr Opin Dent. 1991;1(6):795–801.

63. De Jong MH, Van der Hoeven JS. The growth of oral bacteria on saliva. J Dent Res. 1987;66(2):498–505.

64. Buzalaf MAR, Hannas AR, Kato MT. Saliva and dental erosion. J Appl Oral Sci. 2012;20(5):493–502.

65. Liljemark WF, Bloomquist CG, Coulter MC, Fenner LJ, Skopek RJ, Schachtele CF. Utilization of a continuous streptococcal surface to measure interbacterial adherence in vitro and in vivo. J Dent Res. 1988;67(12):1455–60.

66. Skopek RJ, Liljemark WF. The influence of saliva on interbacterial adherence. Oral Microbiol Immunol. 1994;9(1):19–24.

67. Dibdin GH, Dawes C. A mathematical model of the influence of salivary urea on the pH of fasted dental plaque and on the changes occurring during a cariogenic challenge. Caries Res. 1998;32(1):70–4.

68. Dawes C, Dibdin GH. Salivary concentrations of urea released from a chewing gum containing urea and how these affect the urea content of gel-stabilized plaques and their pH after exposure to sucrose. Caries Res. 2001;35(5):344–53.

69. Bardow A, Moe D, Nyvad B, Nauntofte B. The buffer capacity and buffer systems of human whole saliva measured without loss of CO2. Arch Oral Biol. 2000;45(1):1–12.

70. Ship JA, Fox PC, Baum BJ. How much saliva is enough? "Normal" function defined. J Am Dent Assoc. 1991;122(3):63–9.

71. Javed F, Utreja A, Bello Correa FO, Al-Askar M, Hudieb M, Qayyum F, et al. Oral health status in children with acute lymphoblastic leukemia. Crit Rev Oncol Hematol. 2012;83(3):303–9.

72. Areias C, Sampaio-Maia B, Pereira MDL, Azevedo A, Melo P, Andrade C, et al. Reduced salivary flow and colonization by mutans streptococci in children with Down syndrome. Clin (Sao Paulo). 2012; 67(9):1007–11.

73. Bardow A, Nyvad B, Nauntofte B. Relationships between medication intake, complaints of dry mouth, salivary flow rate and composition, and the rate of tooth demineralization in situ. Arch Oral Biol. 2001; 46(5):413–23.

74. Navazesh M, Mulligan RA, Kipnis V, Denny PA, Denny PC. Comparison of whole saliva flow rates and mucin concentrations in healthy Caucasian young and aged adults. J Dent Res. 1992;71(6):1275–8.

75. Imanguli MM, Atkinson JC, Harvey KE, Hoehn GT, Ryu OH, Wu T, et al. Changes in salivary proteome following allogeneic hematopoietic stem cell transplantation. Exp Hematol. 2007;35(2):184–92.

76. Khalili S, Faustman DL, Liu Y, Sumita Y, Blank D, Peterson A, et al. Treatment for salivary gland hypofunction at both initial and advanced stages of Sjögren-like disease: a comparative study of bone marrow therapy versus spleen cell therapy with a 1-year monitoring period. Cytotherapy. 2014;16(3): 412–23.

77. Proctor GB, Carpenter GH. Regulation of salivary gland function by autonomic nerves. Auton Neurosci. 2007;133(1):3–18.

78. González S, Sung H, Sepúlveda D, González M, Molina C. Oral manifestations and their treatment in Sjögren's syndrome. Oral Dis. 2014;20(2):153–61.

79. Jensdottir T, Buchwald C, Nauntofte B, Hansen HS, Bardow A. Saliva in relation to dental erosion before and after radiotherapy. Acta Odontol Scand. 2013; 71(3–4):1008–13.

80. MacFarlane TW, Mason DK. Changes in the oral flora in Sjögren's syndrome. J Clin Pathol. 1974;27(5): 416–9.

81. Almståhl A, Wikström M, Kroneld U. Microflora in oral ecosystems in primary Sjögren's syndrome. J Rheumatol. 2001;28(5):1007–13.

82. Psoter WJ, Spielman AL, Gebrian B, St Jean R, Katz RV. Effect of childhood malnutrition on salivary flow and pH. Arch Oral Biol. 2008;53(3):231–7.

83. Bradshaw DJ, Lynch RJM. Diet and the microbial aetiology of dental caries: new paradigms. Int Dent J. 2013;63 Suppl 2:64–72.

84. Witbracht MG, Van Loan M, Adams SH, Keim NL, Laugero KD. Dairy food consumption and meal-induced cortisol response interacted to influence weight loss in overweight women undergoing a 12-week, meal-controlled, weight loss intervention. J Nutr. 2013; 143(1):46–52.

85. Sekine S, Kataoka K, Tanaka M, Nagata H, Kawakami T, Akaji K, et al. Active domains of salivary statherin on apatitic surfaces for binding to Fusobacterium nucleatum cells. Microbiology (Reading, Engl). 2004;150(Pt 7):2373–9.

86. Kolenbrander PE, Palmer RJ, Periasamy S, Jakubovics NS. Oral multispecies biofilm development and the key role of cell-cell distance. Nat Rev Microbiol. 2010;8(7):471–80.

87. Eliasson L, Carlén A. An update on minor salivary gland secretions. Eur J Oral Sci. 2010;118(5): 435–42.

88. Tabak LA. In defense of the oral cavity: structure, biosynthesis, and function of salivary mucins. Annu Rev Physiol. 1995;57:547–64.

89. Bolscher J, Veerman E, Van Nieuw Amerongen A, Tulp A, Verwoerd D. Distinct populations of high-M(r) mucins secreted by different human salivary glands discriminated by density-gradient electrophoresis. Biochem J. 1995;309(Pt 3):801–6.

90. Carlson DM. Salivary proline-rich proteins: biochemistry, molecular biology, and regulation of expression. Crit Rev Oral Biol Med. 1993;4(3–4):495–502.

91. Li T, Khah MK, Slavnic S, Johansson I, Strömberg N. Different type 1 fimbrial genes and tropisms of commensal and potentially pathogenic Actinomyces spp. with different salivary acidic proline-rich protein and statherin ligand specificities. Infect Immun. 2001;69(12):7224–33.

92. Douglas CW. Bacterial-protein interactions in the oral cavity. Adv Dent Res. 1994;8(2):254–62.

93. Offner GD, Troxler RF. Heterogeneity of high-molecular-weight human salivary mucins. Adv Dent Res. 2000;14(1):69–75.

94. Nakamura T, Takada N, Tonozuka T, Sakano Y, Oguma K, Nishikawa A. Binding properties of Clostridium botulinum type C progenitor toxin to mucins. Biochim Biophys Acta. 2007;1770(4): 551–5.

95. Strombeck DR, Harrold D. Binding of cholera toxin to mucins and inhibition by gastric mucin. Infect Immun. 1974;10(6):1266–72.

96. Proctor GB, Carpenter GH. Chewing stimulates secretion of human salivary secretory immunoglobulin A. J Dent Res. 2001;80(3):909–13.

97. Zee KY, Samaranayake LP, Attström R. Salivary immunoglobulin A levels in rapid and slow plaque formers: a pilot study. Microbios. 2001;106 Suppl 2:81–7.

98. Marcotte H, Lavoie MC. Oral microbial ecology and the role of salivary immunoglobulin A. Microbiol Mol Biol Rev. 1998;62(1):71–109.

99. Brandtzaeg P, Berstad AE, Farstad IN, Haraldsen G, Helgeland L, Jahnsen FL, et al. Mucosal immunity–a major adaptive defence mechanism. Behring Inst Mitt. 1997;98:1–23.

100. Loimaranta V, Tenovuo J, Virtanen S, Marnila P, Syväoja EL, Tupasela T, et al. Generation of bovine immune colostrum against Streptococcus mutans and Streptococcus sobrinus and its effect on glucose uptake and extracellular polysaccharide formation by mutans streptococci. Vaccine. 1997;15(11):1261–8.

101. Tenovuo JO. Human saliva: clinical chemistry and microbiology. Boca Raton: CRC Press, Inc.; 1989.

102. Tenovuo J. Antimicrobial function of human saliva – how important is it for oral health? Acta Odontol Scand. 1998;56(5):250–6.

103. Millar MR, Inglis T. Influence of lysozyme on aggregation of Staphylococcus aureus. J Clin Microbiol. 1987;25(9):1587–90.

104. Battino M, Ferreiro MS, Gallardo I, Newman HN, Bullon P. The antioxidant capacity of saliva. J Clin Periodontol. 2002;29(3):189–94.

105. Noble RE. Salivary alpha-amylase and lysozyme levels: a non-invasive technique for measuring parotid vs submandibular/sublingual gland activity. J Oral Sci. 2000;42(2):83–6.

106. Gregory MR, Gregory WW, Bruns DE, Zakowski JJ. Amylase inhibits Neisseria gonorrhoeae by degrading starch in the growth medium. J Clin Microbiol. 1983;18(6):1366–9.

107. Berger U. Inhibition of Neisseria meningitidis by alpha-amylase. Zentralbl Bakteriol Mikrobiol Hyg A. 1984;258(2–3):156–8.

108. Mellersh A, Clark A, Hafiz S. Inhibition of Neisseria gonorrhoeae by normal human saliva. Br J Venereol Dis. 1979;55(1):20–3.

109. Bortner CA, Miller RD, Arnold RR. Effects of alpha-amylase on in vitro growth of Legionella pneumophila. Infect Immun. 1983;41(1):44–9.

110. Veerman EC, van den Keybus PA, Vissink A, Nieuw Amerongen AV. Human glandular salivas: their separate collection and analysis. Eur J Oral Sci. 1996;104(4 (Pt 1)):346–52.

111. Van der Hoeven JS, De Jong MH, Van Nieuw Amerongen A. Growth of oral microflora on saliva from different glands. Microb Ecol Health Dis. 1989;2:171–80.

112. Lingström P, Moynihan P. Nutrition, saliva, and oral health. Nutrition. 2003;19(6):567–9.

113. Mathews SA, Kurien BT, Scofield RH. Oral manifestations of Sjögren's syndrome. J Dent Res. 2008;87(4):308–18.

114. Eliasson L, Carlén A, Almståhl A, Wikström M, Lingström P. Dental plaque pH and micro-organisms during hyposalivation. J Dent Res. 2006;85(4):334–8.

115. Palmer RJ, Gordon SM, Cisar JO, Kolenbrander PE. Coaggregation-mediated interactions of streptococci and actinomyces detected in initial human dental plaque. J Bacteriol. 2003;185(11):3400–9.

116. Palmer RJ, Kazmerzak K, Hansen MC, Kolenbrander PE. Mutualism versus independence: strategies of mixed-species oral biofilms in vitro using saliva as the sole nutrient source. Infect Immun. 2001;69(9):5794–804.

117. Lancy P, Dirienzo JM, Appelbaum B, Rosan B, Holt SC. Corncob formation between Fusobacterium nucleatum and Streptococcus sanguis. Infect Immun. 1983;40(1):303–9.

118. Weiss EI, Kolenbrander PE, London J, Hand AR, Andersen RN. Fimbria-associated proteins of Bacteroides loescheii PK1295 mediate intergeneric coaggregations. J Bacteriol. 1987;169(9):4215–22.

119. Weiss EI, London J, Kolenbrander PE, Kagermeier AS, Andersen RN. Characterization of lectinlike surface components on Capnocytophaga ochracea ATCC 33596 that mediate coaggregation with gram-positive oral bacteria. Infect Immun. 1987;55(5):1198–202.

120. Diaz PI, Chalmers NI, Rickard AH, Kong C, Milburn CL, Palmer RJ, et al. Molecular characterization of subject-specific oral microflora during initial colonization of enamel. Appl Environ Microbiol. 2006;72(4):2837–48.

121. Staat RH, Gawronski TH, Schachtele CF. Detection and preliminary studies on dextranase-producing microorganisms from human dental plaque. Infect Immun. 1973;8(6):1009–16.

122. Koo H, Falsetta ML, Klein MI. The exopolysaccharide matrix: a virulence determinant of cariogenic biofilm. J Dent Res. 2013;92(12):1065–73.

123. Kolenbrander PE, Andersen RN, Moore LV. Intrageneric coaggregation among strains of human oral bacteria: potential role in primary colonization of the tooth surface. Appl Environ Microbiol. 1990;56:3890–4.

124. Rosen G, Nisimov I, Helcer M, Sela MN. Actinobacillus actinomycetemcomitans serotype b lipopolysaccharide mediates coaggregation with Fusobacterium nucleatum. Infect Immun. 2003;71(6):3652–6.

125. Hooper SJ, Crean SJ, Fardy MJ, Lewis MAO, Spratt DA, Wade WG, et al. A molecular analysis of the bacteria present within oral squamous cell carcinoma. J Med Microbiol. 2007;56(12):1651–9.

126. Hooper SJ, Crean SJ, Lewis MAO, Spratt DA, Wade WG, Wilson MJ. Viable bacteria present within oral squamous cell carcinoma tissue. J Clin Microbiol. 2006;44(5):1719–25.

127. Shiga K, Tateda M, Saijo S, Hori T, Sato I, Tateno H, et al. Presence of Streptococcus infection in extra-oropharyngeal head and neck squamous cell carcinoma and its implication in carcinogenesis. Oncol Rep. 2001;8(2):245–8.

128. Narikiyo M, Tanabe C, Yamada Y, Igaki H, Tachimori Y, Kato H, et al. Frequent and preferential infection of Treponema denticola, Streptococcus mitis, and Streptococcus anginosus in esophageal cancers. Cancer Sci. 2004;95(7):569–74.

129. Kostic AD, Chun E, Robertson L, Glickman JN, Gallini CA, Michaud M, et al. Fusobacterium nucleatum potentiates intestinal tumorigenesis and modulates the tumor-immune microenvironment. Cell Host Microbe. 2013;14(2):207–15.

130. Rubinstein MR, Wang X, Liu W, Hao Y, Cai G, Han YW. Fusobacterium nucleatum promotes colorectal carcinogenesis by modulating E-cadherin/β-catenin signaling via its FadA adhesin. Cell Host Microbe. 2013;14(2):195–206.

131. Salazar CR, Sun J, Li Y, Francois F, Corby P, Perez-Perez G, et al. Association between selected oral pathogens and gastric precancerous lesions. PLoS ONE. 2013;8(1):e51604.

132. Salazar CR, Francois F, Li Y, Corby P, Hays R, Leung C, et al. Association between oral health and gastric precancerous lesions. Carcinogenesis. 2012;33(2):399–403.

133. Farrell JJ, Zhang L, Zhou H, Chia D, Elashoff D, Akin D, et al. Variations of oral microbiota are associated with pancreatic diseases including pancreatic cancer. Gut. 2012;61(4):582–8.

134. Okada M, Kawamura M, Oda Y, Yasuda R, Kojima T, Kurihara H. Caries prevalence associated with Streptococcus mutans and Streptococcus sobrinus in Japanese schoolchildren. Int J Paediatr Dent. 2012; 22(5):342–8.

135. Sánchez-Acedo M, Montiel-Company J, Dasí-Fernández F, Almerich-Silla J. Streptococcus mutans and Streptococcus sobrinus detection by polymerase chain reaction and their relation to dental caries in 12 and 15 year-old schoolchildren in Valencia (Spain). Med Oral Patol Oral Cir Bucal. 2013;18(6): e839–45.

136. Palmer EA, Nielsen T, Peirano P, Nguyen AT, Vo A, Nguyen A, et al. Children with severe early childhood caries: pilot study examining mutans streptococci genotypic strains after full-mouth caries restorative therapy. Pediatr Dent. 2012;34(2):e1–10.

137. Crossner C. Salivary lactobacillus counts in the prediction of caries activity. Community Dent Oral Epidemiol. 1981;9(4):182–90.

138. Wolff D, Frese C, Maier-Kraus T, Krueger T, Wolff B. Bacterial biofilm composition in caries and caries-free subjects. Caries Res. 2013;47(1):69–77.

139. Roeters FJM, Van der Hoeven JS, Burgersdijk RCW, Schaeken MJM. Lactobacilli, mutans streptococci and dental caries: a longitudinal study in 2-year-old children up to the age of 5 years. Caries Res. 1995;29(4):272–9.

140. Stecksén-Blicks C. Salivary counts of lactobacilli and Streptococcus mutans in caries prediction. Eur J Oral Sci. 1985;93(3):204–12.

141. Okada M, Soda Y, Hayashi F, Doi T, Suzuki J, Miura K, et al. PCR detection of Streptococcus mutans and S. sobrinus in dental plaque samples from Japanese pre-school children. J Med Microbiol. 2002;51(5): 443–7.

142. Köhler B, Persson M. Salivary levels of mutans streptococci and lactobacilli in dentate 80- and 85-year-old Swedish men and women. Community Dent Oral Epidemiol. 1991;19(6):352–6.

143. Petersson GH, Isberg P, Twetman S. Caries risk profiles in schoolchildren over 2 years assessed by Cariogram. Int J Paediatr Dent. 2010;20(5):341–6.

144. Fure S. Ten-year cross-sectional and incidence study of coronal and root caries and some related factors in elderly Swedish individuals. Gerodontology. 2004; 21(3):130–40.

145. Belstrøm D, Fiehn N, Nielsen CH, Holmstrup P, Kirkby N, Klepac-Ceraj V, et al. Altered bacterial profiles in saliva from adults with caries lesions: a case-cohort study. Caries Res. 2014;48(5):368–75.

146. Ashimoto A, Chen C, Bakker I, Slots J. Polymerase chain reaction detection of 8 putative periodontal pathogens in subgingival plaque of gingivitis and advanced periodontitis lesions. Oral Microbiol Immunol. 1996;11(4):266–73.

147. Van Winkelhoff AJ, Loos BG, van der Reijden WA, Van der Velden U. Porphyromonas gingivalis, bacteroides forsythus and other putative periodontal pathogens in subjects with and without periodontal destruction. J Clin Periodontol. 2002;29(11): 1023–8.

148. Slots J, Slots H. Bacterial and viral pathogens in saliva: disease relationship and infectious risk. Periodontology 2000. 2011;55(1):48–69.

149. Saygun I, Kubar A, Sahin S, Sener K, Slots J. Quantitative analysis of association between herpesviruses and bacterial pathogens in periodontitis. J Periodont Res. 2008;43(3):352–9.

150. Imbronito AV, Okuda OS, de Freitas Maria N, Moreira Lotufo RF, Nunes FD. Detection of herpesviruses and periodontal pathogens in subgingival plaque of patients with chronic periodontitis, generalized aggressive periodontitis, or gingivitis. J Periodontol. 2008;79(12):2313–21.

151. Ito T, Yasuda M, Kaneko H, Sasaki H, Kato T, Yajima Y. Clinical evaluation of salivary periodontal pathogen levels by real-time polymerase chain reaction in patients before dental implant treatment. Clin Oral Implants Res. 2014;25:977–82.

152. Ebersole JL, Holt SC, Hansard R, Novak MJ. Microbiologic and immunologic characteristics of periodontal disease in Hispanic americans with type 2 diabetes. J Periodontol. 2008;79(4):637–46.

153. Lalla E, Cheng B, Lal S, Tucker S, Greenberg E, Goland R, et al. Periodontal changes in children and adolescents with diabetes: a case-control study. Diabetes Care. 2006;29(2):295–9.

154. Kuo L, Polson AM, Kang T. Associations between periodontal diseases and systemic diseases: a review of the inter-relationships and interactions with diabetes, respiratory diseases, cardiovascular diseases and osteoporosis. Public Health. 2008;122(4): 417–33.

155. Zambon JJ, Reynolds H, Fisher JG, Shlossman M, Dunford R, Genco RJ. Microbiological and immunological studies of adult periodontitis in patients with noninsulin-dependent diabetes mellitus. J Periodontol. 1988;59(1):23–31.

156. Mashimo PA, Yamamoto Y, Slots J, Park BH, Genco RJ. The periodontal microflora of juvenile diabetics: culture, immunofluorescence, and serum antibody studies. J Periodontol. 1983;54(7):420–30.

157. Casarin RCV, Barbagallo A, Meulman T, Santos VR, Sallum EA, Nociti FH, et al. Subgingival biodiversity in subjects with uncontrolled type-2 diabetes and chronic periodontitis. J Periodontal Res. 2013;48(1):30–6.

158. Said HS, Suda W, Nakagome S, Chinen H, Oshima K, Kim S, et al. Dysbiosis of salivary microbiota in inflammatory bowel disease and its association with oral immunological biomarkers. DNA Res. 2014;21(1):15–25.

159. Grössner-Schreiber B, Fetter T, Hedderich J, Kocher T, Schreiber S, Jepsen S. Prevalence of dental caries and periodontal disease in patients with inflammatory bowel disease: a case-control study. J Clin Periodontol. 2006;33(7):478–84.

160. Leung KCM, McMillan AS, Cheung BPK, Leung WK. Sjögren's syndrome sufferers have increased oral yeast levels despite regular dental care. Oral Dis. 2008;14(2):163–73.

161. Leung KCM, Leung WK, McMillan AS. Supragingival microbiota in Sjögren's syndrome. Clin Oral Investig. 2007;11(4):415–23.

162. Ergun S. Oral Aspects of Sjogren's Syndrome. In: Harrison A, editor. Insights and perspectives in rheumatology. InTech; 2012. p. 149–71.

163. Abraham CM, al-Hashimi I, Haghighat N. Evaluation of the levels of oral Candida in patients with Sjögren's syndrome. Oral Surg Oral Med Oral Pathol Oral Radiol Endod. 1998;86(1):65–8.

164. Thomas DM, Mirowski GW. Nutrition and oral mucosal diseases. Clin Dermatol. 2010;28(4):426–31.

165. Timmerman MF, Abbas F, Loos BG, Van der Weijden GA, Van Winkelhoff AJ, Winkel EG, et al. Java project on periodontal diseases: the relationship between vitamin C and the severity of periodontitis. J Clin Periodontol. 2007;34(4):299–304.

166. Kreth J, Merritt J, Qi F. Bacterial and host interactions of oral streptococci. DNA Cell Biol. 2009;28(8):397–403.

167. Kalfas S, Andersson M, Edwardsson S, Forsgren A, Naidu AS. Human lactoferrin binding to Porphyromonas gingivalis, Prevotella intermedia and Prevotella melaninogenica. Oral Microbiol Immunol. 1991;6(6):350–5.

168. Vestman NR, Timby N, Holgerson PL, Kressirer CA, Claesson R, Domellöf M, et al. Characterization and in vitro properties of oral lactobacilli in breast-fed infants. BMC Microbiol. 2013;13:193.

169. Miyakawa H, Nakazawa F. Role of asaccharolytic anaerobic gram-positive rods on periodontitis. J Oral Biosci. 2010;52(3):240–4.

170. Amerongen AVN, Veerman ECI. Saliva–the defender of the oral cavity. Oral Dis. 2002;8(1):12–22.

171. Ghasempour M, Rajabnia R, Irannejad A, Hamzeh M, Ferdosi E, Bagheri M. Frequency, biofilm formation and acid susceptibility of streptococcus mutans and streptococcus sobrinus in saliva of preschool children with different levels of caries activity. Dent Res J (Isfahan). 2013;10(4):440–5.

172. Fozo EM, Kajfasz JK, Quivey RG. Low pH-induced membrane fatty acid alterations in oral bacteria. FEMS Microbiol Lett. 2004;238(2):291–5.

173. Hamada S, Ooshima T. Production and properties of bacteriocins (mutacins) from streptococcus mutans. Arch Oral Biol. 1975;20(10):641–8. IN5.

174. Holmberg K, Hallander HO. Production of bactericidal concentrations of hydrogen peroxide by Streptococcus sanguis. Arch Oral Biol. 1973;18(3):423–34. IN7.

175. Geiger T, Kästle B, Gratani FL, Goerke C, Wolz C. Two small (p)ppGpp synthases in Staphylococcus aureus mediate tolerance against cell envelope stress conditions. J Bacteriol. 2014;196(4):894–902.

176. Santiago B, Marek M, Faustoferri RC, Quivey RG. The Streptococcus mutans aminotransferase encoded by ilvE is regulated by CodY and CcpA. J Bacteriol. 2013;195(16):3552–62.

177. Marsh PD. Dental plaque as a biofilm and a microbial community – implications for health and disease. BMC Oral Health. 2006;6 Suppl 1:S14.

178. Brown LJ, Löe H. Prevalence, extent, severity and progression of periodontal disease. Periodontology 2000. 1993;2(1):57–71.

179. Brown LJ, Brunelle JA, Kingman A. Periodontal status in the United States, 1988–1991: prevalence, extent, and demographic variation. J Dent Res. 1996;75(Spec No):672–83.

180. LÖE H, Ånerud Å, Boysen H. The natural history of periodontal disease in man: prevalence, severity, and extent of gingival recession. J Periodontol. 1992;63(6):489–95.

181. Krzyściak W, Jurczak A, Kościelniak D, Bystrowska B, Skalniak A. The virulence of Streptococcus mutans and the ability to form biofilms. Eur J Clin Microbiol Infect Dis. 2014;33(4):499–515.

182. Svensäter G, Larsson U, Greif ECG, Cvitkovitch DG, Hamilton IR. Acid tolerance response and survival by oral bacteria. Oral Microbiol Immunol. 1997;12(5):266–73.

183. Hughes JA, West NX, Parker DM, van den Braak MH, Addy M. Effects of pH and concentration of citric, malic and lactic acids on enamel, in vitro. J Dent. 2000;28(2):147–52.

184. Takahashi N, Nyvad B. The role of bacteria in the caries process: ecological perspectives. J Dent Res. 2011;90(3):294–303.

185. Byun R, Nadkarni MA, Chhour KL, Martin FE, Jacques NA, Hunter N. Quantitative analysis of diverse lactobacillus species present in advanced dental caries. J Clin Microbiol. 2004;42(7):3128–36.

186. Bradshaw DJ, Mckee AS, Marsh PD. Effects of carbohydrate pulses and pH on population shifts within oral microbial communities in vitro. J Dent Res. 1989;68(9):1298–302.

187. Zeng L, Burne RA. Comprehensive mutational analysis of sucrose-metabolizing pathways in Streptococcus mutans reveals novel roles for the sucrose phosphotransferase system permease. J Bacteriol. 2013;195(4):833–43.

188. Mo S, Bao W, Lai G, Wang J, Li M. The microfloral analysis of secondary caries biofilm around class I and class II composite and amalgam fillings. BMC Infect Dis. 2010;10:241.
189. Marsh PD. Role of the oral microflora in health. Microb Ecol Health Dis. 2000;12(3):130–7.
190. Okada M, Soda Y, Hayashi F, Doi T, Suzuki J, Miura K, et al. Longitudinal study of dental caries incidence associated with Streptococcus mutans and Streptococcus sobrinus in pre-school children. J Med Microbiol. 2005;54(Pt 7):661–5.
191. Rosema NAM, Timmerman MF, Piscaer M, Strate J, Warren PR, Van der Velden U, et al. An oscillating/pulsating electric toothbrush versus a high-frequency electric toothbrush in the treatment of gingivitis. J Dent. 2005;33 Suppl 1:29–36.
192. Versteeg PA, Timmerman MF, Rosema NAM, Warren PR, Van der Velden U, Van der Weijden GA. Sonic-powered toothbrushes and reversal of experimental gingivitis. J Clin Periodontol. 2005;32(12):1236–41.
193. Berezow AB, Darveau RP. Microbial shift and periodontitis. Periodontology 2000. 2011;55(1):36–47.
194. Consensus report periodontal diseases: pathogenesis and microbial factors. Ann Periodontol. 2014;1(1):926–32.
195. Field EA, Speechley JA, Rugman FR, Varga E, Tyldesley WR. Oral signs and symptoms in patients with undiagnosed vitamin B12 deficiency. J Oral Pathol Med. 1995;24(10):468–70.
196. Mager DL, Haffajee AD, Socransky SS. Effects of periodontitis and smoking on the microbiota of oral mucous membranes and saliva in systemically healthy subjects. J Clin Periodontol. 2003;30(12):1031–7.
197. Cortelli JR, Aquino DR, Cortelli SC, Nobre Franco GC, Fernandes CB, Roman-Torres CVG, et al. Detection of periodontal pathogens in oral mucous membranes of edentulous individuals. J Periodontol. 2008;79(10):1962–5.
198. Papaioannou W, Gizani S, Haffajee AD, Quirynen M, Mamai-Homata E, Papagiannoulis L. The microbiota on different oral surfaces in healthy children. Oral Microbiol Immunol. 2009;24(3):183–9.
199. Umeda M, Contreras A, Chen C, Bakker I, Slots J. The utility of whole saliva to detect the oral presence of periodontopathic bacteria. J Periodontol. 1998;69(7):828–33.
200. Umeda M, Chen C, Bakker I, Contreras A, Morrison JL, Slots J. Risk indicators for harboring periodontal pathogens. J Periodontol. 1998;69(10):1111–8.
201. Albandar JM. Global risk factors and risk indicators for periodontal diseases. Periodontology 2000. 2002;29(1):177–206.
202. Könönen E, Paju S, Pussinen PJ, Hyvönen M, Di Tella P, Suominen-Taipale L, et al. Population-based study of salivary carriage of periodontal pathogens in adults. J Clin Microbiol. 2007;45(8):2446–51.
203. Zhang L, Henson BS, Camargo PM, Wong DT. The clinical value of salivary biomarkers for periodontal disease. Periodontology 2000. 2009;51:25–37.
204. Ramseier CA, Kinney JS, Herr AE, Braun T, Sugai JV, Shelburne CA, et al. Identification of pathogen and host-response markers correlated with periodontal disease. J Periodontol. 2009;80(3):436–46.
205. Paju S, Pussinen PJ, Suominen-Taipale L, Hyvönen M, Knuuttila M, Könönen E. Detection of multiple pathogenic species in saliva is associated with periodontal infection in adults. J Clin Microbiol. 2009;47(1):235–8.
206. Giannobile WV, Beikler T, Kinney JS, Ramseier CA, Morelli T, Wong DT. Saliva as a diagnostic tool for periodontal disease: current state and future directions. Periodontology 2000. 2009;50:52–64.
207. Ghannoum MA, Jurevic RJ, Mukherjee PK, Cui F, Sikaroodi M, Naqvi A, et al. Characterization of the oral fungal microbiome (mycobiome) in healthy individuals. PLoS Pathog. 2010;6(1):e1000713.
208. Phalane KG, Kriel M, Loxton AG, Menezes A, Stanley K, van der Spuy GD, et al. Differential expression of host biomarkers in saliva and serum samples from individuals with suspected pulmonary tuberculosis. Mediat Inflamm. 2013;2013:981984.
209. Nakao K, Imoto I, Ikemura N, Shibata T, Takaji S, Taguchi Y, et al. Relation of lactoferrin levels in gastric mucosa with Helicobacter pylori infection and with the degree of gastric inflammation. Am J Gastroenterol. 1997;92(6):1005–11.
210. Lau C, Kim Y, Chia D, Spielmann N, Eibl G, Elashoff D, et al. Role of pancreatic cancer-derived exosomes in salivary biomarker development. J Biol Chem. 2013;288(37):26888–97.
211. Lamster IB, Lalla E, Borgnakke WS, Taylor GW. The relationship between oral health and diabetes mellitus. J Am Dent Assoc. 2008;139(5):19S–24.
212. Kampoo K, Teanpaisan R, Ledder RG, McBain AJ. Oral bacterial communities in individuals with type 2 diabetes who live in southern Thailand. Appl Environ Microbiol. 2014;80(2):662–71.
213. Karjalainen KM, Knuuttila MLE. The onset of diabetes and poor metabolic control increases gingival bleeding in children and adolescents with insulin-dependent diabetes mellitus. J Clin Periodontol. 1996;23(12):1060–7.
214. Chi AC, Neville BW, Krayer JW, Gonsalves WC. Oral manifestations of systemic disease. Am Fam Physician. 2010;82(11):1381–8.
215. Taylor G, Borgnakke W. Periodontal disease: associations with diabetes, glycemic control and complications. Oral Dis. 2008;14(3):191–203.
216. Tsai C, Hayes C, Taylor GW. Glycemic control of type 2 diabetes and severe periodontal disease in the US adult population. Community Dent Oral Epidemiol. 2002;30(3):182–92.
217. Kumar P, Natarajan K, Shanmugam N. High glucose driven expression of pro-inflammatory cytokine and chemokine genes in lymphocytes: molecular mechanisms of IL-17 family gene expression. Cell Signal. 2014;26(3):528–39.
218. Graves DT, Liu R, Alikhani M, Al-Mashat H, Trackman PC. Diabetes-enhanced inflammation and

apoptosis–impact on periodontal pathology. J Dent Res. 2006;85(1):15–21.

219. Martin M, Schifferle RE, Cuesta N, Vogel SN, Katz J, Michalek SM. Role of the Phosphatidylinositol 3 Kinase-AKT pathway in the regulation of IL-10 and IL-12 by porphyromonas gingivalis lipopolysaccharide. J Immunol. 2003;171(2):717–25.

220. Salvi GE, Yalda B, Collins JG, Jones BH, Smith FW, Arnold RR, et al. Inflammatory mediator response as a potential risk marker for periodontal diseases in insulin-dependent diabetes mellitus patients. J Periodontol. 1997;68(2):127–35.

221. Botero JE, Contreras A, Parra B. Profiling of inflammatory cytokines produced by gingival fibroblasts after human cytomegalovirus infection. Oral Microbiol Immunol. 2008;23(4):291–8.

222. Kim J, Amar S. Periodontal disease and systemic conditions: a bidirectional relationship. Odontology. 2006;94(1):10–21.

223. Taylor JJ. Cytokine regulation of immune responses to Porphyromonas gingivalis. Periodontology 2000. 2010;54(1):160–94.

224. Sfakianakis A, Barr CE, Kreutzer DL. Localization of the chemokine interleukin-8 and interleukin-8 receptors in human gingiva and cultured gingival keratinocytes. J Periodontol Res. 2002;37(2):154–60.

225. Mirbod SM, Ahing SI, Pruthi VK. Immunohistochemical study of vestibular gingival blood vessel density and internal circumference in smokers and non-smokers. J Periodontol. 2001; 72(10):1318–23.

226. Tilg H, Moschen AR. Inflammatory mechanisms in the regulation of insulin resistance. Mol Med. 2008;14(3–4):222–31.

227. Guggenheimer J, Moore PA, Rossie K, Myers D, Mongelluzzo MB, Block HM, et al. Insulin-dependent diabetes mellitus and oral soft tissue pathologies. I. Prevalence and characteristics of non-candidal lesions. Oral Surg Oral Med Oral Pathol Oral Radiol Endod. 2000;89(5):563–9.

228. Guggenheimer J, Moore PA, Rossie K, Myers D, Mongelluzzo MB, Block HM, et al. Insulin-dependent diabetes mellitus and oral soft tissue pathologies: II. Prevalence and characteristics of candida and candidal lesions. Oral Surg Oral Med Oral Pathol Oral Radiol Endod. 2000;89(5):570–6.

229. Laass MW, Roggenbuck D, Conrad K. Diagnosis and classification of Crohn's disease. Autoimmun Rev. 2014;13(4–5):467–71.

230. Mays JW, Sarmadi M, Moutsopoulos NM. Oral manifestations of systemic autoimmune and inflammatory diseases: diagnosis and clinical management. J Evid Based Dent Pract. 2012;12(3 Supplement):265–82.

231. Harty S, Fleming P, Rowland M, Crushell E, McDermott M, Drumm B, et al. A prospective study of the oral manifestations of Crohn's disease. Clin Gastroenterol Hepatol. 2005;3(9):886–91.

232. Chiodini RJ, Dowd SE, Davis B, Galandiuk S, Chamberlin WM, Kuenstner JT, et al. Crohn's disease may be differentiated into 2 distinct biotypes based on the detection of bacterial genomic sequences and virulence genes within submucosal tissues. J Clin Gastroenterol. 2013;47(7):612–20.

233. Michailidou E, Arvanitidou S, Lombardi T, Kolokotronis A, Antoniades D, Samson J. Oral lesions leading to the diagnosis of Crohn disease: report on 5 patients. Quintessence Int. 2009;40(7):581–8.

234. Kuo S. The interplay between fiber and the intestinal microbiome in the inflammatory response. Adv Nutr. 2013;4(1):16–28.

235. Martin J, Geisel T, Maresch C, Krieger K, Stein J. Inadequate nutrient intake in patients with celiac disease: results from a German dietary survey. Digestion. 2013;87(4):240–6.

236. Delaleu N, Immervoll H, Cornelius J, Jonsson R. Biomarker profiles in serum and saliva of experimental Sjögren's syndrome: associations with specific autoimmune manifestations. Arthritis Res Ther. 2008;10(1):R22.

237. Al-Ahmad A, Roth D, Wolkewitz M, Wiedmann-Al-Ahmad M, Follo M, Ratka-Krüger P, et al. Change in diet and oral hygiene over an 8-week period: effects on oral health and oral biofilm. Clin Oral Investig. 2010;14(4):391–6.

238. Humphrey LT, De Groote I, Morales J, Barton N, Collcutt S, Bronk Ramsey C, et al. Earliest evidence for caries and exploitation of starchy plant foods in Pleistocene hunter-gatherers from Morocco. Proc Natl Acad Sci U S A. 2014;111(3):954–9.

239. Scardina GA, Messina P. Good oral health and diet. J Biomed Biotechnol. 2012;2012:720692.

240. Saarela RKT, Soini H, Hiltunen K, Muurinen S, Suominen M, Pitkälä K. Dentition status, malnutrition and mortality among older service housing residents. J Nutr Health Aging. 2014;18(1):34–8.

241. Moynihan PJ, Lingström P, Touger-Decker R, Sirois DA, Mobley CC. Oral consequences of compromised nutritional well-being. Humana Press; 2004. ISBN: 978-953-307-846-5, Available from: http://www.intechopen.com/books/insights-and-perspectives-in-rheumatology/oral-aspects-of-sjo-gren-ssyndrome

242. Sajantila A. Major historical dietary changes are reflected in the dental microbiome of ancient skeletons. Investig Genet. 2013;4(1):10.

243. Dawes C. Estimates, from salivary analyses, of the turnover time of the oral mucosal epithelium in humans and the number of bacteria in an edentulous mouth. Arch Oral Biol. 2003;48(5):329–36.

244. Creamer B, Shorter RG, Bamforth J. The turnover and shedding of epithelial cells: part I the turnover in the gastro-intestinal tract. Gut. 1961;2(2):110–6.

245. Greenberg MS. Clinical and histologic changes of the oral mucosa in pernicious anemia. Oral Surg Oral Med Oral Pathol. 1981;52(1):38–42.

246. Drummond JF, White DK, Damm DD. Megaloblastic anemia with oral lesions: a consequence of gastric bypass surgery. Oral Surg Oral Med Oral Pathol. 1985;59(2):149–53.

247. Hjorting-Hansen E, Bertram U. Oral aspects of pernicious anaemia. Br Dent J. 1968;125(6):266–70.

248. Sweeney MP, Bagg J, Fell GS, Yip B. The relationship between micronutrient depletion and oral health in geriatrics. J Oral Pathol Med. 1994;23(4):168–71.

249. Arslan SY, Leung KP, Wu CD. The effect of lactoferrin on oral bacterial attachment. Oral Microbiol Immunol. 2009;24(5):411–6.

250. Paradkar PN, De Domenico I, Durchfort N, Zohn I, Kaplan J, Ward DM. Iron depletion limits intracellular bacterial growth in macrophages. Blood. 2008;112(3):866–74.

251. Berlutti F, Pilloni A, Pietropaoli M, Polimeni A, Valenti P. Lactoferrin and oral diseases: current status and perspective in periodontitis. Ann Stomatol (Roma). 2011;2(3–4):10–8.

252. Tang R, Huang M, Huang S. Relationship between dental caries status and anemia in children with severe early childhood caries. Kaohsiung J Med Sci. 2013;29(6):330–6.

253. Ross AC. Diet in vitamin A research. Methods Mol Biol. 2010;652:295–313.

254. Sessle BJ. Irreversibility of retarded incisor eruption in the vitamin A-deficient rat. J Oral Ther Pharmacol. 1968;4(5):395–7.

255. Naidu KA. Vitamin C in human health and disease is still a mystery? An overview. Nutr J. 2003;2:7.

256. Pfeffer F, Casanueva E, Kamar J, Guerra A, Perichart O, Vadillo-Ortega F. Modulation of 72-kilodalton type IV collagenase (matrix metalloproteinase-2) by ascorbic acid in cultured human amnion-derived cells. Biol Reprod. 1998;59(2):326–9.

257. Gerster H. Human vitamin C requirements. Z Ernahrungswiss. 1987;26(2):125–37.

258. Jemal A, Bray F, Center MM, Ferlay J, Ward E, Forman D. Global cancer statistics. CA Cancer J Clin. 2011;61(2):69–90.

259. Tighe D, Kwok A, Putcha V, McGurk M. Identification of appropriate outcome indices in head and neck cancer and factors influencing them. Int J Oral Maxillofac Surg. 2014;43:1047–53.

260. Jessri M, Farah CS. Next generation sequencing and its application in deciphering head and neck cancer. Oral Oncol. 2014;50(4):247–53.

261. Zafereo M. Surgical salvage of recurrent cancer of the head and neck. Curr Oncol Rep. 2014;16(5):386.

262. Meurman JH. Oral microbiota and cancer. J Oral Microbiol. 2010;2. doi:10.3402/jom.v2i0.5195.

263. Choudhary K, Gandhi N, Rajeev R, Panda S. Role of bacteria in oral carcinogenesis. South Asian J Cancer. 2012;1(2):78–83.

264. Sasaki M, Yamaura C, Ohara-Nemoto Y, Tajika S, Kodama Y, Ohya T, et al. Streptococcus anginosus infection in oral cancer and its infection route. Oral Dis. 2005;11(3):151–6.

265. Tateda M, Shiga K, Saijo S, Sone M, Hori T, Yokoyama J, et al. Streptococcus anginosus in head and neck squamous cell carcinoma: implication in carcinogenesis. Int J Mol Med. 2000;6(6):699–703.

266. Yu X, Shahir A, Sha J, Feng Z, Eapen B, Nithianantham S, et al. Short-chain fatty acids from periodontal pathogens suppress histone deacetylases, EZH2, and SUV39H1 to promote Kaposi's sarcoma-associated herpesvirus replication. J Virol. 2014;88(8):4466–79.

267. Ahn J, Chen CY, Hayes RB. Oral microbiome and oral and gastrointestinal cancer risk. Cancer Causes Control. 2012;23(3):399–404.

268. Han YW. Oral bacteria as drivers for colorectal cancer. J Periodontol. 2014;85:1155–7.

269. Song H, Michel A, Nyrén O, Ekström A, Pawlita M, Ye W. A CagA-independent cluster of antigens related to the risk of noncardia gastric cancer: associations between helicobacter pylori antibodies and gastric adenocarcinoma explored by multiplex serology. Int J Cancer. 2014;134(12):2942–50.

270. Perrais M, Rousseaux C, Ducourouble M, Courcol R, Vincent P, Jonckheere N, et al. Helicobacter pylori urease and flagellin alter mucin gene expression in human gastric cancer cells. Gastric Cancer. 2014;17(2):235–46.

271. Corey L, Wald A, Celum CL, Quinn TC. The effects of herpes simplex virus-2 on HIV-1 acquisition and transmission: a review of two overlapping epidemics. J Acquir Immune Defic Syndr. 2004;35(5):435–45.

272. Sarid O, Anson O, Yaari A, Margalith M. Epstein-Barr virus specific salivary antibodies as related to stress caused by examinations. J Med Virol. 2001;64(2):149–56.

273. Yap LF, Ahmad M, Zabidi MMA, Chu TL, Chai SJ, Lee HM, et al. Oncogenic effects of WNT5A in Epstein-Barr virus-associated nasopharyngeal carcinoma. Int J Oncol. 2014;44(5):1774–80.

274. Cimino PJ, Zhao G, Wang D, Sehn JK, Lewis JS, Duncavage EJ. Detection of viral pathogens in high grade gliomas from unmapped next-generation sequencing data. Exp Mol Pathol. 2014;96:310–5.

275. Mirghani H, Amen F, Moreau F, Guigay J, Hartl DM, Hartl DM, Lacau St Guily J. Oropharyngeal cancers: relationship between epidermal growth factor receptor alterations and human papillomavirus status. Eur J Cancer. 2014;50(6):1100–11.

276. Rajendra S, Sharma P. Barrett's esophagus. Curr Treat Options Gastroenterol. 2014;12(2):169–82.

277. Dayama A, Srivastava V, Shukla M, Singh R, Pandey M. Helicobacter pylori and oral cancer: possible association in a preliminary case control study. Asian Pac J Cancer Prev. 2011;12(5):1333–6.

278. Fernando N, Jayakumar G, Perera N, Amarasingha I, Meedin F, Holton J. Presence of Helicobacter pylori in betel chewers and non betel chewers with and without oral cancers. BMC Oral Health. 2009;9:23.

279. Lalla E, Kaplan S, Chang SJ, Roth GA, Celenti R, Hinckley K, et al. Periodontal infection profiles in type 1 diabetes. J Clin Periodontol. 2006;33(12):855–62.

280. Lax AJ, Thomas W. How bacteria could cause cancer: one step at a time. Trends Microbiol. 2002;10(6):293–9.

281. Sheu B. Cytokine regulation networks in the cancer microenvironment. Front Biosci. 2008;13:6255.

282. Katz J, Wallet S, Cha S. Periodontal disease and the oral-systemic connection: "is it all the RAGE?". Quintessence Int. 2010;41(3):229–37.

283. Tezal M, Sullivan MA, Reid ME, Marshall JR, Hyland A, Loree T, et al. Chronic periodontitis and the risk of tongue cancer. Arch Otolaryngol Head Neck Surg. 2007;133(5):450–4.

284. Michaud DS. Role of bacterial infections in pancreatic cancer. Carcinogenesis. 2013;34(10):2193–7.

285. Ferlay J, Shin H, Bray F, Forman D, Mathers C, Parkin DM. Estimates of worldwide burden of cancer in 2008: GLOBOCAN 2008. Int J Cancer. 2010;127(12):2893–917.

286. Dharmani P, Strauss J, Ambrose C, Allen-Vercoe E, Chadee K. Fusobacterium nucleatum infection of colonic cells stimulates MUC2 mucin and tumor necrosis factor alpha. Infect Immun. 2011;79(7):2597–607.

287. Grivennikov SI, Wang K, Mucida D, Stewart CA, Schnabl B, Jauch D, et al. Adenoma-linked barrier defects and microbial products drive IL-23/IL-17-mediated tumour growth. Nature. 2012;491(7423):254–8.

288. Keku TO, McCoy AN, Azcarate-Peril AM. Fusobacterium spp. and colorectal cancer: cause or consequence? Trends Microbiol. 2013;21(10):506–8.

289. Peinado H, Alečković M, Lavotshkin S, Matei I, Costa-Silva B, Moreno-Bueno G, et al. Melanoma exosomes educate bone marrow progenitor cells toward a pro-metastatic phenotype through MET. Nat Med. 2012;18(6):883–91.

290. Somasundaram R, Herlyn M. Melanoma exosomes: messengers of metastasis. Nat Med. 2012;18(6):853–4.

291. O'Connor BP, Eun S, Ye Z, Zozulya AL, Lich JD, Moore CB, et al. Semaphorin 6D regulates the late phase of CD4+ T cell primary immune responses. Proc Natl Acad Sci U S A. 2008;105(35):13015–20.

292. Rehman M, Tamagnone L. Semaphorins in cancer: biological mechanisms and therapeutic approaches. Semin Cell Dev Biol. 2013;24(3):179–89.

293. Zhao X, Chen L, Xu Q, Li Y. Expression of semaphorin 6D in gastric carcinoma and its significance. WJG. 2006;12(45):7388–90.

294. Lin F, Fukuoka Y, Spicer A, Ohta R, Okada N, Harris CL, et al. Tissue distribution of products of the mouse decay-accelerating factor (DAF) genes. Exploitation of a Daf1 knock-out mouse and site-specific monoclonal antibodies. Immunology. 2001;104(2):215–25.

295. Kimura KD, Tissenbaum HA, Liu Y, Ruvkun G. daf-2, an insulin receptor-like gene that regulates longevity and diapause in Caenorhabditis elegans. Science. 1997;277(5328):942–6.

296. Garsin DA. Long-lived C, elegans daf-2 mutants are resistant to bacterial pathogens. Science. 2003;300(5627):1921.

297. Kenon C, Chang J, Gensch E, Rudner A, Tabtiang R. A C. elegans mutant that lives twice as long as wild type. Nature. 1993;366(6454):461–4.

298. Kalamajski S, Aspberg A, Lindblom K, Heinegård D, Oldberg A. Asporin competes with decorin for collagen binding, binds calcium and promotes osteoblast collagen mineralization. Biochem J. 2009;423(1):53–9.

299. Martínez-Gil M, Romero D, Kolter R, Espinosa-Urgel M. Calcium causes multimerization of the large adhesin LapF and modulates biofilm formation by Pseudomonas putida. J Bacteriol. 2012;194(24):6782–9.

300. Abraham NM, Jefferson KK. Staphylococcus aureus clumping factor B mediates biofilm formation in the absence of calcium. Microbiology. 2012;158(Pt 6):1504–12.

301. Shukla SK, Rao TS. Effect of calcium on Staphylococcus aureus biofilm architecture: a confocal laser scanning microscopic study. Colloids Surf B Biointerfaces. 2013;103:448–54.

302. Cruz LF, Cobine PA, La Fuente DL. Calcium increases Xylella fastidiosa surface attachment, biofilm formation, and twitching motility. Appl Environ Microbiol. 2012;78(5):1321–31.

303. Samaranayake LP, Keung Leung W, Jin L. Oral mucosal fungal infections. Periodontology 2000. 2009;49:39–59.

304. Williams DW, Kuriyama T, Silva S, Malic S, Lewis MAO. Candida biofilms and oral candidosis: treatment and prevention. Periodontology 2000. 2011;55(1):250–65.

305. Fichtenbaum CJ, Koletar S, Yiannoutsos C, Holland F, Pottage J, Cohn SE, et al. Refractory mucosal candidiasis in advanced human immunodeficiency virus infection. Clin Infect Dis. 2000;30(5):749–56.

306. Bruatto M, Vidotto V, Marinuzzi G, Raiteri R, Sinicco A. Candida albicans biotypes in human immunodeficiency virus type 1-infected patients with oral candidiasis before and after antifungal therapy. J Clin Microbiol. 1991;29(4):726–30.

307. Feigal DW, Katz MH, Greenspan D, Westenhouse J, Winkelstein W, Lang W, et al. The prevalence of oral lesions in HIV-infected homosexual and bisexual men: three San Francisco epidemiological cohorts. AIDS. 1991;5(5):519–25.

308. McCarthy GM, Mackie ID, Koval J, Sandhu HS, Daley TD. Factors associated with increased frequency of HIV-related oral candidiasis. J Oral Pathol Med. 1991;20(7):332–6.

309. Boriollo MFG, Bassi RC, Santos Nascimento dos CMG, Feliciano LM, Francisco SB, Barros LM, et al. Distribution and hydrolytic enzyme characteristics of Candida albicans strains isolated from diabetic patients and their non-diabetic consorts. Oral Microbiol Immunol. 2009;24(6):437–50.

310. Schloissnig S, Arumugam M, Sunagawa S, Mitreva M, Tap J, Zhu A, et al. Genomic variation landscape of the human gut microbiome. Nature. 2013;493(7430):45–50.

311. Wesolowski LG, MacKellar DA, Facente SN, Dowling T, Ethridge SF, Zhu JH, et al. Post-marketing surveillance of OraQuick whole blood

and oral fluid rapid HIV testing. AIDS. 2006; 20(12):1661–6.

312. Raggam RB, Wagner J, Michelin BDA, Putz-Bankuti C, Lackner A, Bozic M, et al. Reliable detection and quantitation of viral nucleic acids in oral fluid: liquid phase-based sample collection in conjunction with automated and standardized molecular assays. J Med Virol. 2008;80(9):1684–8.

313. Slots J. Herpesviral-bacterial interactions in periodontal diseases. Periodontology 2000. 2010; 52(1):117–40.

314. Goyal A, Shaikh NJ, Kinikar AA, Wairagkar NS. Oral fluid, a substitute for serum to monitor measles IgG antibody? Indian J Med Microbiol. 2009;27(4):351–3.

315. Williams SCP. The other microbiome. Proc Natl Acad Sci U S A. 2013;110(8):2682–4.

316. Orlova EV. How viruses infect bacteria? EMBO J. 2009;28(7):797–8.

317. Reyes A, Haynes M, Hanson N, Angly FE, Heath AC, Rohwer F, et al. Viruses in the faecal microbiota of monozygotic twins and their mothers. Nature. 2010;466(7304):334–8.

318. Minot S, Sinha R, Chen J, Li H, Keilbaugh SA, Wu GD, et al. The human gut virome: inter-individual variation and dynamic response to diet. Genome Res. 2011;21(10):1616–25.

319. Willner D, Furlan M, Haynes M, Schmieder R, Angly FE, Silva J, et al. Metagenomic analysis of respiratory tract DNA viral communities in cystic fibrosis and non-cystic fibrosis individuals. PLoS ONE. 2009;4(10):e7370.

320. McElvania TeKippe E, Wylie KM, Deych E, Sodergren E, Weinstock G, Storch GA. Increased prevalence of anellovirus in pediatric patients with fever. PLoS ONE. 2012;7(11):e50937.

321. Celum CL. The interaction between herpes simplex virus and human immunodeficiency virus. Herpes. 2004;11 Suppl 1:36A–45.

322. Stoopler ET. Oral herpetic infections (HSV 1–8). Dent Clin N Am. 2005;49(1):15–29, vii.

323. Slots J. Human viruses in periodontitis. Periodontology 2000. 2010;53:89–110.

324. Slots J. Oral viral infections of adults. Periodontology 2000. 2009;49:60–86.

325. Shirtcliff EA, Coe CL, Pollak SD. Early childhood stress is associated with elevated antibody levels to herpes simplex virus type 1. Proc Natl Acad Sci U S A. 2009;106(8):2963–7.

326. Mehta SK, Cohrs RJ, Forghani B, Zerbe G, Gilden DH, Pierson DL. Stress-induced subclinical reactivation of varicella zoster virus in astronauts. J Med Virol. 2004;72(1):174–9.

327. Mehta SK, Pierson DL, Cooley H, Dubow R, Lugg D. Epstein-Barr virus reactivation associated with diminished cell-mediated immunity in antarctic expeditioners. J Med Virol. 2000;61(2):235–40.

328. Pierson DL, Stowe RP, Phillips TM, Lugg DJ, Mehta SK. Epstein-Barr virus shedding by astronauts during space flight. Brain Behav Immun. 2005;19(3): 235–42.

329. Payne DA, Mehta SK, Tyring SK, Stowe RP, Pierson DL. Incidence of Epstein-Barr virus in astronaut saliva during spaceflight. Aviat Space Environ Med. 1999;70(12):1211–3.

330. Uchakin PN, Stowe RP, Paddon-Jones D, Tobin BW, Ferrando AA, Wolfe RR. Cytokine secretion and latent herpes virus reactivation with 28 days of horizontal hypokinesia. Aviat Space Environ Med. 2007;78(6):608–12.

331. Sarid O, Anson O, Yaari A, Margalith M. Human cytomegalovirus salivary antibodies as related to stress. Clin Lab. 2002;48(5–6):297–305.

332. Sarid O, Anson O, Yaari A, Margalith M. Academic stress, immunological reaction, and academic performance among students of nursing and physiotherapy. Res Nurs Health. 2004;27(5):370–7.

333. Cohrs RJ, Mehta SK, Schmid DS, Gilden DH, Pierson DL. Asymptomatic reactivation and shed of infectious varicella zoster virus in astronauts. J Med Virol. 2008;80(6):1116–22.

334. Brown ZA, Selke S, Zeh J, Kopelman J, Maslow A, Ashley RL, et al. The acquisition of herpes simplex virus during pregnancy. N Engl J Med. 1997; 337(8):509–15.

335. Miller CS, Cunningham LL, Lindroth JE, Avdiushko SA. The efficacy of valacyclovir in preventing recurrent herpes simplex virus infections associated with dental procedures. J Am Dent Assoc. 2004;135(9): 1311–8.

336. Breuer J, Whitley R. Varicella zoster virus: natural history and current therapies of varicella and herpes zoster. Herpes. 2007;14 Suppl 2:25–9.

337. Ongrádi J, Várnai G, Bendinelli M, Kulcsár G, Dán P, Nász I. Carriage, transfer and interaction of oral viruses and bacteria. Acta Microbiol Hung. 1993;40(3):201–16.

338. Liu YG, Lerner UH, Teng YA. Cytokine responses against periodontal infection: protective and destructive roles. Periodontology 2000. 2010;52(1): 163–206.

339. Carlsson G, Wahlin Y, Johansson A, Olsson A, Eriksson T, Claesson R, et al. Periodontal disease in patients from the original Kostmann family with severe congenital neutropenia. J Periodontol. 2006;77(4):744–51.

340. Wu Y, Yan J, Ojcius DM, Chen L, Gu Z, Pan J. Correlation between infections with different genotypes of human cytomegalovirus and Epstein-Barr virus in subgingival samples and periodontal status of patients. J Clin Microbiol. 2007;45(11):3665–70.

341. Sahin S, Saygun I, Kubar A, Slots J. Periodontitis lesions are the main source of salivary cytomegalovirus. Oral Microbiol Immunol. 2009;24(4):340–2.

342. Slots J. Herpesviruses, the missing link between gingivitis and periodontitis? J Int Acad Periodontol. 2004;6(4):113–9.

343. Grenier G, Gagnon G, Grenier D. Detection of herpetic viruses in gingival crevicular fluid of patients suffering from periodontal diseases: prevalence and effect of treatment. Oral Microbiol Immunol. 2009;24(6):506–9.

344. Saygun I, Kubar A, Ozdemir A, Slots J. Periodontitis lesions are a source of salivary cytomegalovirus and Epstein-Barr virus. J Periodont Res. 2005;40(2):187–91.

345. Contreras A, Umeda M, Chen C, Bakker I, Morrison JL, Slots J. Relationship between herpesviruses and adult periodontitis and periodontopathic bacteria. J Periodontol. 1999;70(5):478–84.

346. Sharma R, Padmalatha O, Kaarthikeyan G, Jayakumar ND, Varghese S, Sherif K. Comparative analysis of presence of Cytomegalovirus (CMV) and Epsteinbarr virus -1 (EBV-1) in cases of chronic periodontitis and aggressive periodontitis with controls. Indian J Dent Res. 2012;23(4):454–8.

347. Das S, Krithiga GSP, Gopalakrishnan S. Detection of human herpes viruses in patients with chronic and aggressive periodontitis and relationship between viruses and clinical parameters. J Oral Maxillofac Pathol. 2012;16(2):203–9.

348. McMillan BC, Golubjatnikov R, Hanson RP, Sinha SK. A study of Cytomegalovirus, Epstein-Barr virus and Herpesvirus hominis (types 1 and 2) antibody in institutionalized and non-institutionalized children. Health Lab Sci. 1977;14(4):261–8.

349. Idesawa M, Sugano N, Ikeda K, Oshikawa M, Takane M, Seki K, et al. Detection of Epstein-Barr virus in saliva by real-time PCR. Oral Microbiol Immunol. 2004;19(4):230–2.

350. Abiko Y, Ikeda M, Hondo R. Secretion and dynamics of herpes simplex virus in tears and saliva of patients with Bell's palsy. Otol Neurotol. 2002;23(5):779–83.

351. Furuta Y, Aizawa H, Ohtani F, Sawa H, Fukuda S. Varicella-zoster virus DNA level and facial paralysis in Ramsay Hunt syndrome. Ann Otol Rhinol Laryngol. 2004;113(9):700–5.

352. Furuta Y, Ohtani F, Sawa H, Fukuda S, Inuyama Y. Quantitation of varicella-zoster virus DNA in patients with Ramsay Hunt syndrome and zoster sine herpete. J Clin Microbiol. 2001;39(8):2856–9.

353. Brown EL, Wald A, Hughes JP, Morrow RA, Krantz E, Mayer K, et al. High risk of human immunodeficiency virus in men who have sex with men with herpes simplex virus type 2 in the EXPLORE study. Am J Epidemiol. 2006;164(8):733–41.

354. Gray RH, Wawer MJ, Sewankambo NK, Serwadda D, Li C, Moulton LH, et al. Relative risks and population attributable fraction of incident HIV associated with symptoms of sexually transmitted diseases and treatable symptomatic sexually transmitted diseases in Rakai District, Uganda. Rakai Project Team. AIDS. 1999;13(15):2113–23.

355. Reynolds SJ, Risbud AR, Shepherd ME, Zenilman JM, Brookmeyer RS, Paranjape RS, et al. Recent herpes simplex virus type 2 infection and the risk of human immunodeficiency virus type 1 acquisition in India. J Infect Dis. 2003;187(10):1513–21.

356. Holmberg SD, Stewart JA, Gerber AR, Byers RH, Lee FK, O'Malley PM, et al. Prior herpes simplex virus type 2 infection as a risk factor for HIV infection. JAMA. 1988;259(7):1048–50.

357. Wald A, Corey L. How does herpes simplex virus type 2 influence human immunodeficiency virus infection and pathogenesis? J Infect Dis. 2003;187(10):1509–12.

358. Golden MP, Kim S, Hammer SM, Ladd EA, Schaffer PA, DeLuca N, et al. Activation of human immunodeficiency virus by herpes simplex virus. J Infect Dis. 1992;166(3):494–9.

359. Hanookai D, Nowzari H, Contreras A, Morrison JL, Slots J. Herpesviruses and periodontopathic bacteria in Trisomy 21 periodontitis. J Periodontol. 2000;71(3):376–84.

360. do Canto CL, Granato CF, Garcez E, Villas Boas LS, Fink MC, Estevam MP, et al. Cytomegalovirus infection in children with Down syndrome in a day-care center in Brazil. Rev Inst Med Trop Sao Paulo. 2000;42(4):179–83.

361. Rhinow K, Schmidt-Westhausen AM, Ellerbrok H, Pauli G, Schetelig J, Siegert W. Quantitative determination of CMV-DNA in saliva of patients with bone marrow and stem cell transplantation using TaqMan-PCR. Mund Kiefer Gesichtschir. 2003;7(6):361–4.

362. Kilian M, Frandsen EVG, Haubek D, Poulsen K. The etiology of periodontal disease revisited by population genetic analysis. Periodontology 2000. 2006;42:158–79.

363. Michalowicz BS, Ronderos M, Camara-Silva R, Contreras A, Slots J. Human herpesviruses and Porphyromonas gingivalis are associated with juvenile periodontitis. J Periodontol. 2000;71(6):981–8.

364. Teughels W, Sliepen I, Quirynen M, Haake SK, Van Eldere J, Fives-Taylor P, et al. Human cytomegalovirus enhances A. actinomycetemcomitans adherence to cells. J Dent Res. 2007;86(2):175–80.

365. Stern J, Shai E, Zaks B, Halabi A, Houri-Haddad Y, Shapira L, et al. Reduced expression of gamma interferon in serum and marked lymphoid depletion induced by Porphyromonas gingivalis increase murine morbidity and mortality due to cytomegalovirus infection. Infect Immun. 2004;72(10):5791–8.

366. Traylen CM, Patel HR, Fondaw W, Mahatme S, Williams JF, Walker LR, et al. Virus reactivation: a panoramic view in human infections. Futur Virol. 2011;6(4):451–63.

367. Qiu X, Chen D, Liu C, Mauk MG, Kientz T, Bau HH. A portable, integrated analyzer for microfluidic – based molecular analysis. Biomed Microdevices. 2011;13(5):809–17.

368. Raggam RB, Wagner J, Bozic M, Michelin BDA, Hammerschmidt S, Homberg C, et al. Detection and quantitation of Epstein-Barr virus (EBV) DNA in EDTA whole blood samples using automated sample preparation and real time PCR. Clin Chem Lab Med. 2010;48(3):413–8.

Development of Nanoparticle-Enabled Protein Biomarker Discovery: Implementation for Saliva-Based Traumatic Brain Injury Detection

Shane V. Caswell, Nelson Cortes, Kelsey Mitchell, Lance Liotta, and Emanuel F. Petricoin

Abstract

In this chapter we will discuss a new approach for amplifying low-abundance proteins for biomarker discovery and how this new approach can be applied to identifying new markers for the detection of traumatic brain injury (TBI) and concussion. Of particular focus is the discovery of non-subjective, sensitive, and specific biomarkers for early detection of TBI/concussion that can be quantified accurately and which can be measured in an easily obtainable biofluid. We propose that such a method can be applied to TBI detection in saliva—a biofluid that heretofore has not been considered for this application.

S.V. Caswell, PhD, ATC (✉) • N. Cortes, PhD
Sports Medicine Assessment, Research and Testing Laboratory, George Mason University,
Manassas, VA, USA
e-mail: epetrico@gmu.edu; ncortes@gmu.edu

K. Mitchell, BS
Sports Medicine Assessment, Research and Testing Laboratory, George Mason University,
Manassas, VA, USA

Center for Applied Proteomics and Molecular Medicine, George Mason University,
Manassas, VA, USA

L. Liotta, MD, PhD
Center for Applied Proteomics and Molecular Medicine, George Mason University,
Manassas, VA, USA

E.F. Petricoin, PhD
Center for Applied Proteomics and Molecular Medicine, George Mason University,
Manassas, VA, USA

School of Systems Biology, George Mason University, Manassas, VA, USA

Introduction

Currently, the diagnosis of mild traumatic brain injury/concussion relies mainly upon clinicians' ability to accurately interpret a patient's self-reported (and subjective) signs and symptoms [1]. Consequently, concussion diagnosis can be challenging due to the variability in the neuro-physiological and cognitive manifestations that a patient may present. Indeed, many concussion symptoms commonly present with patients who have sleep disturbances, depression, or attention deficit disorder. Commonly used diagnostic tools include self-reported symptoms, neuropsychological testing, and dynamic stability (balance) assessment [2, 3], which are impacted by coincident occurrences of trauma, fatigue, and environmental or psychological conditions [1]. New classes of diagnostic imaging such as computed

C.F. Streckfus (ed.), *Advances in Salivary Diagnostics*,
DOI 10.1007/978-3-662-45399-5_6, © Springer-Verlag Berlin Heidelberg 2015

tomography (CT) or magnetic resonance imaging (MRI) can be used to rule out more severe injuries, but due to cost and interpretive incongruence, especially for mild concussions, these technologies have limited clinical impact at present [4–6]. Thus, of critical importance is the development of new approaches and technologies that can overcome these current limitations. MRI diffusion tensor imaging [6, 7], quantitative electroencephalogram [8], visual tracking [9], and serum-based biomarkers of brain injury [10] hold potential to aid clinicians in objectively diagnosing concussion and are currently under intense evaluation [11].

Of particular focus is the discovery of nonsubjective, sensitive, and specific biomarkers for early detection of TBI/concussion that can be quantified accurately and which can be measured in an easily obtainable biofluid. A recent report by the National Academy of Sciences on Sports-Related Concussions in Youth [12] discusses that the current lack of reliable biomarkers and a reliance on subjective symptom-based diagnosis is a significant barrier to early TBI detection as well as the "return to play" determination [12]. Furthermore, a recent US Department of Defense report described the critical importance of biochemical markers of brain injury to inform clinical decision-making and test the efficacy of new potential treatments [13].

Since proteins are the biochemical effectors of cellular function and comprise the enzymes and structural molecules of the cell, many current biomarkers for detecting disease and organ dysfunction are proteins, not genes. This realization has led to rapid growth in the field of proteomics, a branch of biotechnology focused on analyzing and characterizing at the multiplexed level all of the proteins found in a particular cell, tissue, or organism [14]. In this chapter we will discuss a new approach for amplifying low-abundance proteins for biomarker discovery and how this new approach can be applied to identifying new markers for the detection of TBI/concussion. Finally we propose that such a method can be applied to TBI detection in saliva—a biofluid that heretofore has not been considered for this application.

Proteomic Approaches for Concussion Detection

Global proteomic profiling, so-called "unbiased" analysis for discovery-oriented applications, uses mass spectrometry (MS) as the central workhorse platform for nearly every investigator. MS can measure thousands of proteins at once without the need for antibodies or other protein detection reagent [15]. Certainly, the application of MS-based analysis has shown great promise for diseases such as cancer, for which several MS discovered biomarkers are now used for clinical purposes [16–18]. Once MS has uncovered the differential protein expression, investigators then use immuno-based technologies (e.g., enzyme-linked immunosorbent assay [ELISA]) for more routine clinical measurement. The applications of proteomic approaches have found biomarkers that may have important applications for neurological disorders. Recent studies have found that decreased levels of alpha-syn and DJ-1 are associated with Parkinson's disease [19]. Altered expression of GFAP, Aβ(beta)42, and Aβ(beta)40 proteins has been identified in Alzheimer's patients [20]. These successes provide increased confidence that proteomics technologies can uncover biomarkers of brain trauma and TBI. Indeed there are a number of existing proteins such as S100B [21–30], GFAP [22, 31–35], NSE [36–41], and UCHL1 [23, 42–44] that are promising candidates for TBI and mild concussion detection. Protein breakdown products may also be potential biomarkers for concussion. Spectrin N-terminal fragment [45]; spectrin breakdown products 120, 145, and 150 [46–48]; collapsin response mediation [49]; and synaptotagmin breakdown product [49] have all been implicated recently. The presence of these proteins and protein fragments/peptides provides increasing confidence that the implementation of discovery-based proteomics, using ever-increasing sophisticated and high-resolution mass spectrometry, may identify new protein maker candidates with the highest levels of sensitivity and specificity for concussion diagnosis and monitoring. However, despite this potential, significant challenges and barriers exist that are preventing overarching success for the field of proteomics to identify new clinically relevant biomarkers for TBI/mild concussion detection and monitoring.

Current Limitations and Barriers for Protein Biomarker Discovery Research

Blood-Brain Barrier Permeability Can Influence the Presence of Any TBI Marker in the Periphery

Any biomarker that is related to brain trauma must overcome the blood-brain barrier (BBB) in order for it to be measured in a peripheral body fluid such as blood, saliva, sweat, etc. Concussion causes disruption of the BBB, which allows permeability between the brain tissue and cerebrospinal fluid (CSF), leading to elevated presence of particular biomarkers in blood [21, 50]. Once in the blood, the markers can then circulate and be found in other body fluids such as saliva, tears, sweat, etc., albeit at much lower inherent concentrations than what is found in the blood due to the distal nature of these fluids in relation to the location of the trauma.

Coincident Traumatic Events Can Confound TBI-Specific Marker Discovery

Another potential challenge to developing clinically applicable biomarkers for concussion is the presence of polytrauma. Many patients in which a concussion marker would be useful to definitively rule in or rule out TBI also present with other trauma, including musculoskeletal injury [51]. Injury to these other tissues and organs also releases markers into the bloodstream, and so the search for brain trauma-specific markers may be complicated by coincident injuries that may complicate the clinical application of individual markers to concussion diagnosis [52, 53].

Most Biomarkers for Early Detection of TBI are Low-Abundance Biomarkers

Despite recent technological advances in mass spectrometry and sample fractionation methods, analytical and physiological barriers currently hinder biological marker discovery. By definition, most biomarkers associated with the earliest changes in normal pathophysiology are found in very low abundances, with concentrations likely in the sub-nanogram per milliliter range, well below the detection limits of even the most sophisticated mass spectrometry instrumentation. This is because the production of the marker at the initiating stages of disease/trauma will be low and the resulting concentration in peripheral body fluids also at the lowest levels. Additionally, the abundance of endogenous high-molecular-weight proteins such as albumin and immunoglobulins may be one billion or more times abundant than these low-abundance trauma-specific proteins. Moreover, due to the resultant mass action kinetics, any low-abundance TBI-specific biomarkers are very likely non-covalently and endogenously associated with resident proteins that account for >95 % of circulating proteins, making it difficult to isolate and characterize them [14, 15, 54].

Uncontrolled Sample Collection Methods Can Result in Biomarker Loss

Field-based environments, whether on the playing field, battlefield, etc., present significant logistical challenges to sample collection and analysis. These settings are often in geographically remote regions, often without power, and unable to store collected biospecimens in a controlled environment. Moreover, designing point-of-care diagnostic methods/instrumentation wherein any biomarker is directly measured in the field, and which could obviate the need for transporting, deployment, and operation of sensitive and bulky testing platforms—such as standard enzyme-linked immunosorbent assay

(ELISA)—also have a number of serious limitations as a point-of-care diagnostic tool [1]. In addition, these harsh environments present significant technical barriers to the collection of commonly used body fluids such as blood, CSF, or urine. For example, blood and cerebrospinal fluid collections are invasive and carry a risk of infection. Urine collection is intrusive and has associated privacy issues. A biofluid that may represent a new and underutilized principal source for biomarker discovery and measurement is saliva. Saliva holds the potential to solve a number of the aforementioned issues since it is one the least invasive biofluids to collect, is safe, and would not involve costly transport or storage methods.

Saliva Biology and Use as a Concussion Biomarker Source

We now know that saliva is a complex and dynamic biological fluid and that numerous compounds can be measured in saliva, such as drugs, pollutants, and hormones, but also biomarkers of bacterial, viral, and systemic disease [55]. Since saliva protein content may be reflective of whole body health, protein changes caused by TBI/concussion could be reflected within the salivary proteome. The key advantage of saliva as a diagnostic tool is that sample collection is low cost, easily deployed in most settings, and noninvasive [56].

Salivary gland output is a combination of serous and mucous and is controlled by the autonomic nervous system. When the sympathetic nervous system is activated by bodily stress, such as a TBI, the stimulation may cause protein concentration changes in serous-rich saliva. Saliva biomarker discovery has been used to detect pathophysiological conditions such as Sjögren's syndrome [57–59], non-Hodgkin's lymphoma [60], head and neck squamous cell carcinoma [60], lung cancer [18], pancreatic cancer [61], gastric cancer [62], and neurodegenerative diseases [20, 63–67]. Beyond the ease of collection of saliva compared to a CSF, which often precludes the routine clinical implementation of any marker, saliva has other key advantages because

whole saliva collection can be obtained within a few minutes compared to much longer times for CSF or serum/blood collection methods. By immediately placing collected saliva samples on dry ice and directly transporting and depositing them in a –80 °C freezer, degradation of proteins in saliva and bacterial growth can be minimized. Protein has been reported to be stable at six months after freezing at –80 °C [56].

Development and Implementation of Nanoparticle-Based Biomarker Capture and Preservation for TBI Marker Research in Saliva

While concussion biomarker research has achieved new levels of success and new marker candidates being evaluated, and there have been significant technical improvements in MS instrumentation and proteomic technology development, there are many impediments that remain. However, each of these impediments provides opportunities for innovative approaches to overcome these challenges. Until now, most scientists have focused on making technical improvements in the detection platforms wherein new chemistries or engineering has been developed to detect proteins at lower and lower levels of analytical sensitivity. Unfortunately, as one increases the analytical sensitivity of any detection platform, inherently process variance increases as limits of detection are approached. An untapped area of focus that could have immediate and substantial impact on biomarker research is the upfront sample collection step. If one could increase the starting concentration of any marker at the sample collection/preparation step, then inherently the downstream measurement devices benefit immediately.

A recent exciting new technological innovation has been the development of core-shell hydrogel nanoparticles that have been engineered to rapidly concentrate and preserve extremely small quantities of biomarkers in bodily fluids [14]. This novel technology provides new opportunities for field-based diagnostic tools for implementation in conditions and

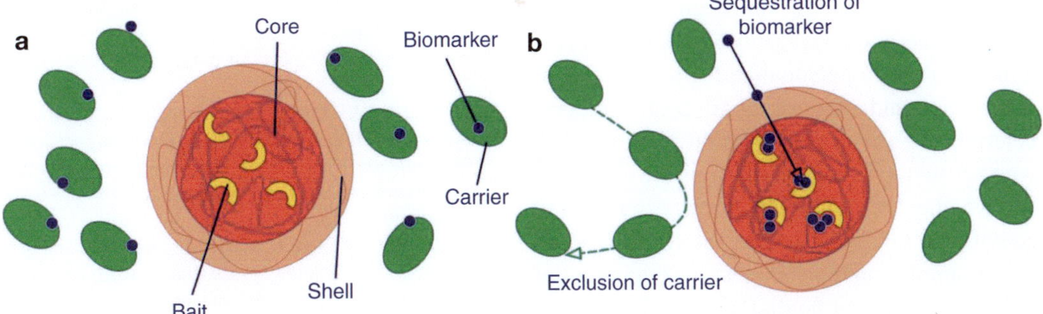

Fig. 6.1 Core-shell hydrogel nanoparticles for low-abundance biomarker capture and amplification. Nanoparticles are engineered with a polymer shell with pore sizes constructed to eliminate high-abundance high-molecular-weight proteins from low-abundance low-molecular-weight TBI biomarkers through size sieving and high-affinity chemical bait dye molecule within the core that binds biomarkers. Due to mass action kinetics, most low-abundance protein markers exist pre-bound to high-abundance carrier proteins such as albumin that exist in billions of fold molar excess. Panel (**a**) Biomarkers are complexed to high-abundance proteins when nanoparticles are introduced into the saliva. Panel (**b**) Within seconds, the biomarkers are collected and concentrated within the nanoparticle as the high-affinity dye molecule out-competes the carrier protein for biomarker binding

environments where existing methodologies are not feasible. In one step in solution, these core-shell hydrogel nanoparticles perform a rapid and complete sequestration of the biomarker archive while simultaneously size sieving high-abundance and high-molecular-weight proteins away from the captured milieu—thereby simultaneously enriching and concentrating the low-molecular-weight (LMW) biomarkers archive (Fig. 6.1) [14, 68–70]. The nanoparticles are engineered with high-affinity dye molecule "bait" molecules that are covalently linked to the core moiety, which bind tightly to any protein/peptide that gets through the nanoparticle shell that has a pore size MW cutoff. The shell acts as a sieve, excluding high-molecular-weight, high-abundance proteins (Fig. 6.1). Once nanoparticles are applied to the sample, the proteins become stable at room temperature for long periods of time [68–70]. The nanoparticles effectively act as a biomarker "vacuum" wherein the biomarker content within 10 ml of collected saliva is concentrated to a 10 µl volume, which would result in a 1,000× increase in the biomarker concentration. Thus, the use of biomarker harvesting nanoparticles coupled with salivary-based biomarker detection workflows represents an entirely novel and new approach for TBI marker discovery and resultant concussion detection and

monitoring. Such an approach serves to replace the current status quo of invasive biofluid-based input (e.g., CSF and/or blood) for TBI marker analysis using workflows fraught with uncontrolled sample collection times, labile marker degradation, etc. to one of a simple one-step biomarker collection device using a noninvasive saliva sample as the input for TBI marker measurements.

Conclusion

A View to the Future for Nanoparticle-Based Salivary TBI Diagnostics

In addition to the potential for the saliva proteome as a new untapped archive for TBI-specific biomarkers, the use of nanoparticle-based biomarker harvesting could provide a new opportunity to characterize the potential aggregate neurodegenerative effects of chronic sub-concussive blows suffered by athletes and by soldiers in the military [71–74]. A salivary-based protein biomarker-profiling tool could provide a facile means to record an individual's unique baseline biomarker signature and then serially track this profile for subtle changes longitudinally over time since saliva collection is so noninvasive. The result of this new opportunity could be a personalized approach to TBI diagnostics and monitoring to help clinicians determine when activity should be restricted, whether therapeutic interventions are effective, and whether the individual is ready to return to activity. In this view to the future, a baseline saliva sample could be taken at the beginning of a football player or soldier's career and then a biomarker profile determined using nanoparticle-harvesting agents. This baseline salivary protein fingerprint could then be compared to subsequent saliva proteomic profiles measured at predetermined intervals for overall monitoring either in a pre- or post-concussion state and provide quantitative information to aid the clinician in managing any short- and long-term effects of TBI.

Acknowledgments

Disclosures
Emanuel Petricoin is a coinventor on issued patents relating to the nanoparticle technology described in this chapter and can receive royalties from the licenses taken. He is an equity interest holder, consultant, and cofounder of Ceres Nanosciences Inc., which has licensed the nanoparticle technology described in this chapter.

Funding
This project was made possible in part by nonrestrictive funding from the Potomac Health Foundation and the generous support of the College of Science and the College of Education and Human Development.

References

1. Schmid KE, Tortella FC. The diagnosis of traumatic brain injury on the battlefield. Front Neurol. 2012;3:90.
2. Jinguji TM, Bompadre V, Harmon KG, Satchell EK, Gilbert K, Wild J, Eary JF. Sport concussion assessment tool–2: baseline values for high school athletes. Br J Sports Med. 2012;46:365–70.
3. Mansell JL, Tierney RT, Higgins M, McDevitt J, Toone N, Glutting J. Concussive signs and symptoms following head impacts in collegiate athletes. Brain Inj. 2010;24:1070–4.
4. Chastain CA, Oyoyo UE, Zipperman M, Joo E, Ashwal S, Shutter LA, Tong KA. Predicting outcomes of traumatic brain injury by imaging modality and injury distribution. J Neurotrauma. 2009;26:1183–96.
5. Mondello S, Papa L, Buki A, Bullock MR, Czeiter E, Tortella FC, Wang KK, Hayes RL. Neuronal and glial markers are differently associated with computed tomography findings and outcome in patients with severe traumatic brain injury: a case control study. Crit Care. 2011;15:R156.
6. Prabhu SP. The role of neuroimaging in sport-related concussion. Clin Sports Med. 2011;30:103.
7. Kumar R, Husain M, Gupta RK, Hasan KM, Haris M, Agarwal AK, Pandey CM, Narayana PA. Serial changes in the white matter diffusion tensor imaging metrics in moderate traumatic brain injury and correlation with neuro-cognitive function. J Neurotrauma. 2009;26:481–95.
8. Nuwer MR, Hovda DA, Schrader LM, Vespa PM. Routine and quantitative EEG in mild traumatic brain injury. Clin Neurophysiol. 2005;116:2001–25.
9. Maruta J, Suh M, Niogi SN, Mukherjee P, Ghajar J. Visual tracking synchronization as a metric for concussion screening. J Head Trauma Rehabil. 2010;25:293–305.
10. Dash PK, Zhao J, Hergenroeder G, Moore AN. Biomarkers for the diagnosis, prognosis, and evaluation of treatment efficacy for traumatic brain injury. Neurotherapeutics. 2010;7:100–14.
11. Marion DW. Current diagnostic and therapeutic challenges. Trauma Brain Inj. 2012:313–23.
12. Graham R, Rivara FP, Ford MA, Mason Spicer C. Eds. Treatment and management of prolonged symptoms and post-concussion syndrome. In: Sports-related concussions in youth: Improving the science, changing the culture. Institute of Medicine of the National Academies, The National Academies Press, Washington, DC, 2013. Available at http://www.iom.edu/Reports/2013/Sports-Related-Concussions-in-Youth-Improving-the-Science-Changing-the-Culture.aspx. Accessed November 13, 2013
13. Diaz-Arrastia R, Kochanek PM, Bergold P, Kenney K, Marx C, Grimes J, Loh Y, Adam G, Oskvig DB, Curley K. Pharmacotherapy of traumatic brain injury: state of the science and the road forward report of the Department of Defense Neurotrauma Pharmacology Workgroup. J Neurotrauma. 2013;31:135–58.
14. Luchini A, Longo C, Espina V, Petricoin III EF, Liotta LA. Nanoparticle technology: addressing the fundamental roadblocks to protein biomarker discovery. J Mater Chem. 2009;19:5071–7.
15. Liotta LA, Petricoin EF. Omics and cancer biomarkers: link to the biological truth or bear the consequences. Cancer Epidemiol Biomarkers Prev. 2012;21:1229–35.

16. Casanova-Salas I, Rubio-Briones J, Fernández-Serra A, López-Guerrero JA. miRNAs as biomarkers in prostate cancer. Clin Transl Oncol. 2012;14:803–11.

17. Siena S, Sartore-Bianchi A, Di Nicolantonio F, Balfour J, Bardelli A. Biomarkers predicting clinical outcome of epidermal growth factor receptor–targeted therapy in metastatic colorectal cancer. J Natl Cancer Inst. 2009;101:1308–24.

18. Socinski MA. The emerging role of biomarkers in advanced non–small-cell lung cancer. Clin Lung Cancer. 2010;11:149–59.

19. Devic I, Hwang HJ, Edgar JS, Izutsu K, Presland R, Pan C, Goodlett DR, Wang Y, Armaly J, Tumas V. Salivary alpha-synuclein and DJ-1: potential biomarkers for Parkinson's disease. Brain. 2011;134:e178.

20. Patel S, Shah RJ, Coleman P, Sabbagh M. Potential peripheral biomarkers for the diagnosis of Alzheimer's disease. Int J Alzheimers Dis. 2011;2011:1–9.

21. Readnower RD, Chavko M, Adeeb S, Conroy MD, Pauly JR, McCarron RM, Sullivan PG. Increase in blood–brain barrier permeability, oxidative stress, and activated microglia in a rat model of blast-induced traumatic brain injury. J Neurosci Res. 2010;88: 3530–9.

22. Ingebrigtsen T, Romner B. Biochemical serum markers of traumatic brain injury. J Trauma Acute Care Surg. 2002;52:798–808.

23. Berger RP, Hayes RL, Richichi R, Beers SR, Wang KKW. Serum concentrations of ubiquitin C-terminal hydrolase-L1 and αII-spectrin breakdown product 145 kDa correlate with outcome after pediatric TBI. J Neurotrauma. 2012;29:162–7.

24. Korfias S, Papadimitriou A, Stranjalis G, Bakoula C, Daskalakis G, Antsaklis A, Sakas DE. Serum biochemical markers of brain injury. Mini Rev Med Chem. 2009;9:227–34.

25. Savola O, Pyhtinen J, Leino TK, Siitonen S, Niemelä O, Hillbom M. Effects of head and extracranial injuries on serum protein S100B levels in trauma patients. J Trauma Acute Care Surg. 2004;56:1229–34.

26. Townend W, Dibble C, Abid K, Vail A, Sherwood R, Lecky F. Rapid elimination of protein S-100B from serum after minor head trauma. J Neurotrauma. 2006;23:149–55.

27. Bazarian JJ, Zemlan FP, Mookerjee S, Stigbrand T. Serum S-100B and cleaved-tau are poor predictors of long-term outcome after mild traumatic brain injury. Brain Inj. 2006;20:759–65.

28. Berger RP, Pierce MC, Wisniewski SR, Adelson PD, Kochanek PM. Serum S100B concentrations are increased after closed head injury in children: a preliminary study. J Neurotrauma. 2002;19:1405–9.

29. Müller K, Townend W, Biasca N, Undén J, Waterloo K, Romner B, Ingebrigtsen T. S100B serum level predicts computed tomography findings after minor head injury. J Trauma. 2007;62:1452.

30. Undén J, Romner B. A new objective method for CT triage after minor head injury-serum S100B. Scand J Clin Lab Invest. 2009;69:13–7.

31. Nylen K, Öst M, Csajbok LZ, Nilsson I, Blennow K, Nellgård B, Rosengren L. Increased serum-GFAP in patients with severe traumatic brain injury is related to outcome. J Neurol Sci. 2006;240:85–91.

32. Nylén K, Csajbok LZ, Öst M, Rashid A, Blennow K, Nellgård B, Rosengren L. Serum glial fibrillary acidic protein is related to focal brain injury and outcome after aneurysmal subarachnoid hemorrhage. Stroke. 2007;38:1489–94.

33. Eng LF, Vanderhaeghen JJ, Bignami A, Gerstl B. An acidic protein isolated from fibrous astrocytes. Brain Res. 1971;28:351.

34. Herrmann M, Vos P, Wunderlich MT, de Bruijn CHMM, Lamers KJB. Release of glial tissue–specific proteins after acute stroke a comparative analysis of serum concentrations of protein S-100B and glial fibrillary acidic protein. Stroke. 2000;31:2670–7.

35. Missler U, Wiesmann M, Wittmann G, Magerkurth O, Hagenström H. Measurement of glial fibrillary acidic protein in human blood: analytical method and preliminary clinical results. Clin Chem. 1999;45:138–41.

36. Ergün R, Bostanci U, Akdemir G, Beşkonakli E, Kaptanoğlu E, Gürsoy F, Taşkin Y. Prognostic value of serum neuron-specific enolase levels after head injury. Neurol Res. 1998;20:418.

37. Ross SA, Cunningham RT, Johnston CF, Rowlands BJ. Neuron-specific enolase as an aid to outcome prediction in head injury. Br J Neurosurg. 1996;10: 471–6.

38. Yamazaki Y, Yada K, Morii S, Kitahara T, Ohwada T. Diagnostic significance of serum neuron-specific enolase and myelin basic protein assay in patients with acute head injury. Surg Neurol. 1995;43:267–71.

39. Marangos PJ, Schmechel DE. Neuron specific enolase, a clinically useful marker for neurons and neuroendocrine cells. Annu Rev Neurosci. 1987;10:269–95.

40. McKeating EG, Andrews PJ, Mascia L. Relationship of neuron specific enolase and protein S-100 concentrations in systemic and jugular venous serum to injury severity and outcome after traumatic brain injury. Acta Neurochir Suppl. 1998;71:117.

41. Woertgen CH, Rothoerl RD, Holzschuh M, Metz C, Brawanski A. Comparison of serial S-100 and NSE serum measurements after severe head injury. Acta Neurochir (Wien). 1997;139:1161–5.

42. Blyth BJ, Farahvar A, He H, Nayak A, Yang C, Shaw G, Bazarian JJ. Elevated serum ubiquitin carboxy-terminal hydrolase L1 is associated with abnormal blood–brain barrier function after traumatic brain injury. J Neurotrauma. 2011;28:2453–62.

43. Papa L, Akinyi L, Liu MC, Pineda JA, Tepas III JJ, Oli MW, Zheng W, Robinson G, Robicsek SA, Gabrielli A. Ubiquitin C-terminal hydrolase is a novel biomarker in humans for severe traumatic brain injury*. Crit Care Med. 2010;38:138.

44. Setsuie R, Wada K. The functions of UCH-L1 and its relation to neurodegenerative diseases. Neurochem Int. 2007;51:105–11.

45. Siman R, Toraskar N, Dang A, McNeil E, McGarvey M, Plaum J, Maloney E, Grady MS. A panel of neuron-enriched proteins as markers for traumatic brain injury in humans. J Neurotrauma. 2009;26:1867–77.

46. Weiss ES, Wang KKW, Allen JG, Blue ME, Nwakanma LU, Liu MC, Lange MS, Berrong J, Wilson MA, Gott VL, Troncoso JC, Hayes RL, Johnston MV, Baumgartner WA. Alpha II-spectrin breakdown products serve as novel markers of brain injury severity in a canine model of hypothermic circulatory arrest. Ann Thorac Surg. 2009;88:543–50.

47. Mondello S, Robicsek SA, Gabrielli A, Brophy GM, Papa L, Tepas III J, Robertson C, Buki A, Scharf D, Jixiang M. αII-spectrin breakdown products (SBDPs): diagnosis and outcome in severe traumatic brain injury patients. J Neurotrauma. 2010;27:1203–13.

48. Brophy GM, Pineda JA, Papa L, Lewis SB, Valadka AB, Hannay HJ, Heaton SC, Demery JA, Liu MC, Tepas III JJ. αII-spectrin breakdown product cerebrospinal fluid exposure metrics suggest differences in cellular injury mechanisms after severe traumatic brain injury. J Neurotrauma. 2009;26:471–9.

49. Kobeissy FH, Ottens AK, Zhang Z, Liu MC, Denslow ND, Dave JR, Tortella FC, Hayes RL, Wang KK. Novel differential neuroproteomics analysis of traumatic brain injury in rats. Mol Cell Proteomics. 2006;5:1887–98.

50. Blyth BJ, Farhavar A, Gee C, Hawthorn B, He H, Nayak A, Stocklein V, Bazarian JJ. Validation of serum markers for blood-brain barrier disruption in traumatic brain injury. J Neurotrauma. 2009;26:1497–507.

51. Keel M, Trentz O. Pathophysiology of polytrauma. Injury. 2005;36:691–709.

52. Jeter CB, Hergenroeder GW, Hylin MJ, Redell JB, Moore AN, Dash PK. Biomarkers for the diagnosis and prognosis of mild traumatic brain injury/concussion. J Neurotrauma. 2013;30:657–70.

53. Pham N, Fazio V, Cucullo L, Teng Q, Biberthaler P, Bazarian JJ, Janigro D. Extracranial sources of S100B do not affect serum levels. PLoS One. 2010;5:e12691.

54. Liotta LA, Ferrari M, Petricoin E. Clinical proteomics: written in blood. Nature. 2003;425:905.

55. Chiappin S, Antonelli G, Gatti R, De Palo EF. Saliva specimen: a new laboratory tool for diagnostic and basic investigation. Clin Chim Acta. 2007;383:30–40.

56. Navazesh M. Methods for collecting saliva. Ann N Y Acad Sci. 2006;694:72–7.

57. Hu S, Wang J, Meijer J, Ieong S, Xie Y, Yu T, Zhou H, Henry S, Vissink A, Pijpe J. Salivary proteomic and genomic biomarkers for primary Sjögren's syndrome. Arthritis Rheum. 2007;56:3588–600.

58. Baldini C, Giusti L, Bazzichi L, Lucacchini A, Bombardieri S. Proteomic analysis of the saliva: a clue for understanding primary from secondary Sjögren's syndrome? Autoimmun Rev. 2008;7:185–91.

59. Higashi K, Yoshida M, Igarashi A, Ito K, Wada Y, Murakami S, Kobayashi D, Nakano M, Sohda M, Nakajima T, Narita I, Toida T, Kashiwagi K, Igarashi K. Intense correlation between protein-conjugated acrolein and primary Sjögren's syndrome. Clin Chim Acta. 2010;411:359–63.

60. Righini CA, De Fraipont F, Timsit JF, Faure C, Brambilla E, Reyt E, Favrot MC. Tumor-specific methylation in saliva: a promising biomarker for early detection of head and neck cancer recurrence. Clin Cancer Res. 2007;13:1179–85.

61. Zhang L, Farrell JJ, Zhou H, Elashoff D, Akin D, Park NH, Chia D, Wong DT. Salivary transcriptomic biomarkers for detection of resectable pancreatic cancer. Gastroenterology. 2010;138:949–57.

62. Lin L-L, Huang H-C, Juan H-F. Discovery of biomarkers for gastric cancer: a proteomics approach. J Proteomics. 2012;75:3081–97.

63. Martins-de-Souza D, Harris LW, Guest PC, Turck CW, Bahn S. The role of proteomics in depression research. Eur Arch Psychiatry Clin Neurosci. 2010;260:499–506.

64. Shi M, Caudle WM, Zhang J. Biomarker discovery in neurodegenerative diseases: a proteomic approach. Neurobiol Dis. 2009;35:157–64.

65. Blennow K, Hampel H, Weiner M, Zetterberg H. Cerebrospinal fluid and plasma biomarkers in Alzheimer disease. Nat Rev Neurol. 2010;6:131–44.

66. Hu WT, Chen-Plotkin A, Arnold SE, Grossman M, Clark CM, Shaw LM, McCluskey L, Elman L, Karlawish J, Hurtig HI, Siderowf A, Lee VM-Y, Soares H, Trojanowski JQ. Biomarker discovery for Alzheimer's disease, frontotemporal lobar degeneration, and Parkinson's disease. Acta Neuropathol (Berl). 2010;120:385–99.

67. King A, Sweeney F, Bodi I, Troakes C, Maekawa S, Al-Sarraj S. Abnormal TDP-43 expression is identified in the neocortex in cases of dementia pugilistica, but is mainly confined to the limbic system when identified in high and moderate stages of Alzheimer's disease. Neuropathology. 2010;30:408–19.

68. Luchini A, Geho DH, Bishop B, Tran D, Xia C, Dufour RL, Jones CD, Espina V, Patanarut A, Zhou W, Ross MM, Tessitore A, Petricoin 3rd EF, Liotta LA. Smart hydrogel particles: biomarker harvesting: one-step affinity purification, size exclusion, and protection against degradation. Nano Lett. 2008;8:350–61.

69. Tamburro D, Fredolini C, Espina V, Douglas TA, Ranganathan A, Ilag L, Zhou W, Russo P, Espina BH, Muto G, Petricoin 3rd EF, Liotta LA, Luchini A. Multifunctional core-shell nanoparticles: discovery of previously invisible biomarkers. J Am Chem Soc. 2011;133:19178–88.

70. Longo C, Patanarut A, George T, Bishop B, Zhou W, Fredolini C, Ross MM, Espina V, Pellacani G, Petricoin 3rd EF, Liotta LA, Luchini A. Core-shell hydrogel particles harvest, concentrate and preserve

labile low abundance biomarkers. PLoS One. 2009;4: e4763.

71. Halstead ME, Walter KD. Sport-related concussion in children and adolescents. Pediatrics. 2010;126: 597–615.

72. McKee AC, Cantu RC, Nowinski CJ, Hedley-Whyte ET, Gavett BE, Budson AE, Santini VE, Lee H-S, Kubilus CA, Stern RA. Chronic traumatic encephalopathy in athletes: progressive tauopathy following repetitive head injury. J Neuropathol Exp Neurol. 2009;68:709.

73. Gavett BE, Stern RA, McKee AC. Chronic traumatic encephalopathy: a potential late effect of sport-related concussive and subconcussive head trauma. Clin Sports Med. 2011;30:179. xi.

74. Saulle M, Greenwald BD. Chronic traumatic encephalopathy: a review. Rehabil Res Pract. 2012;2012: 816069.

Saliva Diagnostics for Oral Diseases

Xi Zhang, Arutha Kulasinghe, Rafid Shahriyar Karim, and Chamindie Punyadeera

Abstract

Oral diseases, or stomatognathic diseases, denote the diseases of the mouth ("stoma") and jaw ("gnath"). Dental caries and periodontal diseases have been traditionally considered as the most important global oral health burdens. It is important to note that in oral diagnostics, the greatest challenges are determining the clinical utility of potential biomarkers for screening (in asymptomatic people), predicting the early onset of disease (prognostic tests), and evaluating the disease activity and the efficacy of therapy through innovative diagnostic tests. An oral diagnostic test, in principle, should provide valuable information for differential diagnosis, localization of disease, and severity of infection. This information can then be incorporated by the physician when planning treatments and will provide means for assessing the effectiveness of therapy.

X. Zhang, BPharm, MBiotech
A. Kulasinghe, BSC (Hons) Medical Microbiology
R.S. Karim, BSc/MBBS – Year 5
Saliva Translational Research Group,
The University of Queensland Diamantina
Institute, The University of Queensland,
Woolloongabba, QLD, Australia
e-mail: x78.zhang@hdr.qut.edu.au;
arutha.kulasinghe@qut.edu.au;
rafid.karim@uqconnect.edu.au

C. Punyadeera, PhD (✉)
Saliva Translational Research Group,
The University of Queensland Diamantina Institute,
Woolloongabba, QLD, Australia
e-mail: chamindie.punyadeera@qut.edu.au

Introduction

Oral diseases, or stomatognathic diseases, denote the diseases of the mouth ("stoma") and jaw ("gnath") [1]. Oral diseases are known by various synonyms such as "oral and maxillofacial pathology" (as used by the American Dental Association) or "diseases of oral cavity, salivary glands and jaws" (as used by the World Health Organization). Despite great achievements in population-based oral health globally, problems still remain in many communities all over the world—particularly among underprivileged people in developing countries. Dental caries and periodontal diseases have traditionally been

C.F. Streckfus (ed.), *Advances in Salivary Diagnostics*,
DOI 10.1007/978-3-662-45399-5_7, © Springer-Verlag Berlin Heidelberg 2015

considered as the most important global oral health burdens. It is important to note that in oral diagnostics, the greatest challenges are determining the clinical utility of potential biomarkers for screening (in asymptomatic people), predicting the early onset of disease (prognostic tests) and monitoring the disease activity and the efficacy of therapy through innovative diagnostic tests. An oral diagnostic test, in principle, should provide valuable information for differential diagnosis, localization of disease, and severity of infection. This information then can be incorporated by the physician when planning treatments and will provide a means for assessing the effectiveness of therapy.

Human saliva has gained attention as an alternative diagnostic medium for detecting oral and systemic diseases. Saliva, a multi-constituent oral fluid, has demonstrated high potential for the surveillance of general health and disease. Saliva is also now considered as an important cancer biofluid by the National Cancer Institute in the USA [2]. Recently, the National Institutes of Health (NIH) granted USD five million to develop saliva-based tests to diagnose stomach cancer. It is not surprising that saliva can be used as a biological medium because it harbors proteins, nucleic acids, electrolytes, and hormones originating from multiple local and systemic sources, and it is now known to contain approximately 30 % of biomolecules that are found in blood [3]. This—along with its ease of collection without the need for medical staff or hypodermic needles, coupled with robust sample collection from individuals even in remote areas such as the Australian Outback and developing countries, and the ability to be stored in stabilizing solutions and posted several days later to the testing centers—means that saliva sample collection has significantly lower physiological and psychological impacts on the donor than blood collection and makes saliva an attractive fluid for decentralized and/or home testing. Saliva has two additional properties that confer advantages over blood and in particular: (1) it does not clot and, therefore, does not require anticoagulation treatment after collection [4], and (2) it is less likely to transmit diseases than blood through contact or needle-stick injury making

it safer for handing by health-care professionals. Therefore, saliva is an appealing diagnostic medium for large population-based screening programs [3, 5]. In addition, due to its dynamic nature, saliva can reflect the status of biochemical and physiological changes in real time.

Saliva has multiple functions within the oral cavity. It facilitates the chewing, tasting, and swallowing of food and initiates carbohydrate and lipid digestion by salivary α(alpha)-amylase and lipase, respectively. It also lubricates the oral cavity, aids in speech, facilitates teeth enamel mineralization, assists in wound healing, and maintains oral hygiene through antimicrobial properties [6]. In general, an adult produces approximately 0.5–1.5 L of saliva per day from the parotid, submandibular, sublingual, and minor salivary glands in the oral cavity [7]. These glands are composed of acinar and ductal epithelial cells. The former produce, store, and secrete salivary granules, while the latter modify salivary content [7, 8]. Within the salivary ducts, K^+ is actively secreted into saliva, while Na^+ is actively absorbed; at the same time Cl^- is passively absorbed and HCO3- is secreted into saliva, giving saliva a pH of 6.2–7.4. Saliva contains 99 % water and 1 % proteins and salts [7], with an average protein concentration ranging from 0.5 to 2 mg/mL in healthy adults [6].

Multiple studies utilizing mass spectrometry (MS) have shown the presence of hundreds to thousands of different types of proteins in human whole saliva [9–14], with the highest number discovered thus far being 2,340 [14]. However, these contents are not limited to the local products of salivary glands. Many of the proteins are thought to come from surrounding blood capillaries through the processes of passive diffusion, ultrafiltration, and/or active transport [3, 4] (Fig. 7.1). One of the bottlenecks to the advancement of saliva diagnostics is that saliva contains analytes at lower concentrations (pg/mL) than in blood [4, 15]. Unlike blood, which is quite stable, salivary composition is known to vary in response to many factors [16] such as age [17, 18], gender [18], and genetic [19] differences, which cannot be controlled, resulting in interindividual variation in the molecular makeup of saliva. Balance

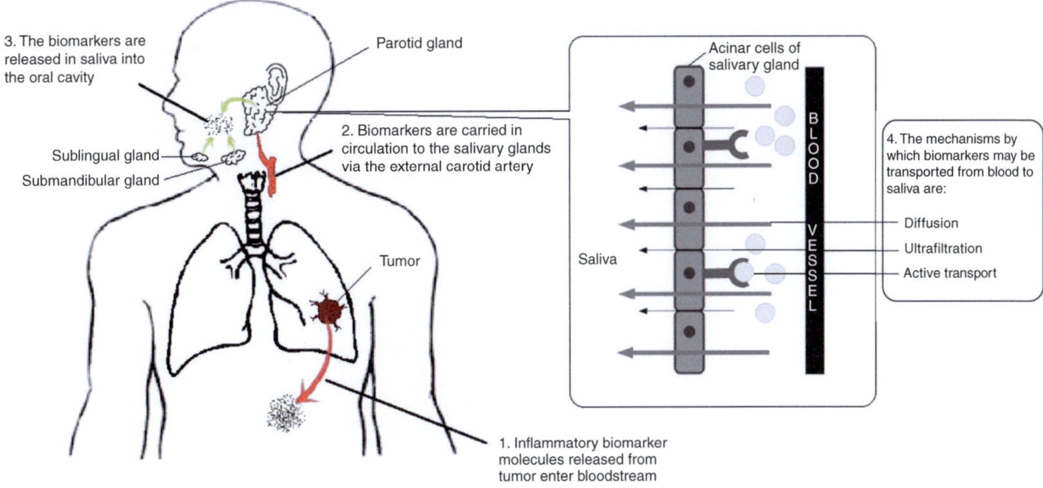

Fig. 7.1 Illustration of biomolecular transport across salivary cells and blood endothelial cells

of sympathetic and parasympathetic nervous system activity can result in the variation of salivary flow rate [20–22] and viscosity [23]. Salivary flow can be induced either through chemical (acid) or mechanical (chewing, biting) stimuli [24]. The flow rate and composition of saliva vary between stimulated versus unstimulated saliva, as well as with the type, intensity, and duration of the stimulus [7, 24]. Therefore, it is important to take these variables into account when measuring and reporting analytes in saliva.

The method of sample collection has also been shown to affect protein concentrations in saliva [24, 25]. This poses a challenge in standardizing saliva collection prior to developing diagnostic assays. Further difficulty is posed by factors that can cause intraindividual variations due to circadian fluctuations [26, 27]. As an example, salivary growth hormone levels are relatively higher in the morning compared with measurements made at night/evening/nightly?. Inherently these causes of intraindividual variation can lead to exacerbation of interindividual variations. A standardized protocol for collecting saliva specimens, which specifies the time and method of collection and restricts dietary intake for a fixed period before collection, could be used to minimize the effects of some of the variables causing intraindividual variation. Yet, it is not realistic to control certain other factors that affect saliva, such as prescribed

drugs [3] that people may be taking to control other illnesses. Even differences in the normal bacterial flora in the oral cavity can cause changes to the protein content of saliva between or within individuals because bacterial enzymes catalyze reactions involving salivary proteins [28]. More so, saliva is susceptible to blood contamination: if there is a microscopic bleed in the oral cavity that contaminates saliva with blood, the direct mixing of serum proteins could lead to artificially raised protein levels in saliva [6]. This will obviously impact the measurement of salivary biomolecular profiles and must be taken into consideration in the development of saliva-based tests. However, the advancement of technology, particularly MS and nanotechnology, has greatly increased our ability to detect trace amounts of salivary constituents [4], making the prospect of developing salivary diagnostics a reality.

There are numerous saliva-based kits in the market to measure an array of biomolecules either relevant in disease or to detect contraband drugs, and these include cortisol (steroid), DHEA (adrenal gland secretion), estradiol, estriol (steroid sex hormone), estrone, progesterone (steroid hormone), testosterone (steroid hormone), SIgA (secretory immunoglobulin A), alpha-amylase, cotinine (nicotine exposure), C-reactive protein, human immunodeficiency virus (HIV), and drugs of abuse. Table 7.1 illustrates a catalog of some

Table 7.1 Saliva tests and manufacturers

Application	Product name	Manufacturer	Web site
Drugs of abuse	Oral Stat	American Bio Medica Corporation	www.abmc.com
	DDS®2 Mobile Test System	Alere	www.alere.com
Human immunodeficient virus (HIV)	OraQuick ADVANCE® Rapid HIV-1/2 Antibody Test	OraSure Technologies	www.orasure.com
Hepatitis C	OraQuick® HCV Rapid Antibody Test	OraSure Technologies	www.orasure.com
Hormone	Saliva ELISAs	DRG	www.drg-diagnostics.de
Caries	Dentocult® SM/LB	Orion Diagnostica	www.oriondiagnostica.com
Periodontal diseases	MyPerioPath®, MyPerioID®	OralDNA® Labs	www.oraldna.com
Human papillomavirus (HPV)	OraRisk® HPV salivary diagnostic test	OralDNA® Labs	www.oraldna.com
Personal genome service	23andMe's Personal Genome Service	23andMe	https://www.23andme.com
Ovulation test	Ovulation Scope	Quest Products	https://www.quest.com

of the currently available saliva diagnostic tests. (Figure 7.2 shows the devices used in the authors' laboratory [24].)

Biomarkers

A biomarker is "a characteristic that is objectively measured and evaluated as an indicator of normal biological processes, pathogenic processes, or pharmacological responses to a therapeutic intervention," according to the Biomarkers Definitions Working Group of the National Institutes of Health [29]. This definition inherently describes the usefulness of biomarkers for diagnostic purposes by detecting the presence of pathogenic processes or the absence of normal biological processes in disease. It is not just diagnosis, but the potential of earlier diagnosis compared to current methods, that makes biomarkers a promising avenue for research.

The general clinical benefits of early diagnosis are numerous. Catching a disease in its infancy often gives doctors more treatment options to pursue. The increased treatment options plus the additional time afforded to make a decision enable patients to make better, well-considered choices in cooperation with their doctors, thus furthering the ethos of patient autonomy in medical practice. Beginning treatment earlier in the course of disease also often greatly improves its efficacy. All of these factors contribute to better patient outcomes and satisfaction. Biomarkers play important clinical roles in diagnosis, stratification, prognosis, and therapy for many diseases and promise to feature in many more. There are various types of biomarkers, including DNA, RNA, proteins, and cells. In terms of biological processes, they can also be classified as inflammatory biomarkers, cancer biomarkers, etc.

This chapter is dedicated to three main diseases in the oral cavity, dental caries, periodontal diseases, and oral lesions/cancers, which have inflammation as a common etiology factor. Each section is dedicated to highlighting the epidemiology, clinical problem, and the treatment strategies. We also highlight where possible biomarkers that are either clinically used or still within a research phase.

Inflammatory Biomarkers

Inflammatory biomarkers have been identified as candidates for dental caries, periodontal diseases and oral cancer because of the growing evidence of a reciprocal, causal relationship between these diseases and either acute or chronic inflammation [30]. Transcription factors common to both cancer and inflammation have been shown to produce inflammatory mediators that enhance DNA damage, oncogenic activity, immune evasion, angiogenesis, and metastasis, all of which contribute to cancer development [31]. Because of the early

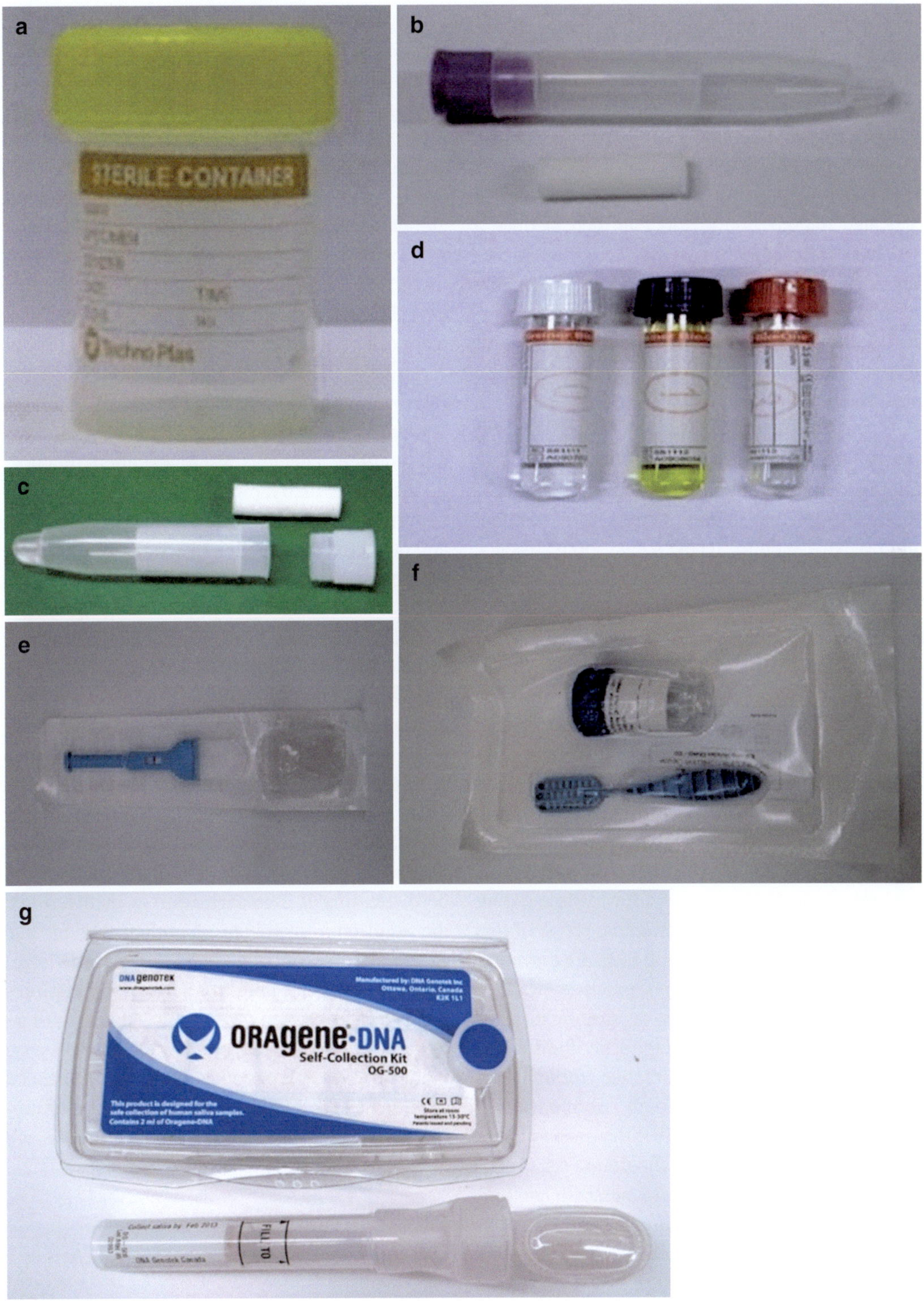

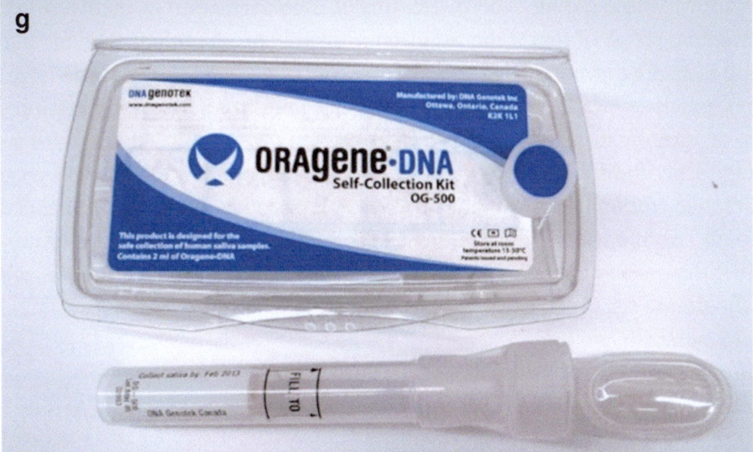

Fig. 7.2 The commercially available saliva collection devices that are used in our laboratory. (**a**) Drool collected in a sterile specimen container [24]. (**b**) Salimetrics® Oral Swab (SOS). (**c**) Salivette. (**d**) Greiner Bio-One, Saliva Collection System® (GBO SCS®). (**e**) Versi-SAL® saliva collection system. (**f**) DNA-SAL™ saliva collection system. (**g**) Oragene® DNA Self-Collection Kit to isolate DNA and RNA from saliva

involvement of host inflammation in the cancer process, inflammatory biomarkers are useful in enabling early detection of cancer [32]. The inflammatory events in oral cancer have many potential triggers: tobacco, alcohol, etc. These triggers cause the activation of inflammatory transcription factors such as NF-κ(kappa)β, STAT3, and AP-1 [31]. The activated transcription factors can then mediate a number of effects: expression of oncogenes, silencing of tumor suppressor genes and the production of inflammatory chemokines, cytokines, and prostaglandins [31]. It is therefore important to investigate inflammatory biomarker changes in a disease state compared with a healthy state.

Body Fluids as Biomarker Sources

Biomarkers can be measured in a wide range of biological media: blood, urine, cerebrospinal fluid (CSF), sputum, feces, saliva, body tissues, etc. Blood testing generally involves sampling of blood from a superficial arm vein by venipuncture. This is one of the most common biological fluids currently used in a clinical laboratory setting. The close contact and subsequent substance exchange of blood with most organs make it ideal for detecting underlying pathology almost anywhere in the body. Blood biomarkers are utilized for a plethora of diseases—CA-125 for ovarian cancer [33], troponin I for myocardial infarction [34], immunoglobulin A for PD, and miRNA-21 for oral cancer [35], to name a few. While listing the uses of blood tests is outside the scope of this chapter, it is evident that blood tests are currently part of the standard clinical practice when it comes to clinical diagnosis or stratification of disease. CSF is another diagnostic fluid often used for standard clinical practice, though perhaps not as frequently as blood. Examination of CSF is the gold standard for the diagnosis of several central nervous system disorders, e.g., meningitis [36, 37], subarachnoid hemorrhage [37, 38] and carcinomatous meningitis [37].

Similar to blood, the use of urine is also extremely common in clinical practice. Urine output measurements for kidney function, urine dipstick tests and urinalysis are all routinely performed in hospitals and clinics. Many biomarkers in urine are derived from blood and serve as a proxy to noninvasively observe systemic events. Proteins are ultrafiltrated in the kidney glomeruli based on size and charge [39] and then mostly reabsorbed in the proximal convoluted tubules [40]. Nevertheless, a large number of blood serum proteins are still present in urine, albeit at a much lower concentration. These serum proteins alongside exosomal apical membrane proteins [41] and exocytosed lysosomal proteins [42] make up a very rich urine proteome—consisting of 1,543 different proteins [43]—with a lot of diagnostic potential.

Urine collection, despite being embarrassing for some, can be done relatively easily, in large amounts and noninvasively if catheterization is not required. This makes it an excellent diagnostic medium. Finally, proximity dictates that urine is particularly suitable for the diagnosis of renal and postrenal pathologies [44–67]. All these factors point toward the inevitable use of urine diagnostic biomarkers in the coming years. Similarly, saliva is used in clinical practice for monitoring and diagnostic purposes. Monitoring roles include that of alcohol, drugs of abuse [68], estrogen [69], progesterone, cholesterol [69, 70], as well as cardiac-specific biomarkers. It is also used to diagnose Cushing's syndrome [71], HIV [72], prostate cancer [69], and breast cancer [73]. Saliva avoids the classic problems associated with urine specimen collection, which can be distressing if catheterization is involved and the additional downside of embarrassment due to violation of privacy. The use of saliva sampling is beneficial not only because it simplifies the testing of poorly compliant patients (e.g., children or psychiatric patients), but also because it improves overall patient compliance. Enhanced compliance for routine, follow-up, and monitoring tests would contribute to better health-care outcomes.

Dental Caries

Dental caries (holes in the teeth), also known as tooth decay or the formation of cavities, is a bacterial infection that causes demineralization and destruction of the hard tissues of the

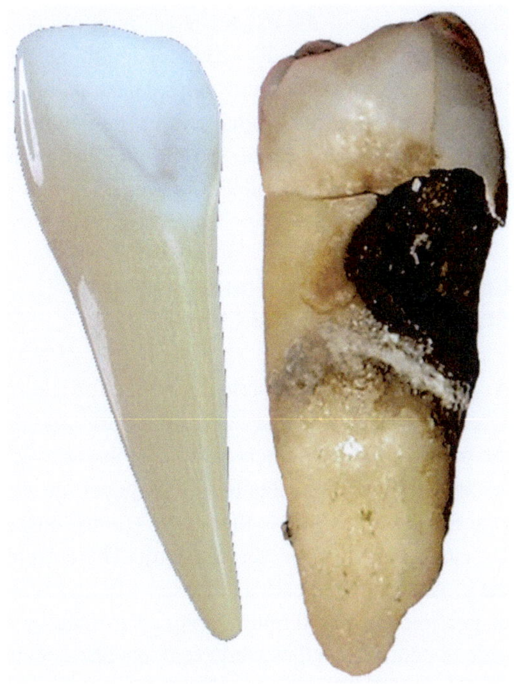

Fig. 7.3 The comparison of a healthy tooth (*left*) and a decayed tooth (*right*)

teeth (enamel, dentin, and cementum) (Fig. 7.3). Dental caries is a result of the production of acid by bacterial fermentation of food debris accumulated on the tooth surface. If tooth demineralization exceeds remineralization (the latter is driven by factors such as the amounts of calcium and fluoride present in toothpaste or in the drinking water), this then promotes hard tissues to progressively break down, producing dental caries. Depending on the extent of tooth destruction, various treatments can be used to restore tooth function and aesthetics, but there is no known method to regenerate large amounts of demineralized tooth structure. Instead, dental health organizations advocate preventive and prophylactic measures, such as regular oral hygiene examinations by professional dental staff and dietary modifications to avoid dental caries.

Epidemiology

Dental caries is one of the most common diseases in the modern world. About 36 % of the global population (2.43 billion people worldwide) have been diagnosed with dental caries or have had teeth removed due to dental caries [74]. Overall, the prevalence of dental caries is relatively low in the developed countries compared with developing countries due to the availability of preventive measures and better oral hygiene practices. Countries in Latin America and in the Middle East have the highest rates of dental caries, while China has the lowest rate of dental caries because of mandatory addition of fluoride to the water supply. However, the excess addition of fluoride has caused other dental problem such as fluorosis [75].

Causes, Signs, and Symptoms

Prior to the establishment of modern dentistry, dental caries was believed to be caused by "tooth worms" in some ancient civilizations [76]. It was not until the seventeenth century that the medical community started to reject the idea that "tooth worms" caused dental caries [77]. Due to the advancements in technology (improved microscopy), scientists began to realize the real cause of dental caries. During the golden age of microbiology in the late nineteenth century, American oral microbiologist Willoughby D. Miller proposed a theory that caries is caused by the acids produced by oral bacteria as a result of the fermentation of sugars [78]. Since mineral is the main component of a tooth, demineralization and remineralization between the teeth and saliva are constantly occurring in our oral cavity, and if demineralization exceeds remineralization, this then leads to dental cavities. The pits and fissures of the teeth and other regions that are hard to clean with either saliva or a toothbrush are hot spots for caries, since residues of food accumulate easily, giving the bacteria more nutrition to live on. Certain types of bacteria can ferment carbohydrates (e.g., sucrose, glucose, and fructose) which are left in the oral cavity through a glycolytic process and produce acid that will lower the pH and promote demineralization. Among all the bacteria present within the oral cavity, those which can produce a high level of acid through sugar fermentation have the ability to survive in a low pH environment and cause dental caries. *Streptococcus mutans* and *Lactobacilli* are believed to be the two main bacteria involved in the formation of caries. When they colonize the teeth and gum area, they form a biofilm called plaque. Plaques serve as the frontier of demineralization. At the initial stage of caries, there is often a white-spot lesion on the surface of the enamel. This white spot is a sign of extensive demineralization of the tooth. As the demineralization continues, the white spot may turn brown before the decay becomes an irreversible cavitation. The cavity will become more obvious as the decay carries on. The color and texture of the affected areas of the tooth will get darker and softer. Sharp pain will occur when the decay passes through enamel and dentin and reaches the pulp where the blood vessels and nerves are located. If left untreated, the bacteria will eventually overwhelm the pulp tissue and cause infection.

Pathophysiology

Virulence factors released from various oral bacteria residing either in the tooth or in the oral cavity cause degradation of host tissue by directly or indirectly activating host immune response. The latter initiates the release of biological mediators from host cells, leading to the host tissue destruction [79]. A number of bacteria-derived enzymes, such as collagen-degrading enzymes, elastase-like enzymes, trypsin-like proteases, aminopeptidases, and dipeptidyl peptidases, are recognized as important players in tissue destruction. Therefore, host and bacteria-derived enzymes, proteins, and other inflammatory mediators hold great promise as salivary biomarkers for the diagnosis of dental caries. Salivary phosphopeptides appear to be involved in the remineralization processes, delaying the loss of tooth structure [80]. As an example, when the demineralization is caused by acid on the outer part of the tooth enamel, there is no regeneration of this structure due to the lack of cells with enamel-producing ability (ameloblasts). But when the decay penetrates the enamel, dentin can react to the

caries because of the existence of odontoblasts, which can continuously produce dentin at the border between dentin and pulp. These salivary proteins serve as key biomarkers in the development of pathogenic process: inflammation, collagen degradation, and bone turnover.

Current Diagnostics and Treatment Strategies for Dental Caries

As dental caries is reversible before the formation of cavity, early diagnosis of dental caries holds the promise for early interventions. However, caries are often unnoticeable until they penetrate the enamel and cause pain to the patients, hence making early identification very difficult. The current diagnosis for dental caries relies heavily on visual inspection and dental radiography performed by a trained dentist, and these requirements have made diagnostics challenging in some developing countries due to the associated costs.

A tooth extraction may be the most traditional treatment option for dental caries since it requires minimal equipment to perform. In the modern day dental practice, removal of the decayed tooth is performed if the tooth has been destroyed by the decay and will lead to further complications in the future. Dental restoration is now a more common treatment option for most dental caries. After removal of large portions of the decayed part of an infected tooth, restorative materials such as dental amalgam, composite resin, porcelain, or gold may be used to fill in the decayed area.

Saliva Proteomics for Dental Caries

The salivary defense system includes salivary proteins, which play important roles in maintaining the health of the oral cavity and preventing caries, as stated by Mazengo et al. [81]. Saliva surrounds soft and hard oral tissues and is in direct contact with the teeth. This gives saliva the advantage of proximity to serve as a diagnostic medium for dental caries. Currently, there is no established saliva-based method to diagnose dental caries in a clinical setting. However, saliva can be easily used to monitor the risk of caries [82]. An increase in salivary phosphopeptide levels (PRP1/3, histatin-1, and statherin) was associated with the absence of dental caries, emphasizing the importance of these peptides in the maintenance of tooth integrity [80]. In a study investigating early childhood caries, it was found that a higher number of proline-rich proteins correlated with caries-free individuals, substantiating the protective role of this type of protein [80]. Tulunoglui et al. demonstrated that salivary calcium concentrations are significantly decreased in children and teenagers who previously have had dental caries [83]. They also found that the total protein concentrations and antioxidant concentrations were higher in people with underlying caries compared with individuals with no previous history of caries. Ayad et al. demonstrated that IB-7 (a phenotype of proline-rich proteins) was higher in the saliva of caries-free individuals than in people who had previously suffered from caries [84]. Due to the fact that dental caries is mainly caused by *mutans streptococci*, the level of salivary *mutans streptococci* was also used to evaluate the caries risk. The association between salivary *mutans streptococci* and dental caries varied between studies [85–87]. Zhang *et al.* demonstrated that in children aged 6–7 years of age, salivary *mutans streptococci* counts were a good indicator for dental caries [87], while another study had a different conclusion [86]. A possible reason for conflicting data may be due to the fact that besides *mutans streptococci,* there are other bacteria that can cause caries, which may vary between individuals studied. Table 7.2 gives an overview of the salivary biomarkers that are used in a research phase to diagnose dental caries [83]. Further laboratory and clinical studies are required to truly understand the clinical utility of these salivary biomarkers before they can be implemented in a standard dental practice.

Future Perspective

The current diagnosis for dental caries is largely based on visual inspection and often not made

Table 7.2 Salivary biomarkers in a research phase to diagnose dental caries

Saliva sample type	Findings	Reference
Acid-stimulated parotid gland saliva	No differences in the salivary levels of proline-rich, parotid acidic, and double-band parotid proteins were found between subjects with and without caries	[88]
Unstimulated whole-mouth saliva	The total protein concentrations increased (0.65 g/dL vs. 0.35 g/dL) in boys aged 7–10 years with caries compared with boys without caries	[83]
Unstimulated whole saliva	A 17 kDa protein was found to be (not characterized) increased in patients with dental caries	[89]
Tongue surface scrape	Salivary *mutans streptococci* concentration was increased in people with dental caries	[85]

until caries become irreversible, warranting reliable early diagnostic methods. As the medium that is in direct contact with the teeth, naturally saliva has a strong potential to be used in dental caries. The noninvasive nature of saliva collection provides another advantage in contrast to the traditional method (dental explorer) in which the pressure from the dental explorer can create a cavity even if the demineralization may still be reversible. Diagnostic tests that utilize oligosaccharide biomarkers in saliva to predict caries formation in children are under development [90].

Periodontal Disease

After dental caries, the most common oral disease is periodontal disease. Gingivitis and periodontal disease may affect 80 % of the adult population, making it one of the most prevalent oral diseases. Periodontal is a combination of two meanings derived from the Greek language, "peri" for around and "odontal" for the teeth. Hence, this is a disease of the structures surrounding the teeth, which include the gums, the cement, the periodontal ligament, and the alveolar bone. Teeth are embedded in the bone and cushioned in the socket by the periodontal ligament; the ligament spans from the bone to the root of the tooth where there are some ligament fibers above the bone, which hold the gums tightly to the tooth.

Periodontitis presents in three ways: initially the pocket depth increases due to swelling and bone loss, followed by the bleeding of the gums, and finally supporting bone is reduced around the tooth. The first stage of periodontal disease is gingivitis, the infection of the gums. In infected patients, plaque (a sticky, colorless bacterial deposit) and tartar (a crusty deposit) cause irritation of the gums and bone loss; this leads to the loss of tooth support structure. This can ultimately lead to the loss of teeth, which is readily seen in adult populations around the world. The bone and gum should ideally fit snugly around the teeth; however, when periodontal disease is present, the supporting tissue and bone is destroyed, forming pockets around the teeth. Over time, these pockets deepen.

Epidemiology

As of 2010, chronic periodontitis affected more than 750 million people or about 11 % of the global population. In the USA, one in two American adults aged 30 years and above has periodontal disease, according to the Centers for Disease Control and Prevention (CDC) [91]. It was documented that 47.2 % or nearly 65 million American adults have early, moderate, or severe periodontitis. In adults over the age of 65 years, the prevalence was 70 %. The disease was more prevalent in men than in women, with the distribution 56.4 and 38.4 %, respectively. Other factors that were found to correlate with high prevalence were the patients' smoking status, whether they lived below the poverty line, and whether they had a high school education.

Approximately 800,000 dental implants are used in the USA annually, with this steadily increasing at a rate of 25 % as of 2006 [92]. Smoking, diabetes, hormonal changes in women, medications, and genetic susceptibility are a few of the risk factors that predispose people to periodontal disease. There seems to be increasing evidence that chronic periodontal disease may be associated with smoking, since the risk has also been found to be elevated in smokers [93, 94]. Diabetes affects the body's ability to use blood sugar, thereby making diabetic patients more susceptible for developing infections that do not readily heal. Hormonal changes in women, which occur during puberty, monthly menstruation, pregnancy, and menopause, can make gums sensitive, whereby increasing the risk for gingivitis. Furthermore, illnesses that may compromise the immune system such as AIDS and cancer may affect the condition of the gums. Not forgetting, poor oral hygiene is a contributing factor, and one has to brush and floss on a daily basis using the correct technique to reduce the chance of gingivitis. Family history of dental disease also plays an important role in oral health. There is evidence that stress is associated with periodontal disease, and certain lifestyle events, such as emotional and financial stressors [95] are associated with increased disease susceptibility. In recent studies, it has been found that people with gum disease are more likely to develop heart disease or type 2 diabetes. Furthermore, it has been found that women with gum disease are more likely to deliver preterm babies with lower birth weights than women without gum disease. When the body's immune system is triggered due to periodontal disease, the body releases prostaglandins, which, at increased levels, can cross the threshold and induce labor [96, 97].

Causes, Signs, and Symptoms

Numerous factors give rise to periodontal disease, such as bacteria and dental plaques. It has been estimated that approximately 600 different bacteria are capable of colonizing our mouths. The bacteria associated with periodontal diseases are predominantly gram-negative anaerobic

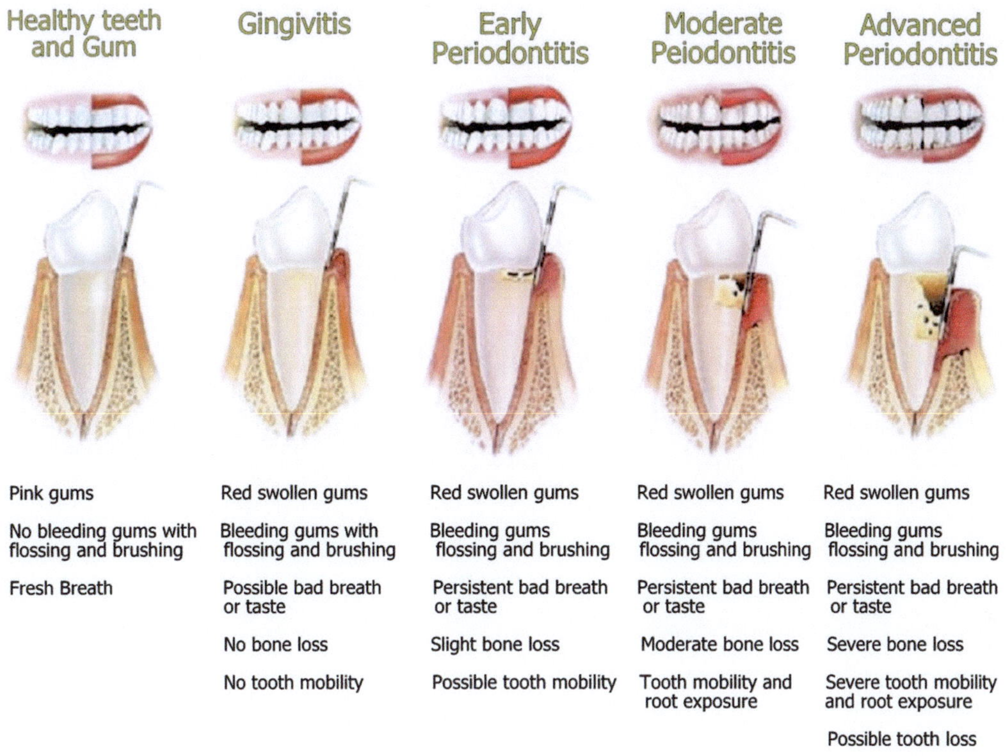

Fig. 7.4 The different stages highlighting the progression of periodontal disease (Reprinted with permission from the Advanced Institute of Oral Health, Brentwood, TN)

bacteria, which can include *Porphyromonas gingivalis* and *Aggregatibacter actinomycetemcomitans*. The bacteria possess virulence factors that allow for colonization to occur in the oral cavity as well as produce harmful by-products that cause tissue damage [98].

A sticky, soft film forms on the surface of the teeth and matures over the duration of a day. This accumulation and eventual hardening results in the formation of calculus or tartar. The dispensation of calculi in the teeth helps form uneven and rough surfaces, further encouraging the bacteria to grow. The unevenness and irregularity of these surfaces are niches that are ideal for the growth of bacterial colonies. Over time, these irritants will destroy the tissues that attach the gums to the teeth, allowing the gums to move away and forming small pockets that can undergo further plaque accumulation. These processes ultimately lead to bone destruction unless interventions occur.

Signs of periodontal disease include red, inflamed, and tender gums that bleed easily. In addition, bad odors, loose and sensitive teeth, pus, teeth depressed into sockets, and teeth that seem to move over time are noteworthy signs. Figure 7.4 presents the clinical manifestation of gum disease over time. The left side is the healthy gums, whereas the right side shows the diseased conditions. The periodontal probe is shown in black, which is adjacent to the teeth (Fig. 7.5). The tip of the instrument is placed into the gingival sulcus, which is the region between the tooth and surrounding tissue. The probe is kept parallel to the contours of the root of the tooth and inserted to the base of the pocket to measure the depth. The average healthy pocket depth is around 3 mm with no bleeding upon probing. It can be seen that

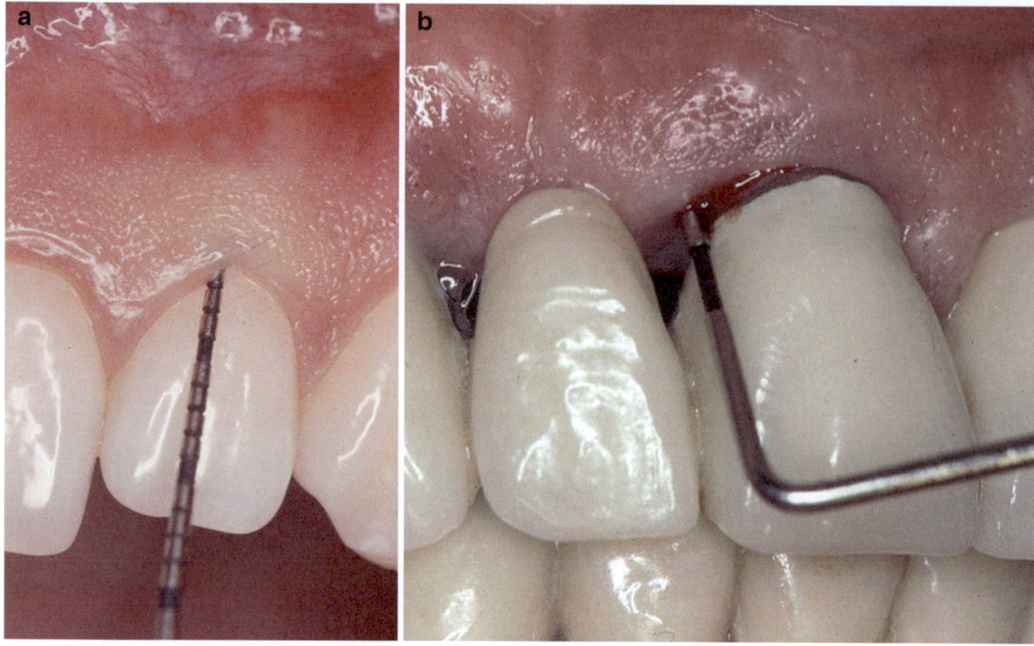

Fig. 7.5 The clinical evaluation of periodontal disease by probing. (**a**) Healthy gum and (**b**) diseased gum, bleeding upon probing (Reprinted with permission from the *Journal of the California Dental Association*, 2013 February; 41(2):119–24)

the pocket depth gets deeper as the stage of periodontitis progresses toward the advanced stage.

There are four stages in the progression of gum disease, each with its own characteristic signs and symptoms. These stages are gingivitis, early periodontal disease followed by moderate and severe periodontal disease. Gingivitis is the initial and reversible stage of gum disease caused by inflammation. Normal, healthy gums are pink, tight, and smooth, allowing food to pass and move into the space between our teeth and cheek. When a person has gingivitis, the gums become red and inflamed and bleed easily, which is particularly noticeable during brushing. When the gums are inflamed, food can be seen to accumulate around the gums and pack in and around the teeth. The characteristic redness and swelling of the gums is due to an increased blood supply, which is the body's immune response against an influx of bacteria. If gingivitis is left untreated and uncontrolled, there is progression to early periodontal disease, which is irreversible. This stage is classically shown by 4–5 mm pockets, early bone loss, and the loss of attachment of the gums around the tooth, which may be seen by X-ray. The importance of the root of the tooth is that it receives its blood supply from the ligament. When the ligament is detached during periodontal disease, the blood supply is lost, causing the root to die. The root surface becomes rough and is prone to bacterial infection and accumulation over time. Moderate periodontal disease is characterized by 5–6 mm pockets as well as bone loss, which is visible on X-ray. Other signs include separation of the front teeth, pus, and bad odors, to name a few. Ultimately, this leads to severe periodontal disease characterized by pockets 6 mm and larger as well as little or no bone structure supporting the teeth.

Pathophysiology

Following microbial plaque formation, an acute exudative inflammatory response begins within a few days, causing gingival fluid and neutrophils to increase locally. Fibrin deposits destroy collagen at these initial stages. Early lesions are

Table 7.3 Salivary biomarkers associated with periodontal disease

Biomarkers	Mode of action	Type of periodontal disease	Reference
Immunoglobulins (IgA, IgM, IgG)	Interfere in adherence and bacterial metabolism	Chronic, aggressive	[80, 81]
Mucins	Interferes with bacterial colonization	Aggressive	[81, 87]
Lysozyme	Regulates biofilm accumulation	Chronic	[81, 87]
Lactoferrin	Inhibits microbial growth	Aggressive	[81, 87]
Histatin	Neutralizes lipopolysaccharides	Chronic, aggressive	[81, 87]
Peroxidase	Interferes with biofilm accumulation	Chronic	[81, 87]
C-reactive protein	Increased concentrations found in serum and saliva of PD patients	Chronic, aggressive	[81, 87]

noticeable by the infiltration of lymphocytic cells as well as monocytes and plasma cells. Over time, these lesions become chronic with noticeable presence of plasma cells and B lymphocytes. With this progression, pockets are formed where the gingiva separates from the tooth. The depth of the pockets increases with brushing, flossing, and chewing. If continued inflammation persists, the periodontal ligaments break down, which leads to the destruction of the local alveolar bone, resulting to teeth falling out.

There appears to be a general consensus that periodontal destruction is host-mediated through the release of pro-inflammatory cytokines by tissues and immune cells in response to bacterial infection, products, or metabolites. Interleukin-1 beta (IL-1β[beta]) and tumor necrosis factor alpha (TNF-α[alpha]) have shown increased levels in periodontal sites during inflammation and tissue destruction. There is also a marked decrease in these biomarkers following periodontal therapy when gums return to a healthy state.

Current Diagnostic Strategies and Treatments for Periodontal Disease

One sign that dentists look for in periodontal disease is bleeding upon probing. A visual assessment is made of the gingival tissue and sulcus by pocket probing. The absence of bleeding is indicative of the absence of periodontal disease, whereas the presence of bleeding upon probing is used as a predictor of the disease. Currently, there are two salivary diagnostic kits that can detect the

bacteria causing periodontal disease [99]. The first test identifies the type and concentration of specific periodontal pathogenic microbes in the patients' saliva sample, which then allows the clinician to determine the appropriate antimicrobial therapy. The second test detects genetic susceptibility in individuals to periodontitis by analyzing genetic variations that affect the production of inflammatory cytokines, i.e., interleukin-1a and b. Both tests use DNA polymerase chain reaction (PCR) to analyze the samples and require a few days to process and analyze before the patient obtains the results. A pitfall of these combined methods is the duration for turnaround time and the fact that they lack the ability to determine when periodontal disease will occur.

Human saliva contains biomarkers that are specific for the unique physiological aspects of periodontitis (Table 7.3), and qualitative changes in the composition of these biomarkers could provide diagnostic opportunities [80, 81, 87]. As an example, saliva holds a number of periodontal proteomic markers from immunoglobulins to bone remodeling proteins. Immunoglobulins (Ig) are antibodies produced by the immune system, which help defend against a number of pathogens. They are not only present in blood but also in saliva. IgA, IgG, and IgM subtypes found in the mouth affect the microbes by interfering with the adherence of bacteria or by inhibiting their metabolism. Patients presenting with periodontal disease have higher salivary concentrations of these immunoglobulin subtypes. Post-periodontal treatment, these levels are notably reduced. Therefore, the use of IgA, in particular, has been brought to the fore, as it provides a clinical means to identify individuals who have the potential to develop periodontal disease as well as to determine the treatment response.

Mucins are glycoproteins produced by a number of salivary glands. The function of these mucins (MG1 and MG2) include that of lubrication, protection from dehydration, and cytoprotection. MG2 is known to affect the adherence and aggregation of bacteria with known interactions with the periodontal pathogen *Aggregatibacter actinomycetemcomitans*. A decrease in these mucins may play a role in increasing colonization by these bacteria.

Lactoferrin is an iron-binding glycoprotein produced by the salivary glands; it inhibits microbe growth by using up the iron present in the environment thereby depriving the bacteria of an essential nutrient that is required for growth. It has been found that lactoferrin is elevated in mucosal secretions and is present in high concentrations in saliva of patients with periodontal disease [100].

Early detection is the key to the prevention of periodontal disease. The dentist, periodontist, or oral hygienist can remove plaque through deep-cleaning techniques such as scaling and root planing. Scaling involves the removal of calculus from above and below the gum line, whereas root planing removes rough areas, which are prone to bacterial accumulation. Medications can also be used with scaling and root planing, but they cannot replace surgery. Medications include antimicrobial mouth rinse, antiseptic "chip," antibiotic gels, antibiotic microspheres, as well as enzyme suppressants. Surgeries such as flap surgery may be needed if the inflammation and deep pockets remain after treatment. The flap surgery removes tartar deposits in deep pockets or reduces the pockets to make it easier to keep clean. This common surgery involves lifting the back gums, removing the tartar, and suturing it back in place so that the tissue fits well around the tooth. Another surgical procedure that is currently undertaken is bone and tissue grafting in addition to flap surgery. The latter replaces and encourages the new growth of bone or gum tissue that previously has been destroyed by periodontitis. A mesh is inserted between the gum and bone, which prevents the gum tissue from growing into the area where the bone should be and allows the bone to regrow.

Future Perspective

There remain challenges in the advancement of saliva diagnostics for use in periodontal disease. These include the nonspecific nature of biomarkers, which may not be disease specific, and the tests are not "true" real-time measurements. There have been recent advances in high-throughput transcriptomic studies enabling the profiling of genes that are differentially expressed in saliva of PD patients compared with healthy controls. The recent Food and Drug Administration (FDA) approval of the oral fluid-based HIV antibody test demonstrates that saliva can be used just as well as a blood test.

To date, a large number of periodontal biomarkers have been identified; however, they are yet to be used in a rapid point of care test platform. The field of saliva biomarkers does have vast potential for use in diagnosing PD in the general population in a cost-effective manner. Before a clinical diagnostic test for PD can be launched, one has to take into consideration the need for validation of periodontal diagnostics, which need to be benchmarked with existing standard measures such as alveolar bone height.

Oral Lesions and Oral Cancer

Besides DC and PD, an oral soft tissue lesion is another common condition that dentists encounter in their daily clinical practice. An oral lesion is an abnormality on the mucous membrane of the oral cavity. There are many types of oral lesions, but not all of them will transform into invasive cancer. In 2005, the WHO Collaborating Centre for Oral Cancer/Precancer convened an international working group in London and recommended the term "oral potentially malignant disorders" to describe oral precancerous lesions that have the potential of malignant transformation [101]. The most common types of potentially malignant oral disorders include leukoplakia, erythroplakia, candidiasis, submucous fibrosis, actinic cheilitis, and lichen planus.

Oral cancer (more than 90 % are oral squamous cell carcinomas [OSCCs]) refers to any cancer that is located within the oral cavity and is a subtype of head and neck cancer (HNC). The location of oral cancer can be in the hard palate, gingivae, floor of mouth, inner lip, and tongue. Oral cancer can originate either from these locations or metastasize from a distant site. It may also arise by extension from a neighboring location around the head and neck area, for example, the larynx or nasopharynx.

Epidemiology

Global prevalence of oral potentially malignant disorders is estimated to range from 1 to 5 % [102]. However, there are very wide geographical differences in the prevalence of oral potentially malignant disorders due to the differences in demographic characteristics, pattern of tobacco use, ethnicity, and variations of age distributions. For example, the prevalence of oral potentially malignant disorders in Sweden was recorded to be between 1.9 and 3.6 % [103, 104], while in Southeast Asia and Melanesian countries, the prevalence was reported to be higher than 10 % [105, 106]. Oral cancer is the most common cancer in some Southeast Asian countries such as India, Sri Lanka, and Pakistan. In the developing world, leukoplakia is more common in individuals aged between 30 and 70 years old, while in the developed countries, it is more common in individuals aged between 40 and 70 years old [107]. In general, men are more likely to have oral potentially malignant disorders because of their greater use of tobacco and alcohol.

Oral cancer is the tenth most common cancer in men and, in combination with women, is the ninth most common cancer [108]. Globally, Oral cancer has an average 5-year survival rate of approximately 60 % [109]. This poor survival rate has not improved over the past three decades despite the advancements in therapeutic strategies. The challenge today is to reduce the mortality and morbidity from OSCC by developing novel diagnostic strategies to detect this type of cancer at an early stage combined with targeted treatments. The global incidence and mortality rate for oral and pharynx cancer were estimated to be 8.7 per 100,000 and 5 per 100,000, respectively. Since a significant portion of oral cancer is transformed from preexisting oral potentially malignant disorders, the former shares some of the epidemiology characteristics of oral potentially malignant disorders. The highest incidence rate for oral cancer was found in Melanesia, where the inhabitants have the habit of chewing areca nut and consuming tobacco. Most OSCCs develop in people who are in their 50s or 60s. But there is now a trend that indicates OSCC has become more prominent among young individuals. Various studies have shown that in many parts of the world, the incidence of oropharyngeal cancer among young people has significantly increased without showing signs of stopping [110]. As an example, oropharyngeal SCCs are frequently positive for human papillomavirus (HPV), which suggests that unprotected oral sex may also contribute to the increasing incidence of oral cancer among younger individuals who are nonsmoking and nondrinking.

Causes, Signs, and Symptoms

The exact cellular mechanisms that cause oral potentially malignant disorders or oral cancer are still unknown. However, researchers were able to identify risk factors that increase the likelihood to develop these conditions. Tobacco smoking and chewing betel nut are usually considered the most important risk factors for oral lesions and cancer. Smoking or inhaling smoke is the leading cause of preventable premature death in the world, with tobacco-related illness killing 4.9 million people in 2000 [111]. Tobacco smoke contains more than 60 different types of known carcinogens. Oral mucosa is the immediate point of contact after an individual inhales tobacco smoke. The long-term exposure to carcinogens in the tobacco smoke significantly increases the oxidative stress

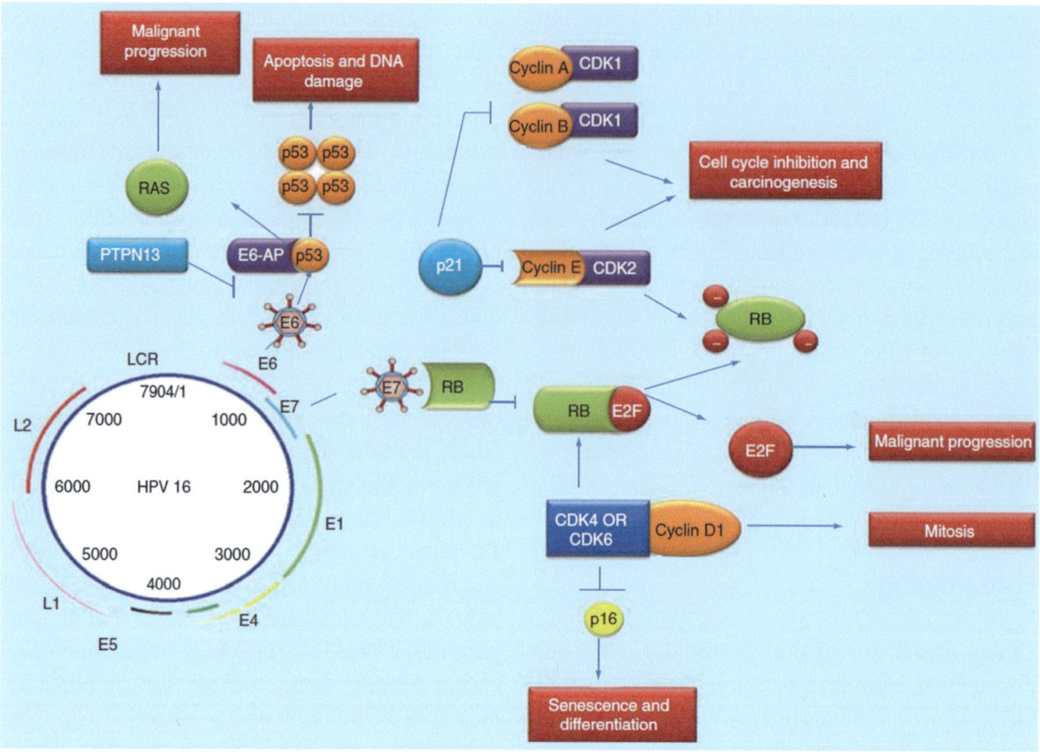

Fig. 7.6 Mechanisms of cell cycle dysregulation via E6 and E7 oncoproteins, adopted from Salazar et al. [128].

to tissues, thus increasing the chance of damaging carbohydrates, lipids, proteins, and DNA within cells. A study showed that tobacco use increased the risk of developing HNC by approximately eight times [112] compared with a nonsmoker.

Certain types of HPV-16/HPV-18 are known to cause cervical cancer can also infect the mucosal regions within the oropharyngeal areas. HPV infects only skin keratinocytes and mucous membranes. A recent study demonstrated that 15–25 % of biopsies collected from HNSCC patients are HPV-16 positive [113]. HPV is a double-stranded DNA virus that has been demonstrated to induce carcinogenesis via the production of the E6 and E7 oncoproteins [114]. It has been demonstrated that both of these viral oncoproteins are responsible for cell cycle dysregulation [114]. The mechanisms of cell cycle dysregulation via E6 and E7 oncoproteins are depicted in Fig. 7.6. There are several checkpoints that must be passed (G2/M and G1/S) in order for replication and proliferation to occur (see Fig. 7.6). In brief, during DNA damage, there

is an upregulation of p53, which in turn upregulates p21; p21 is responsible for the inhibition of the cyclin A-CDK1 and cyclin B-CDK1 complexes (these are the two drivers of progression through the G2/M checkpoint). Therefore, DNA damage will lead to a reduction in progression through the cell cycle [114]. As an oncogene, E6 is responsible for p53 degradation, leading to progression through the G2/M checkpoint. Similarly, E7 binds to retinoblastoma protein pRb, thus preventing the action of pRb and allowing E2F (a key driver through for G1/S checkpoint) to drive cell cycle progression through the G1 checkpoint. Several stimuli act to phosphorylate pRb (thus preventing it binding to E2F), or acting to release the E2F molecules that are bound to pRb. In general, the presence of E6 and E7 within a cell would lead to uncontrolled cell proliferation and, as a consequence, cancer development.

Betel quid chewing is another risk factor that has significantly increased the likelihood of getting OSCC. Unlike tobacco, betel quid is not popular

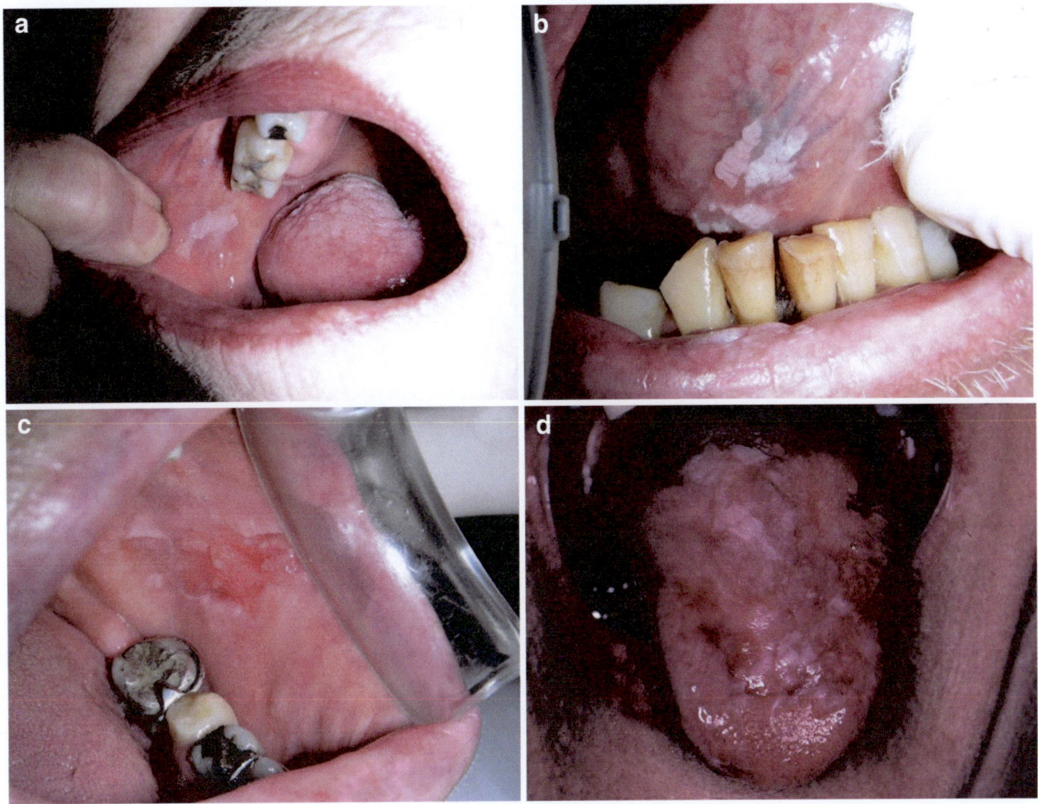

Fig. 7.7 (**a**) Leukoplakia buccal mucosa. (**b**) Leukoplakia on the tongue. (**c**) Erythroplakia buccal mucosa. (**d**) Erythroplakia on the tongue (The images are kindly provided by Dr. Arabelle Clayden)

throughout the world. But in the regions where betel quid consumption is popular, the incidence of OSCC is much higher [115]. Some carcinogens that are found in an excessive amount in betel quid have been shown to induce mutations in the DNA [116].

Alcohol consumption is another important risk factor. The metabolite product of ethanol, acetaldehyde, is considered the main carcinogen in alcohol. Ethanol disrupts the phospholipid cell membranes, making them more permeable. Ethanol also disrupts DNA repair mechanisms. Alcohol is also known to relate to epigenetic alternations, e.g., alter the methylation level of certain tumor suppressor genes [117]. So, people who drink and smoke are at a higher risk of developing oral potentially malignant lesions or OSCC than people who indulge in only one of these social habits [118].

Diet has also been shown to affect the incidence rate of oral and pharyngeal cancer within a Swiss community. People who consume mainly red meat, processed meat, and eggs showed significant trends of increased oral and pharyngeal cancer. In contrast, vegetarians seem more resistant to oral and pharyngeal cancer [119].

In general, oral lesions have appearances that differ from the natural pink color of the oral mucosal surface (due to the underlying capillary vessels) (Fig. 7.7). The signs, symptoms, and color of lesions vary between the different types. For instance, leukoplakia, as the name implies, is mostly white but can also have a whitish yellow or gray color, and erythroplakia normally has a fiery red color. Some lesions have homogeneous appearances, which look uniformly flat and thin, and are usually asymptomatic. In contrast, the lesions can also be symptomatic and have a nonhomogeneous look, which may be speckled, nodular, or wrinkled. The size of the lesions can vary between a small patch on the mucosal membrane to a large area across the oral cavity. Pain or discomforts is infrequent, which make the lesions hard to detect when located in areas of the oral cavity that are hard to visualize, e.g., the base of the tongue.

Since oral potential malignant disorders sometimes transform into oral cancer, they can be considered as the early signs of oral cancer. Other signs of oral cancer also include lumps or ulcers in the oral cavity that do not heal. As the cancer advances, initially painless lesions might develop sensations of pain, burning, odd taste, or other discomfort. More invasive tumors can also cause bleeding or numbness in the mouth and present as a swollen piece of tissue that can be palpated. The pathological changes may cause bad breath, difficulty in swallowing and speaking, enlarged lymph glands in the necks, and sore throat.

Currently, beyond conventional clinical oral examination, there are no reliable early detection methods to diagnose precancer lesions and OSCC [109]. The initial diagnosis of oral potentially malignant disorders significantly relies on subjective judgment of dentists or other health-care providers. Dentists classify the lesions based on their appearances. Needle biopsy samples may be useful to rule out other causes of oral mucosa abnormality. The histologic examination can provide information about the presence of any potential malignant deformation such as epithelial dysplasia. However, the invasive nature of biopsy examination makes it less welcome among patients. Currently, the degree of epithelial dysplasia is the best indication of whether the potentially malignant disorders will transform to oral cancer, even though the change is not inevitable. There is a lack of definitive biomarkers to identify oral potentially malignant disorders that will transform into oral cancer.

Currently, oral cancer diagnosis is similar to oral potentially malignant disorders. Common diagnosis procedures for patients suspected with oral cancer include fine-needle aspiration cytology (FNAC) around enlarged cervical lymph nodes or tissue biopsy of the primary tumor. Other routine cancer diagnosis techniques are also used in the diagnosis of oral cancer, e.g., X-ray and ultrasound. Recurrent and metastatic oral diagnoses are usually presaged by patients expressing pain in the head and neck region.

Due to the lack of a clear indication of whether an oral potentially malignant disorder will transform into oral cancer, treatment options for these oral potentially malignant disorders are very limited. There is no standard procedure or guideline that provides dentists with a clear path to follow when they see an oral potentially malignant disorder. There is suggestion that health-care providers should remove the lesions where practical, irrespective of presence or absence of dysplasia. But there is no evidence to indicate that this action can prevent development of oral cancer. Some oral potentially malignant disorders are often left untreated until it transforms to oral cancer.

Oral cancer surgical procedures are based on the tumor, node, and metastasis (TNM) classification system. TNM grouping is a standardized classification used by pathologists to score the severity of the malignancy. Actions are then decided based on mortality rate, treatment effectiveness, and overall quality of life posttreatment. Generally, positive margin surgeries are favored when the magnitude of the tumor exceeds 2 cm to prevent the impairment of vital functions such as speech, chewing, and ingesting. However, positive margin surgeries have a higher mortality rate compared to negative margin surgeries. Hence, a balance between quantity and quality of life must be taken into account before choosing between the surgical options.

The progression of computer science has improved artificial intelligence (AI) in cancer imaging and radiation delivery. Intensity-modulated radiotherapy (IMRT) is the new cutting-edge radiotherapy with precise radiation delivery accuracy. The main concern regarding radiotherapy lies with the potential side effect of xerostomia—dry mouth due to lack of saliva production. Analysis carried out in the UK demonstrated a steep drop of 36 % with patients experiencing xerostomia posttreatment. In radiotherapy, photon rays of ions will be distributed into the cell to react with the water molecules. The reaction causes the release of unstable free radicals into the surrounding area to damage the DNA double-helical structure, forcing the cell into apoptosis. Radiotherapy is usually coupled with HNSCC surgery to decrease the patient mortality rate, especially in positive margin surgeries.

Despite the advancement of cytotoxic chemotherapy in treating HNSCC patients since 1980, the average patient survival rate remains below 12 months to date. Multi-proxy platinum-based cytotoxic antineoplastic drugs are fundamental in HNSCC treatment. Generally, these drugs are able to trigger defects in DNA repair, new DNA synthesis, cell survival, and irreversible apoptosis via inducing DNA cross-link through the formation of DNA adducts. More so, the adverse effects of the drugs also include nephrotoxicity, neurotoxicity, and hemolytic anemia.

Epidermal growth factor receptor (EGFR) plays a major role in governing tumorigenesis in terms of cell persistence, propagation, and metastasis. EGFR is often overexpressed in the tumorigenic site, altering the cellular biology and leading to poor prognosis and cytotoxic chemotherapy resistance development. Cetuximab, an anti-EGFR monoclonal antibody, is designed to target the extracellular domain of EGFR for HNSCC treatment. It works by binding to the EGFR extracellular domain thereby inhibiting the binding of ligand-induced EGFR tyrosine kinase instigation. Ultimately, EGFR phosphorylation and the downstream signaling cascade are impeded. Combination of cytotoxic chemotherapy and anti-EGFR monoclonal antibody treatment increases HNSCC patient survival up to 29 months. Adverse effects of cetuximab include acneiform eruption, hypomagnesemia, and risk of infusion reaction.

The Use of Saliva to Detect Oral Potentially Malignant Disorders and Oral Cancers

Previous studies have shown the promise of salivary assays to detect both oral disease and pre-cancer lesions [35, 120–122]. There are few studies that have focused on utilizing the expression levels of salivary microRNA (miRNA, miR). These are small pieces of noncoding regulatory RNA (19–25 nucleotides), which are often protected from the degradation by RNases as they are present in extracellular vesicles (exosomes). Exosomes are cell-derived vesicles that have diameters between 30 and 120 nm. These were found in saliva [123], and miRNAs were found to be especially stable within them. Thus, exosomes isolated from saliva potentially may be viable in detecting HNSCC.

A set of miRNA (miRNA-21, miRNA-181b, miRNA345) was found to be significantly elevated in leukoplakia regions of the tissue compared to normal tissue [35]. Another two miRNAs, miRNA-205 and Let-7d, were expressed at low levels in the tumor tissue of HNSCC patients who demonstrated a higher propensity of developing a locoregional occurrence leading to shorter survival times [122]. Patients suffering from oral cancer often find it hard to produce saliva, especially when the tumor is located in the salivary glands [124]. Therefore, it is important to have a method that can obtain enough miRNA for diagnosis from a small amount of saliva. Our group has shown that combining a QIAzol method with commercially available miRNA isolation and enrichment kit gave a high yield of miRNA from as little as 200 µL of human whole saliva. Using this method we have identified salivary miRNA-9 and miRNA-191 as potential biomarkers to detect HNSCC patients from a healthy control group (Fig. 7.8, unpublished data). miR-9 and miR-191 provided a good discriminative ability with AUC values of 0.76 and 0.73, respectively ($p < 0.01$) (unpublished data, Fig. 7.8).

DNA methylation and alterations with histone modifications (epigenetics events) are a hallmark of cancer initiation and progression. Hypermethylation of CpG islands within promoters of tumor suppressor genes can turn off the expression of these genes (silencing), thus promoting tumor growth. Researchers have demonstrated that hypermethylation events can be detected in saliva collected from HNSCC patients [121, 125]. Recent work from our group has shown differences in DNA methylation levels in the saliva collected from HNSCC patients compared with saliva collected from healthy controls for DAPK1, RASSF1α(alpha), and p16 gene promoter methylations. Using a sensitive methylation-specific PCR (MSP)

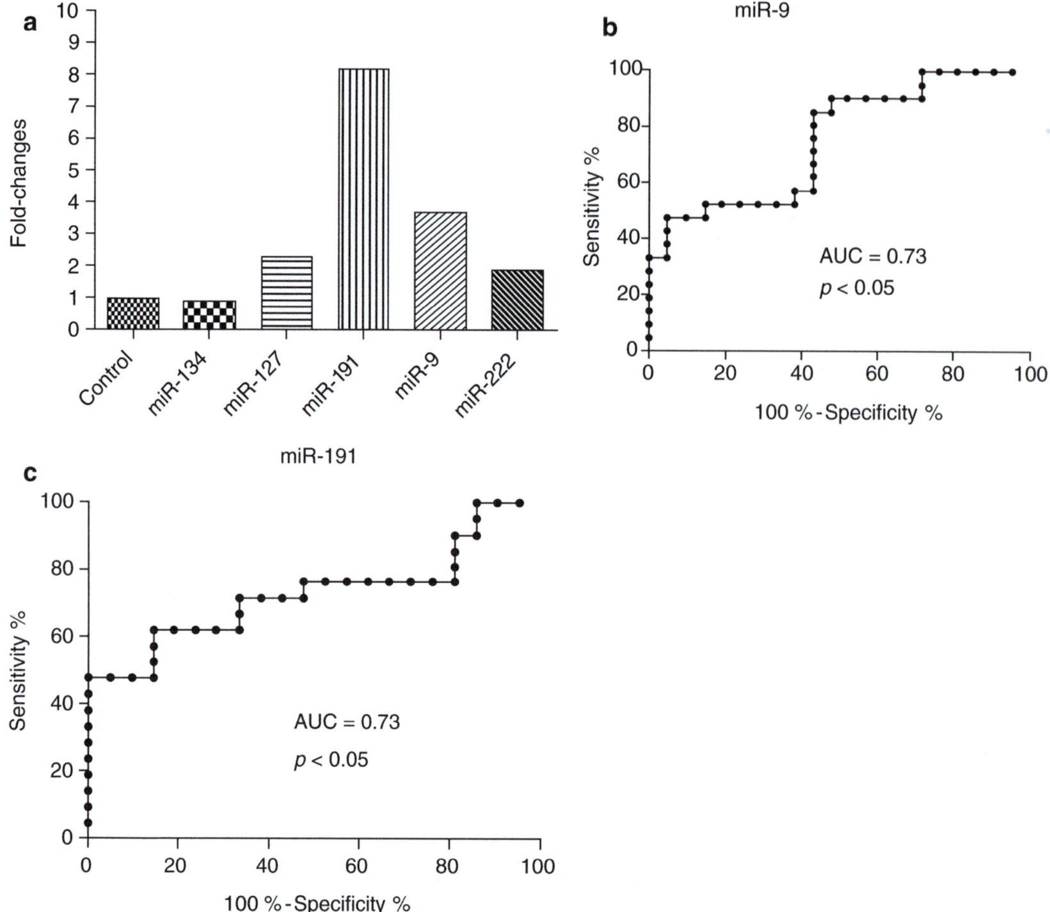

Fig. 7.8 (**a**) The expression levels of miR-222, miR-134, miR-127, miR-9, and miR-191 in saliva collected from HNSCC patients ($n=21$) and healthy controls ($n=21$) by quantitative real-time PCR (RT-PCR). Expression levels of the miRNAs were normalized to SNORD96A. Statistically significant differences were determined using Wilcoxon tests. Statistical significance was obtained for miR-191. Receiver operating curve analysis using saliva (**b**) miR-9 and (**c**) saliva miR-191 for discriminating HNSCC from normal subjects ($p<0.05$)

assay for these three genes, we demonstrated an overall accuracy of 81 % in the DNA isolated from saliva of HNSCC patients ($n=143$) when compared with the healthy nonsmoker controls ($n=31$) (see Fig. 7.9). The specificity for this MSP panel was 87 % and sensitivity was 80 % (with a Fisher's exact test $p<0.0001$). In addition, the test panel performed extremely well in the detection of the early stages of HNSCCs, with a sensitivity of 94 % and specificity of 87 % and a high κ(kappa) value of 0.8, indicating an excellent overall agreement between the presence of HNSCC and a positive MSP panel result. In a nutshell, we have demonstrated the relevance of a compact RASSF1a, DAPK1, and

p16 MSP panel, which can potentially be used to diagnose hypermethylation events in saliva of HNSCC patients.

Future Perspective

Early diagnostic technologies are vital in combating cancer. The increase in survival rates for breast and prostate cancer can be credited to their respective early screening programs [126, 127]. Due to the lack of screening programs, the mortality ratio for HNSCC is still relatively high. Since saliva is in direct contact with the tumors in the oral cavity, it has become an ideal biological fluid for detecting

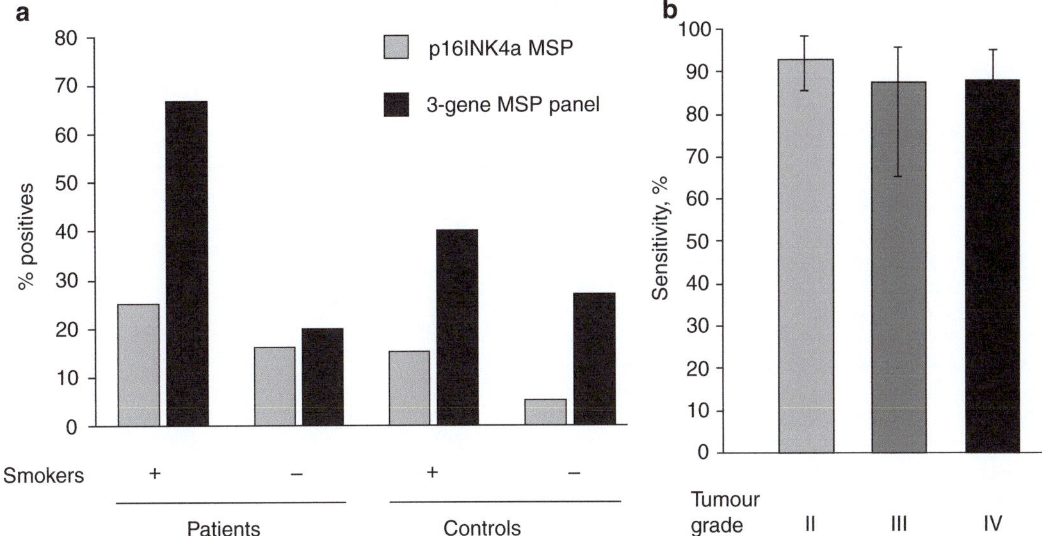

Fig. 7.9 The detection of the promoter hypermethylation events across different sample groups and tumor grades. (**a**) The percentages of samples positive for either whole three-gene MSP panel (*dark gray*) or p16 (*light-gray columns*) in different categories. (**b**) Grade-specific break- down of the detection of hypermethylation in patient saliva samples using the three-gene panel. Notice that detection sensitivity increases with the advancement of the tumor stage. Bars-$p=0.05$ confidence intervals

this type of cancer. The noninvasive nature of saliva collection also makes it an ideal tool for monitoring the progression of oral cancer.

Conclusion

Human saliva has emerged as a promising bio- fluid because of its ability to monitor health status, disease onset, progression, recurrence, and treatment responses in a noninvasive, cost-effective manner, thereby advancing health-care management. It has been demon- strated that saliva can be used to detect both local and systemic diseases, and, as such, recent studies have focused on profiling sali- vary biomolecules for diagnostic and prog- nostic purposes. However, there is an urgent need to translate saliva research from a labora- tory into a clinical setting to detect diseases at an early stage. The strategic plan of the National Institute of Dental and Craniofacial Research as well as the National Cancer Institute has recognized the importance of saliva as a translational fluid.

Currently, saliva is used in a clinical setting to detect dental carries and periodontal disease.

The ability to determine those at risk for bone loss before it occurs, the ability to effectively treat early diseases, and the ability to know when co-management of disease is needed are being defined by salivary diagnostics for peri- odontal disease. However, the use of saliva in detecting oral cancer is still in its infancy. It will be truly revolutionary to use saliva as a proxy medium to provide clinical decision support and inform patient care to those patients with eryth- roplakias in determining who will develop oral cancer.

The sheer number of salivary kits on the market paves the way for other types of saliva- based kits to enter the market. In the next 5 years, there will be saliva-based tests either at the dentist's office or at the general practi- tioner's to determine the health and well-being of individuals both young and old.

Acknowledgments The authors would like to acknowl- edge the financial support from the Queensland Government Smart Futures Co-investment Funding Scheme, University of Queensland Foundation Research Excellence Scheme, and the University of Queensland internal strategic funds. Also, we would like to thank Ms. Anthea Gibbons for her assistance in editing the book chapter.

References

1. Stedman TL. The American heritage Stedman's medical dictionary. Houghton Mifflin Co.; 2004.
2. Phillips C. Rinse and spit: saliva as a cancer biomarker source. NCI Cancer Bull. 2006 [cited 2013 October 25th]; Available from: http://www.cancer.gov/aboutnci/ncicancerbulletin/archive/2005/101105/page4.
3. Pfaffe T, Cooper-White J, Beyerlein P, Kostner K, Punyadeera C. Diagnostic potential of saliva: current state and future applications. Clin Chem. 2011;57(5):675–87.
4. Deepa T, Thirrunavukkarasu N. Saliva as a potential diagnostic tool. Indian J Med Sci. 2010;64(7):293.
5. Mandel ID. Salivary diagnosis: promises, promises. Ann N Y Acad Sci. 1993;694(1 Saliva as a D):1–10.
6. Schulz BL, Cooper-White J, Punyadeera CK. Saliva proteome research: current status and future outlook. Crit Rev Biotechnol. 2013;33(3):246–59.
7. Navazesh M, Kumar SK, University of Southern California School of D. Measuring salivary flow: challenges and opportunities. J Am Dent Assoc. 2008;139(Suppl):35S–40.
8. Turner RJ, Sugiya H. Understanding salivary fluid and protein secretion. Oral Dis. 2002;8(1):3–11.
9. Hu S, Xie Y, Ramachandran P, Ogorzalek Loo RR, Li Y, Loo JA, et al. Large-scale identification of proteins in human salivary proteome by liquid chromatography/mass spectrometry and two-dimensional gel electrophoresis-mass spectrometry. Proteomics. 2005;5(6):1714–28.
10. Huang C-M. Comparative proteomic analysis of human whole saliva. Arch Oral Biol. 2004;49(12):951–62.
11. Wilmarth PA, Riviere MA, Rustvold DL, Lauten JD, Madden TE, David LL. Two-dimensional liquid chromatography study of the human whole saliva proteome. J Proteome Res. 2004;3(5):1017–23.
12. Xie H, Rhodus NL, Griffin RJ, Carlis JV, Griffin TJ. A catalogue of human saliva proteins identified by free flow electrophoresis-based peptide separation and tandem mass spectrometry. Mol Cell Proteomics. 2005;4(11):1826–30.
13. Yan W, Griffin TJ, Hagen F, Hu S, Wolinsky LE, Lee CS, et al. Systematic comparison of the human saliva and plasma proteomes. Proteomics Clin Appl. 2009;3(1):116–34.
14. Bandhakavi S, Stone MD, Onsongo G, Van Riper SK, Griffin TJ. A dynamic range compression and three-dimensional peptide fractionation analysis platform expands proteome coverage and the diagnostic potential of whole saliva. J Proteome Res. 2009;8(12):5590–600.
15. Christodoulides N, Anslyn E, Fox PC, McDevitt JT, Mohanty S, Miller CS, et al. Application of microchip assay system for the measurement of c-reactive protein in human saliva. Lab Chip. 2005;5(3):261.
16. Dawes C. Considerations in the development of diagnostic tests on saliva. Ann N Y Acad Sci. 1993;694(1 Saliva as a D):265–9.
17. Ghezzi EM, Ship JA. Aging and secretory reserve capacity of major salivary glands. J Dent Res. 2003;82(10):844–8.
18. Fleissig Y, Reichenberg E, Redlich M, Zaks B, Deutsch O, Aframian DJ, et al. Comparative proteomic analysis of human oral fluids according to gender and age. Oral Dis. 2010;16(8):831.
19. Oppenheim FG, Salih E, Siqueira WL, Zhang W, Helmerhorst EJ. Salivary proteome and its genetic polymorphisms. Ann N Y Acad Sci. 2007;1098(1):22–50.
20. Proctor GB, Carpenter GH, Garrett JR. Sympathetic decentralization abolishes increased secretion of immunoglobulin a evoked by parasympathetic stimulation of rat submandibular glands. J Neuroimmunol. 2000;109(2):147–54.
21. Edwards AV, Titchen DA. Synergism in the autonomic regulation of parotid secretion of protein in sheep. J Physiol. 1992;451:1–15.
22. Carpenter GH, Proctor GB, Garrett JR. Preganglionic parasympathectomy decreases salivary siga secretion rates from the rat submandibular gland. J Neuroimmunol. 2005;160(1–2):4–11.
23. Navazesh M, Christensen C, Brightman V. Clinical criteria for the diagnosis of salivary gland hypofunction. J Dent Res. 1992;71(7):1363–9.
24. Topkas E, Keith P, Dimeski G, Cooper-White J, Punyadeera C. Evaluation of saliva collection devices for the analysis of proteins. Clin Chim Acta Int J Clin Chem. 2012;413(13–14):1066–70.
25. Michishige F, Kanno K, Yoshinaga S, Hinode D, Takehisa Y, Yasuoka S. Effect of saliva collection method on the concentration of protein components in saliva. J Med Invest. 2006;53(1,2):140–6.
26. Hansen AM, Garde AH, Persson R. Sources of biological and methodological variation in salivary cortisol and their impact on measurement among healthy adults: a review. Scand J Clin Lab Invest. 2008;68(6):448–58.
27. Izawa S, Miki K, Liu X, Ogawa N. The diurnal patterns of salivary interleukin-6 and c-reactive protein in healthy young adults. Brain Behav Immun. 2013;27(1):38–41.
28. Helmerhorst EJ, Oppenheim FG. Saliva: a dynamic proteome. J Dent Res. 2007;86(8):680–93.
29. Houghton JT, Ding Y, Griggs DJ, Noguer M, van der Linden PJ, Dai X, Maskell K, Johnson CA. Climate change 2001: the scientific basis: contribution of working group i to the third assessment report of the intergovernmental panel on climate change. 1st ed. Cambridge University Press, United Kingdom and New York, NY, USA; 2001.
30. Schottenfeld D, Beebe-Dimmer J. Chronic inflammation: a common and important factor in the pathogenesis of neoplasia. CA Cancer J Clin. 2006;56(2):69.
31. Feller L, Altini M, Lemmer J. Inflammation in the context of oral cancer. Oral Oncol. 2013;49(9):887–92.
32. Roy HK, Khandekar JD. Biomarkers for the early detection of cancer: an inflammatory concept. Arch Intern Med. 2007;167(17):1822–4.

33. Anonymous. Early detection of ovarian cancer. Pract Nurse. 2009;37(6):6.
34. Thygesen K, Chaitman B, Clemmensen PM, Dellborg M, Hod H, Porela P, et al. Universal definition of myocardial infarction. Circulation. 2007;116(22): 2634–53.
35. van der Waal I. Potentially malignant disorders of the oral and oropharyngeal mucosa; terminology, classification and present concepts of management. Oral Oncol. 2009;45(4–5):317–23.
36. Welch H, Hasbun R. Lumbar puncture and cerebrospinal fluid analysis. Handb Clin Neurol. 2010;96:31–49.
37. Majed B, Zephir H, Pichonnier-Cassagne V, Yazdanpanah Y, Lestavel P, Valette P, et al. Lumbar punctures: use and diagnostic efficiency in emergency medical departments. Int J Emerg Med. 2009;2(4):227–35.
38. Stewart H, Reuben A, McDonald J. Lp or not lp, that is the question: gold standard or unnecessary procedure in subarachnoid haemorrhage? Emerg Med J. 2013;31(9):720–3.
39. Haraldsson B, Sorensson J. Why do we not all have proteinuria? An update of our current understanding of the glomerular barrier. News Physiol Sci. 2004;19:7–10.
40. Maunsbach AB. Absorption of i125-labeled homologous albumin by rat kidney proximal tubule cells. A study of microperfused single proximal tubules by electron microscopic autoradiography and histochemistry. J Am Soc Nephrol. 1997;8(2):323–51; discussion 327–31.
41. Pisitkun T, Shen RF, Knepper MA. Identification and proteomic profiling of exosomes in human urine. Proc Natl Acad Sci U S A. 2004;101(36):13368–73.
42. Klein D, Bussow H, Fewou SN, Gieselmann V. Exocytosis of storage material in a lysosomal disorder. Biochem Biophys Res Commun. 2005;327(3):663–7.
43. Adachi J, Kumar C, Zhang Y, Olsen JV, Mann M. The human urinary proteome contains more than 1,500 proteins, including a large proportion of membrane proteins. Genome Biol. 2006;7(9):R80.
44. Theodorescu D, Wittke S, Ross MM, Walden M, Conaway M, Just I, et al. Discovery and validation of new protein biomarkers for urothelial cancer: a prospective analysis. Lancet Oncol. 2006;7(3):230–40.
45. Wittke S, Haubitz M, Walden M, Rohde F, Schwarz A, Mengel M, et al. Detection of acute tubulointerstitial rejection by proteomic analysis of urinary samples in renal transplant recipients. Am J Transplant. 2005;5(10):2479–88.
46. Meier M, Kaiser T, Herrmann A, Knueppel S, Hillmann M, Koester P, et al. Identification of urinary protein pattern in type 1 diabetic adolescents with early diabetic nephropathy by a novel combined proteome analysis. J Diabetes Complicat. 2005;19(4):223–32.
47. Mishra J, Dent C, Tarabishi R, Mitsnefes MM, Ma Q, Kelly C, et al. Neutrophil gelatinase-associated lipocalin (ngal) as a biomarker for acute renal injury after cardiac surgery. Lancet. 2005;365(9466):1231–8.
48. Rehman I, Azzouzi AR, Catto JW, Allen S, Cross SS, Feeley K, et al. Proteomic analysis of voided urine after prostatic massage from patients with prostate cancer: a pilot study. Urology. 2004;64(6):1238–43.
49. Zhang YF, Wu DL, Guan M, Liu WW, Wu Z, Chen YM, et al. Tree analysis of mass spectral urine profiles discriminates transitional cell carcinoma of the bladder from noncancer patient. Clin Biochem. 2004;37(9):772–9.
50. Pieper R, Gatlin CL, McGrath AM, Makusky AJ, Mondal M, Seonarain M, et al. Characterization of the human urinary proteome: a method for high-resolution display of urinary proteins on two-dimensional electrophoresis gels with a yield of nearly 1,400 distinct protein spots. Proteomics. 2004;4(4):1159–74.
51. Celis JE, Wolf H, Ostergaard M. Bladder squamous cell carcinoma biomarkers derived from proteomics. Electrophoresis. 2000;21(11):2115–21.
52. Rasmussen HH, Orntoft TF, Wolf H, Celis JE. Towards a comprehensive database of proteins from the urine of patients with bladder cancer. J Urol. 1996;155(6):2113–9.
53. Feng C, Wu Z, Guo T, Jiang H, Guan M, Zhang Y, et al. Blca-4 expression is related to mmp-9, vegf, il-1alpha and il-8 in bladder cancer but not to pedf, tnf-alpha or angiogenesis. Pathol Biol (Paris). 2012;60(3):e36–40.
54. Fujita K, Ewing CM, Isaacs WB, Pavlovich CP. Immunomodulatory il-18 binding protein is produced by prostate cancer cells and its levels in urine and serum correlate with tumor status. Int J Cancer. 2011;129(2):424–32.
55. Idasiak-Piechocka I, Oko A, Pawliczak E, Kaczmarek E, Czekalski S. Urinary excretion of soluble tumour necrosis factor receptor 1 as a marker of increased risk of progressive kidney function deterioration in patients with primary chronic glomerulonephritis. Nephrol Dial Transplant. 2010;25(12):3948–56.
56. Liu BC, Zhang L, Lv LL, Wang YL, Liu DG, Zhang XL. Application of antibody array technology in the analysis of urinary cytokine profiles in patients with chronic kidney disease. Am J Nephrol. 2006;26(5):483–90.
57. Margel D, Pesvner-Fischer M, Baniel J, Yossepowitch O, Cohen IR. Stress proteins and cytokines are urinary biomarkers for diagnosis and staging of bladder cancer. Eur Urol. 2011;59(1):113–9.
58. Meijer E, Boertien WE, Nauta FL, Bakker SJ, van Oeveren W, Rook M, et al. Association of urinary biomarkers with disease severity in patients with autosomal dominant polycystic kidney disease: a cross-sectional analysis. Am J Kidney Dis. 2010;56(5):883–95.
59. Nauta FL, Boertien WE, Bakker SJ, van Goor H, van Oeveren W, de Jong PE, et al. Glomerular and tubular damage markers are elevated in patients with diabetes. Diabetes Care. 2011;34(4):975–81.
60. Ni J, Huang HQ, Lu LL, Zheng M, Liu BC. Influence of irbesartan on the urinary excretion of cytokines

in patients with chronic kidney disease. Chin Med J (Engl). 2012;125(6):1147–52.

61. Nielsen SE, Hansen HP, Jensen BR, Parving HH, Rossing P. Urinary neutrophil gelatinase-associated lipocalin and progression of diabetic nephropathy in type 1 diabetic patients in a four-year follow-up study. Nephron Clin Pract. 2011;118(2):c130–5.

62. Parikh CR, Dahl NK, Chapman AB, Bost JE, Edelstein CL, Comer DM, et al. Evaluation of urine biomarkers of kidney injury in polycystic kidney disease. Kidney Int. 2012;81(8):784–90.

63. Sola-Del Valle DA, Mohan S, Cheng JT, Paragas NA, Sise ME, D'Agati VD, et al. Urinary ngal is a useful clinical biomarker of hiv-associated nephropathy. Nephrol Dial Transplant. 2011;26(7):2387–90.

64. Suen JL, Liu CC, Lin YS, Tsai YF, Juo SH, Chou YH. Urinary chemokines/cytokines are elevated in patients with urolithiasis. Urol Res. 2010;38(2):81–7.

65. Urquidi V, Kim J, Chang M, Dai Y, Rosser CJ, Goodison S. Ccl18 in a multiplex urine-based assay for the detection of bladder cancer. PLoS One. 2012;7(5):e37797. U6 – ctx_ver=Z3988-2004&ctx_enc=info%3Aofi%2Fenc%3AUTF-8&rfr_id=info:sid/summonserialssolutionscom&rft_val_fmt=info:ofi/fmt:kev:mtx:journal&rftgenre=article&rftatitle=CCL18+in+a+multiplex+urine-based+assay+for+the+detection+of+bladder+cancer&rftjtitle=PloS+one&rftau=Urquidi%2C+Virginia&rftau=Kim%2C+Jeongsoon&rftau=Chang%2C+Myron&rftau=Dai%2C+Yunfeng&rftdate=2012&rfteissn=1932-6203&rftvolume=7&rftissue=5&rftspage=e37797&rft_id=info:pmid/22629457&rftexternalDocID=22629457¶mdict=en-US U7 – Journal Article U8 – FETCH-LOGICAL-p1142-ee209faf3c3a88f0d62a1895d4e493102f15aea302bd289c6cce0a55d5b8e1741.

66. Wasilewska A, Taranta-Janusz K, Debek W, Zoch-Zwierz W, Kuroczycka-Saniutycz E. Kim-1 and ngal: new markers of obstructive nephropathy. Pediatr Nephrol. 2011;26(4):579–86.

67. Wasilewska A, Zoch-Zwierz W, Taranta-Janusz K, Kolodziejczyk Z. Urinary monocyte chemoattractant protein-1 excretion in children with glomerular proteinuria. Scand J Urol Nephrol. 2011;45(1):52–9.

68. Dams R, Choo RE, Lambert WE, Jones H, Huestis MA. Oral fluid as an alternative matrix to monitor opiate and cocaine use in substance-abuse treatment patients. Drug Alcohol Depend. 2007;87(2–3):258–67.

69. Kefalides PT. Saliva research leads to new diagnostic tools and therapeutic options. Ann Intern Med. 1999;131(12):991.

70. Karjalainen S, Sewon L, Soderling E, Larsson B, Johansson I, Simell O, et al. Salivary cholesterol of healthy adults in relation to serum cholesterol concentration and oral health. J Dent Res. 1997;76(10):1637–43.

71. Ceccato F, Barbot M, Zilio M, Ferasin S, Occhi G, Daniele A, et al. Performance of salivary cortisol in the diagnosis of cushing's syndrome, adrenal incidentaloma, and adrenal insufficiency. Eur J Endocrinol. 2013;169(1):31–6.

72. Fransen K, Vermoesen T, Beelaert G, Menten J, Hutse V, Wouters K, et al. Using conventional HIV tests on oral fluid. J Virol Methods. 2013;194:46–51.

73. Streckfus C, Bigler L, Dellinger T, Dai X, Kingman A, Thigpen JT. The presence of soluble c-erbb-2 in saliva and serum among women with breast carcinoma: a preliminary study. Clin Cancer Res. 2000;6(6):2363–70.

74. Vos T, Flaxman AD, Naghavi M, Lozano R, Michaud C, Ezzati M, et al. Years lived with disability (ylds) for 1160 sequelae of 289 diseases and injuries 1990–2010: a systematic analysis for the global burden of disease study 2010. Lancet. 2012;380(9859): 2163–96.

75. WHO. The world oral health report: continuous improvement of oral health in the 21st century – the approach of the who global oral health programme. Geneva: World Health Organization; 2003.

76. Suddick RP, Harris NO. Historical perspectives of oral biology: a series. Crit Rev Oral Bio Med. 1990;1(2):135–51.

77. Gerabek WE. The tooth-worm: historical aspects of a popular medical belief. Clin Oral Investig. 1999;3(1):1–6.

78. Miller WD. The human mouth as a focus of infection. Dental Cosmos. 1891;33(9):18.

79. Haffajee AD, Socransky SS. Microbiology of periodontal diseases: introduction. Periodontol 2000. 2005;38:9–12.

80. Vitorino R, Lobo MJ, Duarte JR, Ferrer-Correia AJ, Domingues PM, Amado FM. The role of salivary peptides in dental caries. Biomed Chromatogr. 2005;19(3):214–22.

81. Mazengo MC, Tenovuo J, Hausen H. Dental caries in relation to diet, saliva and cariogenic microorganisms in tanzanians of selected age groups. Community Dent Oral Epidemiol. 1996;24(3):169–74.

82. Streckfus CF, Bigler LR. Saliva as a diagnostic fluid. Oral Dis. 2002;8(2):69–76.

83. Tulunoglu Ö, Demirtas S, Tulunoglu I. Total antioxidant levels of saliva in children related to caries, age, and gender. Int J Paediatr Dent. 2006;16(3):186–91.

84. Ayad M, Van Wuyckhuyse BC, Minaguchi K, Raubertas RF, Bedi GS, Billings RJ, et al. The association of basic proline-rich peptides from human parotid gland secretions with caries experience. J Dent Res. 2000;79(4):976–82.

85. Thibodeau EA, O'Sullivan DM. Salivary mutans streptococci and caries development in the primary and mixed dentitions of children. Community Dent Oral Epidemiol. 1999;27(6):406–12.

86. van Palenstein Helderman WH, Mikx FH, Van't Hof MA, Truin G, Kalsbeek H. The value of salivary bacterial counts as a supplement to past caries experience as caries predictor in children. Eur J Oral Sci. 2001;109(5):312–5.

87. Zhang Q, Bian Z, Fan M, van Palenstein Helderman WH. Salivary mutans streptococci counts as indicators in caries risk assessment in 6–7-year-old chinese children. J Dent. 2007;35(2):177–80.

88. Anderson LC, Mandel ID. Salivary protein polymorphisms in caries-resistant adults. J Dent Res. 1982;61(10):1167–8.

89. Roa NS, Chaves M, Gomez M, Jaramillo LM. Association of salivary proteins with dental caries in a Colombian population. Acta Odontol Latinoam. 2008;21(1):69–75.

90. Denny PC. A saliva-based prognostic test for dental caries susceptibility. Am Dent Hyg Assoc. 2009;83(4):175–6.

91. Research NIoDaC. Periodontal (gum) disease: causes, symptoms and treatments. 2013 [updated August 2012; cited 2013 10/10/2013]; Available from: http://www.nidcr.nih.gov/OralHealth/Topics/GumDiseases/PeriodontalGumDisease.htm.

92. Group MR. Millenium Research Group. Global markets for dental implants 2007. Millenium Research Group: Toronto, Canada, 2008.

93. Preber H, Bergström J. Cigarette smoking in patients referred for periodontal treatment. Scand J Dent Res. 1986;94(2):102.

94. Borojevic T. Smoking and periodontal disease. Materia Socio-Medica. 2012;24(4):274.

95. Anonymous. Emotional stress could cause periodontal disease. 2012 [cited 2013 October 15th]; Available from: http://www.knowyourteeth.com/infobites/abc/article/?abc=G&iid=324&aid=1249.

96. Lieff S, Boggess KA, Murtha AP, Jared H, Madianos PN, Moss K, et al. The oral conditions and pregnancy study: periodontal status of a cohort of pregnant women. J Periodontol. 2004;75(1):116–26.

97. Wilder R, Robinson C, Jared HL, Lieff S, Boggess K. Obstetricians' knowledge and practice behaviors concerning periodontal health and preterm delivery and low birth weight. J Dent Hyg. 2007;81(4):81.

98. Giannobile WV, Beikler T, Kinney JS, Ramseier CA, Morelli T, Wong DT. Saliva as a diagnostic tool for periodontal disease: current state and future direction. Periodontology 2000. 2009;50:52–64.

99. Khashu H, Baiju CS, Bansal SR, Chillar A. Salivary biomarkers: a periodontal overview. J Oral Health Community Dent. 2012;6(1):28–33.

100. Groenink J, Walgreen-Weterings E, Nazmi K, Bolscher JG, Veerman EC, Van Winkelhoff AJ. Salivary lactoferrin and low-mr mucin mg2 in *actinobacillus actinomycetemcomitans*-associated periodontitis. J Clin Periodontol. 1999;26:269–75.

101. Warnakulasuriya S, Johnson NW, Van Der Waal I. Nomenclature and classification of potentially malignant disorders of the oral mucosa. J Oral Pathol Med. 2007;36(10):575–80.

102. Napier SS, Cowan CG, Gregg TA, Stevenson M, Lamey PJ, Toner PG. Potentially malignant oral lesions in Northern Ireland: size (extent) matters. Oral Dis. 2003;9(3):129–37.

103. Axell T. Occurrence of leukoplakia and some other oral white lesions among 20,333 adult Swedish people. Community Dent Oral Epidemiol. 1987;15(1):46–51.

104. Axell T, Rundquist L. Oral lichen planus–a demographic study. Community Dent Oral Epidemiol. 1987;15(1):52–6.

105. Amarasinghe HK, Usgodaarachchi US, Johnson NW, Lalloo R, Warnakulasuriya S. Betel-quid chewing with or without tobacco is a major risk factor for oral potentially malignant disorders in Sri Lanka: a case-control study. Oral Oncol. 2010;46(4):297–301.

106. Chung CH, Yang YH, Wang TY, Shieh TY, Warnakulasuriya S. Oral precancerous disorders associated with areca quid chewing, smoking, and alcohol drinking in southern Taiwan. J Oral Pathol Med. 2005;34(8):460–6.

107. Napier SS, Speight PM. Natural history of potentially malignant oral lesions and conditions: an overview of the literature. J Oral Pathol Med. 2008;37(1):1–10.

108. GLOBOCAN. World cancer report. International Agency for Research on Cancer; 2008 [cited 2011 Feb. 26]; Available from: http://globocan.iarc.fr/factsheets/populations/factsheet.asp?uno=900.

109. Rethman MP, Carpenter W, Cohen EE, Epstein J, Evans CA, Flaitz CM, et al. Evidence-based clinical recommendations regarding screening for oral squamous cell carcinomas. J Am Dent Assoc. 2010;141(5):509–20.

110. Johnson NW, Jayasekara P, Amarasinghe AA. Squamous cell carcinoma and precursor lesions of the oral cavity: epidemiology and aetiology. Periodontol 2000. 2011;57(1):19–37.

111. Warnakulasuriya S, Sutherland G, Scully C. Tobacco, oral cancer, and treatment of dependence. Oral Oncol. 2005;41(3):244–60.

112. Andre K, Schraub S, Mercier M, Bontemps P. Role of alcohol and tobacco in the aetiology of head and neck cancer: a case-control study in the Doubs region of France. Eur J Cancer B Oral Oncol. 1995;31B(5):301–9 [Research Support, Non-U.S. Gov't].

113. Kreimer AR, Clifford GM, Boyle P, Franceschi S. Human papillomavirus types in head and neck squamous cell carcinomas worldwide: a systematic review. Cancer Epidemiol Biomarkers Prev. 2005;14(2):467–75.

114. Leemans CR, Braakhuis BJ, Brakenhoff RH. The molecular biology of head and neck cancer. Nat Rev Cancer. 2011;11(1):9–22.

115. Thomas SJ, Bain CJ, Battistutta D, Ness AR, Paissat D, Maclennan R. Betel quid not containing tobacco and oral cancer: a report on a case-control study in Papua New Guinea and a meta-analysis of current evidence. Int J Cancer J Int Du Cancer. 2007;120(6):1318–23.

116. Jeng JH, Chang MC, Hahn LJ. Role of areca nut in betel quid-associated chemical carcinogenesis: current awareness and future perspectives. Oral Oncol. 2001;37(6):477–92.

117. Ouko LA, Shantikumar K, Knezovich J, Haycock P, Schnugh DJ, Ramsay M. Effect of alcohol consumption on cpg methylation in the differentially

methylated regions of h19 and ig-dmr in male gametes: implications for fetal alcohol spectrum disorders. Alcohol Clin Exp Res. 2009;33(9): 1615–27.

118. Muwonge R, Ramadas K, Sankila R, Thara S, Thomas G, Vinoda J, et al. Role of tobacco smoking, chewing and alcohol drinking in the risk of oral cancer in Trivandrum, India: a nested case-control design using incident cancer cases. Oral Oncol. 2008;44(5):446–54.

119. Levi F, Pasche C, La Vecchia C, Lucchini F, Franceschi S, Monnier P. Food groups and risk of oral and pharyngeal cancer. Int J Cancer J Int Du Cancer. 1998;77(5):705–9.

120. Nagadia R, Pandit P, Coman WB, Cooper-White J, Punyadeera C. Mirnas in head and neck cancer revisited. Cel Oncol (Dordrecht). 2013;36(1):1–7.

121. Ovchinnikov DA, Cooper MA, Pandit P, Coman WB, Cooper-White JJ, Keith P, et al. Tumor-suppressor gene promoter hypermethylation in saliva of head and neck cancer patients. Transl Oncol. 2012;5(5):321–6.

122. Childs G, Fazzari M, Kung G, Kawachi N, Brandwein-Gensler M, McLemore M, et al. Low-level expression of micrornas let-7d and mir-205 are prognostic markers of head and neck squamous cell carcinoma. Am J Pathol. 2009;174(3):736–45.

123. Berckmans RJ, Sturk A, van Tienen LM, Schaap MC, Nieuwland R. Cell-derived vesicles exposing coagulant tissue factor in saliva. Blood. 2011;117(11):3172–80.

124. Redman RS. On approaches to the functional restoration of salivary glands damaged by radiation therapy for head and neck cancer, with a review of related aspects of salivary gland morphology and development. Biotech Histochem. 2008;83(3):103–30.

125. Schussel J, Zhou XC, Zhang Z, Pattani K, Bermudez F, Jean-Charles G, et al. Ednrb and dcc salivary rinse hypermethylation has a similar performance as expert clinical examination in discrimination of oral cancer/dysplasia versus benign lesions. Clin Cancer Res. 2013;19(12):3268–75.

126. Trogdon JG, Ekwueme DU, Subramanian S, Crouse W. Economies of scale in federally-funded state-organized public health programs: Results from the national breast and cervical cancer early detection programs. Health Care Manag Sci. 2014;17:321–30.

127. Ma X, Wang R, Long JB, Ross JS, Soulos PR, Yu JB, et al. The cost implications of prostate cancer screening in the medicare population. Cancer. 2013;120(1):96–102.

128. Salazar C, et al. miRNAs in human papilloma virus associated oral and oropharyngeal squamous cell carcinomas. Exp Rev Mol Diag. 2014;14(8):1033–40.

Salivary Gland Tissue Engineering and Future Diagnostics

Daniel A. Harrington, Mariane Martinez, Danielle Wu, Swati Pradhan-Bhatt, and Mary C. Farach-Carson

Abstract

Our study of salivary gland structure and function relies on our ability to study the organ in its native environment. To scale those needs to a laboratory setting, researchers have created *in vitro* models that replicate the salient features of the gland, but these are inevitably tied to the abilities of current technologies and may require some compromises along the way. In this chapter, we discuss key features of the gland that would be desired in a model and the potential intersection of those needs with advances in the field of tissue engineering. The application of these new technologies, along with improvements in imaging and phenotype reporting, holds the promise of significantly impacting salivary diagnostics through continual improvements in the accuracy and scalability of laboratory models.

D.A. Harrington, PhD (✉)
M. Martinez, PhD candidate • D. Wu, PhD
Department of Biochemistry and Cell Biology,
Rice University, Houston, TX, USA
e-mail: daniel.a.harrington@rice.edu; mariane.
martinez@rice.edu; daniellewu@rice.edu

S. Pradhan-Bhatt, PhD
Department of Biological Sciences,
University of Delaware, Newark, DE, USA

Center for Translational Cancer Research (CTCR),
Helen F. Graham Cancer Center and Research
Institute, Christiana Care Health Systems,
Newark, DE, USA
e-mail: swati@udel.edu

M.C. Farach-Carson, PhD
Department of Biochemistry, Cell Biology
and Bioengineering, Rice University,
Houston, TX, USA
e-mail: farachca@rice.edu

Necessity for an Ex Vivo Testing Platform

The salivary gland is a remarkable exocrine organ whose secretory activity and products reflect the entire metabolic activity of the organism. The ability to monitor metabolism noninvasively offers an, as yet, untapped means for health monitoring and disease diagnosis. As discussed in earlier chapters of this book, the road to development of reliable salivary diagnostics has not been simple, owing to a combination of technical, biological, and regulatory issues. The development of reliable tissue-engineered functional salivary glands can provide an alternative means to accelerate platform development and testing, independent of host variability. This chapter discusses the current status of salivary gland tissue engineering, the opportunities

C.F. Streckfus (ed.), *Advances in Salivary Diagnostics*,
DOI 10.1007/978-3-662-45399-5_8, © Springer-Verlag Berlin Heidelberg 2015

to integrate progress in materials science and cell and matrix biology to create new ex vivo platforms for diagnostic development, and the potential to develop new means for drug screening in three-dimensional (3D)-engineered systems.

Need for Engineered Salivary Glands

As reviewed elsewhere in this volume, saliva has been used for health monitoring for both diseases of the oral cavity, such as periodontitis, caries, salivary hypofunction, viral infections, or oral cancer, and for systemic disruptors such as endocrine disorders, infection, heart disease, or toxin exposure [1, 2]. Additionally, testing of saliva can be used to monitor at-risk populations for use of prohibited substances such as cocaine or opiates [3]. When the three-compartment blind-ended tube was first envisioned as a model for the engineered salivary gland by Dr. Bruce Baum and colleagues, two purposes were described. In addition to the potential to provide clinical relief to some 400,000 head and neck cancer patients worldwide in a year with radiation-induced xerostomia, an ability to engineer a fluid-secreting tube suitable for testing therapeutic interventions such as gene therapies was described [4]. With the advent of high-throughput screening in 3D systems to replace conventional 2D plastic drug testing systems, the opportunity to develop a functional physiologically relevant platform to identify bioactive compounds with the ability to stimulate salivary cells and relieve xerostomia is on the horizon. Likewise, ex vivo cultured glands composed entirely of human cells offer the ability to study salivary cell function under controlled conditions and in the absence of the variables inherent to any human population that have hindered development of the field [5–8]. While such ex vivo systems exist at present, such as the cultured salisphere [9], they often are composed of nonhuman cells that can differ considerably from their human counterparts or are created using nonhuman materials such as Matrigel®.

Successful implementation of an *in vitro*-built salivary gland is a multidisciplinary effort that relies on advances in clinical, biological, and engineering sciences. This chapter will describe the major structural features of the salivary gland at the cell and tissue levels that constitute a minimum model for its function. We will review past biological systems that shaped our understanding of how to integrate multicellular, multidimensional complexity into tissue models and discuss options for integrating nervous and vascular support. We will review investigators' recent efforts to construct systems that incorporate some or all of these features. In the context of contemporary tissue engineering, we will describe the range of biomaterial scaffolds and salivary cell lines available to investigators for building multilayered 3D systems, as well as some modern successes in related tissue systems, such as the mammary gland. Lastly, these individual elements will be explored in the context of modern imaging and assessment methods. Our hope is that the reader will appreciate the untapped range of technologies and platforms available for developing novel models of salivary structure and function, in the context of biological study and diagnostic assessments.

Complexity of the Salivary Gland System and Levels of Gland Structure

The salivary gland is a uniquely accessible secretory organ that offers an opportune model to understand the architecture and behavior of other exocrine structures. To produce an ex vivo model of the gland for diagnostic applications, researchers must recreate the minimum structural and functional criteria that define the gland and include these in their constructions.

Salivary Gland Structure

The mammalian salivary gland system consists of the three major types of bilateral paired glands: the parotid, the submandibular, and the sublingual. Apart from these, there are about 800–1,000 minor salivary glands that are found throughout the submucosa in the oral cavity. Saliva produced by the salivary glands aids in digestion, lubrication, and maintenance of oral homeostasis. Secretory acinar cells release salivary fluid that is either a protein-rich serous fluid or a mucin-rich viscous fluid. The parotid gland is a purely serous gland, whereas the sublingual is a purely mucous gland. The submandibular is a mixed gland with a mixture of both serous and mucous cells [10–13]. Ductal cells modify the ionic composition of the primary saliva and provide a conduit for its entry into the oral cavity [14]. Myoepithelial cells, whose exact function is unknown, wrap around the acini and are postulated to aid in secretion [10, 11, 14].

Salivary glands are composed of multiple branched lobules, each having a terminal secretory acinus and connecting to intralobular and interlobular ducts. Each acinus is composed of a spherical mass of polarized secretory (serous or mucous) cells with a lumen, which is the initial start site of salivary flow. Serous acinar cells have a broad basal plasma membrane facing the basement membrane (BM) and a narrow apical plasma membrane facing the lumen. The nucleus, mitochondria, and endoplasmic reticulum are located at the basal end of serous cells, while the protein-rich secretory granules are located in the apical region of these cells. Mucous-secreting cells are mostly cuboidal in shape with flattened nuclei located at the base of the cells and are usually arranged into tubules rather than acini. These cells secrete hydrophilic glycoproteins (mucins) that help moisten and lubricate the saliva. In the seromucous-secreting glands, the serous cells are arranged into demilunes located at the terminal end of mucous tubules. Secretory acini and proximal ducts are wrapped around with myoepithelial cell processes, located between the basal lamina and the basolateral cell membrane, that are postulated to have a contractile ability, which serves in providing force for the unidirectional secretion of saliva. These basket-like cells help maintain the structural integrity of secretory acini units that constantly experience swelling when the lumen is filled with saliva.

These secretory terminal acini are connected to the oral cavity via intralobular and interlobular ducts. Intralobular ducts are subdivided into intercalated and striated ducts. Saliva is initially secreted into the intercalated ducts due to their proximity to the secretory acini. The intercalated ductal cells are cuboidal epithelial cells that modify saliva by adding bicarbonate and absorbing chloride as it travels along the ductal system. These ducts are usually short in length and merge with other intercalated ducts to form larger striated ducts. Striated ducts consist of columnar cells with radial striations, or infoldings of the basal plasma membrane, that enhance cell surface area. The mitochondria align along the basal membrane and enable ion absorption, as well as electrolyte and water transport. Na^+ and Cl^- are reabsorbed, and K^+ is released into the salivary secretion. Furthermore, saliva is continuously modified while traveling through the ductal system until reaching the oral cavity, where it can aid in functions such as digestion initiation and tooth decay prevention due to its antibacterial and antifungal properties.

Interplay Among Various Cell Types During Development

The developing embryonic salivary gland follows a carefully orchestrated series of events involving its epithelium, mesenchyme, nerves, and endothelial networks [10–12]. The exact order and timing of each of these well-controlled events are a subject of ongoing investigation. The neural crest-derived mesenchyme plays a major role in the initiation of salivary gland development by forming a condensed primordial layer at specific sites throughout the oral epithelium. The mesenchyme imparts signals that generate the placode at embryonic day 11. Mice lacking *Fgf10*, *Fgfr2b*, *Pitx1*, and *p63* are salivary gland deficient, stressing the importance of these genes in salivary gland development [11]. In the submandibular gland, neuronal precursors derived from the neural crest conjoin to form the parasympathetic ganglion. Axons from the parasympathetic ganglion extend with the epithelium during branching morphogenesis and aid in functionality of the gland. Although endothelial cells are major regulators of initiation of organogenesis in the liver and pancreas, their exact role in salivary gland development remains unknown [11, 12, 15]. An ideal salivary gland substitute will have been formed from a template that follows nature's orderly principles to create a fully functional artificial gland that can respond to signals for regulated secretion.

Cell polarity is vital for the proper function of the salivary glands and represents an early-level target for engineered models of the gland.

Therefore, understanding the associated cellular mechanisms required for the establishment and maintenance of cell junctions and polarity is crucial for engineering representative biological models for diagnostics. *In vitro* salivary gland models would provide useful tools to study salivary cell interactions with basement membrane (BM) components and can be manipulated for studying the effects on cell polarity of adding individual or combined BM components to substrates for salivary epithelial cell culture. As discussed later in this chapter, researchers have already initiated multiple strategies for using naturally derived BM as a substrate for 3D acinar culture or integrating BM components into synthetic engineered substrates [5, 6].

Basement Membrane (BM) Formation and Cell Polarity

Salivary glands consist of tightly packed, polarized secretory acinar and absorptive ductal cells, surrounded by myoepithelial cells that are presumed to have contractile forces to ensure the proper unidirectional secretion of saliva. Cell polarization in salivary parenchymal cells is crucial for the tissue-specific function of salivary secretion. Accordingly, the mechanisms involved in establishing and maintaining cell polarity should be followed to establish an accurate biological model of the gland. *In vitro* salivary gland models using customizable hydrogel scaffolds can provide a useful tool for studying cell polarity [16]. Establishment of epithelial cell polarity requires extracellular signals including cell sensing of the basally disposed BM through integrin activation by BM components and cell-cell binding of asymmetrically distributed cadherins and tight junctional components on lateral membranes. Therefore, the extracellular matrix (ECM) is a key driver during organogenesis because of its important functions that include (1) directing and maintaining cell spatial organization via direct interaction with cell receptors; (2) providing flexible mechanical support to tissue; (3) serving as a reservoir of cytokines needed for important cellular functions such as growth, proliferation, migration, organization, and survival; and (4) physically separating cell layers with distinct functions.

The BM is vital for properly organizing epithelial cells during organogenesis; it aids in cell sorting by separating epithelial cells from the surrounding stromal cells in connective tissue, which allows epithelial cells to organize into a highly interconnected, polarized cell monolayer. The BM has a thickness of approximately 100 nm, is located basally to epithelial and endothelial cell monolayers, and is crucial for the development of a functional salivary gland [17, 18]. The four major components of the BM are laminin, type IV collagen, nidogen/entactin, and the heparan sulfate proteoglycan, perlecan/HSPG2. Laminin is a heterotrimer composed of α-, β-, and γ-chains that self-assemble into a polymeric network (lamina lucida) that lies below epithelial cell monolayers and provides binding sites for cell surface laminin receptors [17, 19]. Nonfibrillar type IV collagen also is a heterotrimer that is assembled from six genetically distinct α-chains into collagen IV protomers, which then self-assemble into the lamina densa's mesh-like suprastructure. The triple helical collagenous domain of type IV collagen protomers provides the structural integrity of the BM. Perlecan, a secreted multidomain heparan sulfate proteoglycan, is present both in the BM and in reactive connective tissue [20]. The core protein of perlecan is made of 4,391 amino acids and is approximately 400–450 kDa. Domain I (N-terminus) of perlecan is covalently linked to three glycosaminoglycan (GAG) chains. Its modular structure contains binding sites for collagen IV (domain IV), laminin (HS), and nidogen (IV-1), among other ECM components, which allows perlecan to stabilize the BM framework by bridging the laminin polymeric network with the collagen IV meshwork [20, 21]. Nidogen, a secreted glycoprotein, is a small component of the BM that adds stability to overall network by bridging laminin, type IV collagen, and perlecan.

In the salivary epithelium, cells bind to neighboring cells via tight junctions and anchoring junctions such as adherens junctions and desmosomes. Tight junctions are located in the uppermost region of the lateral plasma membrane and include transmembrane proteins claudins and occludins and anchoring protein zonula occludens-1 (ZO-1) [22, 23]. The intermembrane barrier created by tight junctions maintains cell polarity and establishes transepithelial ion gradients by preventing the lateral diffusion of membrane proteins between the apical and basolateral membrane domains and prohibits the free movement of ions through the paracellular space [16, 22–24]. Adherens junctions provide the gland with mechanical support by connecting the actin belts of neighboring epithelial cells. These junctions are located below tight junctions on the lateral plasma membrane and contain the transmembrane protein E-cadherin and anchoring proteins catenins, α-actinin, and vinculin.

Cell polarity is controlled by evolutionarily conserved complexes, which include the PAR complex, Crumbs complex, and the Scribble complex, all of which are asymmetrically localized to specific areas of the cell membrane. Cell polarization initiates with E-cadherin dimerization of two adjacent epithelial cells and is subsequently followed by the recruitment of adherens junction, tight junction, and cell polarity proteins including the partitioning defective (PAR) complex and the activation of Rho GTPases needed for downstream signaling [25, 26]. BM components also promote cell polarity by providing binding sites for cell surface receptor β_1-integrin, leading to the activation of Rho GTPase RAC1 [27]. Consequently, the cell undergoes cytoskeletal reorganization and organelle positioning required for the differentiation of cells into a secretory epithelial phenotype [28]. The PAR complex assembled from Ser/Thr kinase atypical protein kinase C (aPKC), PAR-3, and PAR-6 is localized to the apical membrane where it inhibits the diffusion of basolateral proteins into the apical domain [16]. T-cell-lymphoma invasion and metastasis-1 (TIAM1) associates with both RAC1-GTP and PAR-3, enabling the activation of aPKC, which can then phosphorylate downstream targets and lead to tight junction formation and apicobasal polarization. The PAR complex and PAR-1b kinase are essential for cell polarity establishment. Through mutual exclusion, the PAR complex and PAR-1b remain localized to and define the apical and basolateral membrane, respectively. PAR-1b kinase activity promotes the proper positioning of laminin in the BM by restricting the localization of laminin receptors (i.e., dystroglycan complex) to the basolateral membrane [29, 30]. Recent studies indicate that Rho-associated coiled-coil-containing kinase 1 (ROCK-1) directs BM positioning and controls cell polarity by regulating PAR-1b kinase activity in developing mouse submandibular glands [31]. Specifically, ROCK-1 promotes PAR-1b activity in the outer epithelial cells responsible for BM production but inhibits PAR-1b activity in the epithelial cells located within the salivary epithelial bud.

As with the PAR complex, the evolutionarily conserved Crumbs protein complex acts as an apical determinant in polarized epithelial cells. The Crumbs protein complex is composed of transmembrane protein Crumbs and scaffolding proteins associated with LIN-7-1 (PALS1) and PALS1-associated tight junction protein (PATJ). Crosstalk between the Crumbs complex and Cdc42 is involved in maintaining tight junctions, but may not be needed to establish them [16, 32]. The Scribble complex is localized in the basolateral domain and comprises Scribble, discs large (DLG), and lethal giant larvae (LGL). There is mutual exclusion of the Scribble complex and apical domain complexes, mediated by phosphorylation of LGL by aPKC, which is crucial for cell polarity in epithelial cells.

Cell Organization and Differentiation in Developing Glands

In vitro salivary gland models must recapitulate the natural *in vivo* tissue organization to accurately study the biology of the gland and be suitable for testing diagnostics. During salivary gland development, intercalated duct cells are believed to be stem cells of ductal, acinar, and myoepithelial cell types [33–35]. A salivary gland regeneration model would allow the assessment of salivary cell phenotype retention, including changes in differentiation status and progenitor-like phenotypes. Markers that are commonly associated with development and with a progenitor state include c-Kit, cytokeratin-5, and Sca-1 (in rodents) [36]. Our lab has seen that human salivary acinar-like cells (HSACs) with these and other markers have an extended proliferation ability *in vitro* compared to typical primary cells. A model using progenitor-like salivary cells can illustrate the pathways associated with the cytodifferentiation of salivary cells or the transdifferentiation of cell types.

Salivary gland development initiates with the ectodermal epithelium thickening into a prebud at embryonic day (E) 11.5 [10]. Interaction with the neighboring neural crest-derived mesenchyme is important for prebud elongation into an initial bud [37–39]. The epithelium at the base of the gland invaginates during bud elongation and becomes the duct at E12.5. Branching morphogenesis of the initial bud begins during the pseudoglandular stage at E13.5–14.5. Branching morphogenesis is the reiterated cycle that epithelial tubes undergo during development to generate multilobed glandular organs. The growing buds secrete matrix metalloproteases to degrade the ECM and allow the elongation of the bud [37]. The surrounding ECM promotes the growth of bud epithelial cells by acting as a reservoir of cytokines and growth factors, which are released when the ECM is degraded. Studies have shown that the interaction between the gland epithelium and the mesenchyme capsule is crucial for the proper branching morphogenesis of the submandibular gland (SMG) and the organization of nerve fibers *in vitro* [39]. During the canalicular stage at E15.5, the gland continues to branch, and the ducts begin to develop lumens due to increased apoptosis of the central cells, which lack ECM signals. The terminal bud stage consists of the cytodifferentiation of the pro-acinar cells into the acinar phenotype and completion of lumen formation throughout the gland. E-cadherin and β-catenin, along with the Rho GTPases, play a key role in establishing and maintaining cell polarity during the cytodifferentiation stage of gland development, which is necessary for creating all the cell types present in a salivary glandular unit [16, 40].

Innervation and Vascularization in Gland Development

Innervation During Gland Development

Innervation of salivary glands is crucial for stimulating the secretion of saliva on demand. As previously mentioned, salivary components are produced and secreted by acinar cells located at the terminal buds. With the help of contractile myoepithelial cells surrounding the acini, saliva travels unidirectionally through the intralobular and interlobular ducts, during which saliva is continuously modified until reaching the oral cavity [22]. Saliva secretion is stimulated by the autonomic nervous system, including both the parasympathetic nervous system (PNS) and the sympathetic nervous system (SNS).

Stimulation by the PNS leads to copious fluid secretion, whereas stimulation by the SNS leads to a protein-rich secretion. Muscarinic receptors on acinar cells are activated by neurotransmitters, such as acetylcholine, which lead to the activation of IP3 and DAG pathways [41]. Subsequently, IP3-specific Ca^{2+} channels on the endoplasmic reticulum are opened, allowing the rapid release of Ca^{2+} into the cytoplasm. Binding of calcium to the apical Cl^- and basal K^+ channels leads to a transepithelial potential difference that drives the paracellular movement of Na^+ and fluid from the interstitium into the lumen. Saliva then travels through the ductal lumen and is modified via reabsorption of Na^+ and Cl^- and addition of $KHCO_3$, resulting in a hypotonic solution. Protein secretion, however, is largely stimulated by sympathetic innervation. Sympathetic ganglions release norepinephrine, which binds to the β-adrenergic receptors present on the basal membrane of acinar cells. Activation of β-adrenergic receptors leads to the activation of a G protein, and that activated G protein activates adenylate cyclase and enables the conversion of ATP into cAMP. Consequently, cAMP-dependent protein kinase A (PKA) is activated and leads to the exocytosis of proteins present in saliva [42].

Nerve Appearance During Development and Influence on Gland Development

The autonomic ganglia are part of the neural crest cell-derived mesenchyme and are crucial for the proper development of the salivary gland. During the development of the parotid gland, the initial bud continues elongating until it has been innervated by otic postganglionic fibers [13]. Preganglionic nerves originate from the inferior salivatory nucleus in the brain stem and travel via the glossopharyngeal nerve (cranial nerve IX) to synapse at the otic ganglion [13]. Otic postganglionic nerve fibers travel by way of the auriculotemporal nerve of cranial nerve V to reach the parotid initial bud, which then undergoes branching morphogenesis. Proper parasympathetic gangliogenesis of the SMG requires an interaction between the developing gland and postganglionic fibers; thus, innervation occurs in conjunction with development [13]. Preganglionic nerve fibers are derived from the superior salivatory nucleus, and they travel to the facial nerve (cranial nerve VII) where they branch off with the chorda tympani nerve. The chorda tympani nerves travel with the lingual nerves until reaching the submandibular ganglion. The SMG and sublingual gland are subsequently innervated by postganglionic fibers derived from the submandibular ganglion. The glial cell-derived neurotrophin factor (GDNF) family (including GDNF, neurturin, artemin, and persephin) plays important roles in the development of the parasympathetic nerve fibers [13, 43]. In particular, the interaction between neurturin and its receptor GDNF family receptor alpha 2 (GFRα2) is crucial for maintaining parasympathetic innervation of the salivary glands [43, 44].

Sympathetic preganglionic fibers originate from the thoracic ganglion and travel through the spinal cord via the paravertebral sympathetic trunk to the superior cervical ganglion [13]. Sympathetic postganglionic nerve fibers from the superior cervical ganglion use the external carotid artery and blood vessels for guidance to the salivary glands, and this innervation seems to occur perinatally. The neurotrophin nerve growth factor is crucial for the abundant sympathetic innervation of the parotid and submandibular salivary glands and is essential for neuronal survival [41, 45]. The sublingual gland lacks expression of neurotrophin, which may explain the presence of sympathetic innervation in that gland when compared to the other major glands. Both parasympathetic and sympathetic postganglionic nerve fibers align into bundles along with guiding Schwann cells until reaching their target cells [46]. Sympathetic innervation is associated with the differentiation of pro-acinar cells and ductal cell precursors into mature acinar and ductal cells, respectively, and thus is crucial for the proper development of salivary glands [41, 45–47]. Also, sympathetic postganglionic nerve fibers are vital for maintaining a functional salivary gland, as shown by sympathetic denervation studies, which lead to a reduction in the weight of the parotid gland, decreased production of proline-rich proteins, and gland hyperplasia [48, 49].

An *in vitro* model of salivary gland cells cocultured with nerve cells would be beneficial for the study of the molecular interactions between salivary gland cells and nerves required for the development of the gland and for proper innervation or for testing drugs targeting these pathways. A recent study showed that neurturin is essential for survival of parasympathetic ganglia in isolated, irradiation-treated SMGs and for the maintenance of a progenitor cell population in the gland [15]. Therefore, a biological model could help illustrate the signaling mechanisms important for neuronal survival after irradiation treatment. Because the innervation of salivary glands plays a major role in the composition and quantity of salivary secretion, it is important to understand all of the interactions between nerves and salivary glands associated with functional and diseased salivary glands. Understanding these interactions could more accurately lead to biomarker discoveries that are essential to salivary diagnostics.

Vasculature During Development and Influence on Gland Development

The salivary gland is surrounded by a dense network of blood vessels that delivers oxygen to salivary cells, removes cellular waste, and provides the gland with the large supply of fluid needed for saliva [41, 50, 51]. The salivary glands are vascularized through angiogenesis or the formation of blood vessels through proliferation and migration of endothelial cells from preformed arteries [51]. Vascular endothelial growth factor (VEGF) is expressed by hypoxic cells to stimulate endothelial proliferation and migration and ultimately the angiogenesis of tissues. The parotid gland is vascularized by the external carotid artery and its branches [52]. Branches of facial and lingual arteries supply the submandibular gland with blood. Finally, the sublingual gland is vascularized by the sublingual and submental arteries. Blood vessels are innervated by both parasympathetic and sympathetic nerve fibers that stimulate vasodilation and vasoconstriction, respectively. Parasympathetically stimulated vasodilation is part of the salivary reflex and is mediated by vasoactive intestinal peptide, acetylcholine, and nitric oxide [13, 41, 50, 53].

Salivary gland vasculature is essential for the development and tissue-specific function of the salivary glands by providing essential nutrients for growth, removing cellular waste, providing fluids for salivary secretion, and influencing the innervation of the glands. Therefore, there is a need to better understand the influence of vascularization on gland development, function, and disease. One important aspect that can be further studied is the signaling involved in the close interaction between vasculature and nerve fibers observed in salivary glands. For example, postganglionic nerve fibers derived from the superior cervical ganglion travel along external carotid arteries and innervate the salivary glands [51]. Artemin, a GDNF, is expressed by smooth muscle cells surrounding blood vessels and seems to play a role in guiding axons along the vessels, but needs to be further studied [51]. Also, the mechanism used by nerves to establish connections with blood vessels or continue extending until reaching other target tissue remains unknown. Another aspect that should be further investigated is the role that vasculature present in the mesenchyme capsule plays on the thickening of the salivary epithelium during early development. The involvement of vasculature on gland development and even gland physiology can be addressed by establishing coculture models of endothelial cells and salivary cells/glands [11].

Building Complex Multicellular Models for Ex Vivo Study

While some of the features described previously are unique to the salivary gland, most aspects of salivary architecture can be found in other similar tissues. This validates the utility of the salivary gland in studying other, less accessible secretory systems, but also suggests that advances in biological models of other systems can be reap-

plied to enhance salivary models. In the following section, we review select models and methods from other tissues, as well as some efforts to build salivary-like structures.

Models of Organogenesis and Disease

In vitro biological studies of organogenesis, tissue-specific functions, and disease are performed more accurately with the use of 3D culture systems. Both traditional organ cultures and more recent tissue-engineered alternatives are vehicles to more accurately recapitulate *in vivo* organization at a cellular and tissue level. Physiologically relevant models enable the biological study of organs, including cellular pathways and cell-ECM interactions, and provide a platform for better diagnostics and discoveries of new therapeutics. Tissue-specific functions and cellular interactions within organs have been studied with many well-established, historical models.

Tissue Recombination Model in the Renal Capsule

In the renal capsule model, developed through multiple publications by Cunha and coworkers, embryonic rudiments are grown and adult tissues are maintained *in vivo* by implanting them under the renal capsule of immunocompromised hosts. The renal capsule is a thin layer of fibrous connective tissue, composed of elastin and collagen, that surrounds the kidney. The kidneys are highly vascularized organs, leading to an almost perfect take rate of grafts. For example, low-grade human prostate cancer (PCa) cells implanted under the renal capsule have an increased take rate when compared to subcutaneously implanted PCa cells [54]. Cunha's renal capsule model has enabled the establishment of human prostate epithelium and mammary gland xenografts, among other tissues [54, 55]. Subrenal capsule grafting of patient-derived prostate cancer tissue in nonobese diabetic/severe combined immunodeficient (NOD/SCID) mice has yielded a metastatic prostate cancer model that has become a useful tool for studying the cellular mechanisms involved in metastasis [56].

The defining series of early studies with this model described the reciprocal interaction between the epithelium and mesenchyme in the urogenital sinus (UGS) [57]. Crosstalk between the UGE and UGM enables the full differentiation of each into epithelial and stromal components, and the details of this interaction were obtained by separating the two layers from the UGS and demonstrating their inability to fully mature without interaction from the other layer. Subsequent studies examined recombination of heterotypic mesenchyme/epithelial sources and delineated the organ-specific factors that were required for prostatic development. Additionally, Cunha's renal capsule model enabled the growth of tissues from lethal knockout models, allowing the study of any knockout phenotype that would otherwise not be observable. In short, the tissue recombination model in the renal capsule provides a highly vascularized environment and, ultimately, yields a model to study the biological mechanisms of disease and organ development *in vivo*. Observations of epithelial-mesenchymal interaction have translated to tissue-engineered systems and have been implemented in similar recombination experiments for the salivary gland.

Ex Vivo Organ Culture of Embryonic SMG

An earlier, but similar, model, using organ culture of embryonic mouse submandibular glands, has enabled complex evaluations of gland development, particularly the evolution of branched structures during these early timepoints in development. Pioneering studies described the method and utility of the techniques, notably the selective removal, exchange, or modification of the mesenchyme and epithelial buds, to identify participant "diffusible and nondiffusible components of inductive processes" that influence the eventual organ morphology [58, 59]. These same methods were extended by multiple investigators to studies in other organ systems, such as the lung, liver, pancreas, mammary gland, and kidney (e.g., [60, 61]). Recent studies in the salivary gland using such methods identified the contribution of multiple signaling molecules—including fibroblast growth factors and their receptors and PI3K—to branching morphogenesis [62, 63].

Important contributions from the ECM have also been demonstrated (e.g., fibronectin deposition at branching points during cleft formation) [64], and most recently, an essential neuronal-epithelial interaction has been shown to guide the maturation of the embryonic progenitors into mature organs [15, 65].

Salivary Cells Grown on Matrigel as a Biological Model

Human submandibular gland (HSG)-derived cell line has been cultured on Matrigel® for the use of a biological model to study morphogenesis, salivary acinar cell formation, cytodifferentiation, gene expression, and physiology of the gland [66]. This method of culturing HSG cells is purely for the purpose of performing biological studies because Matrigel® is tumor derived and thus cannot be used for regenerative therapy. HSG cells grown on Matrigel® form polarized spherical acini-like structures with decreased cell proliferation and increased apoptosis in the lumen. Incorporation of Matrigel® in culture conditions led to an increased expression of acinar cell proteins such as α-amylase, aquaporin-5 (AQ5), cytokeratins, and mucin-1; however, this increased expression was not associated with an increase in transcription. Therefore, the mechanism responsible for increasing the production of acinar cell proteins by HSG cells cultured on Matrigel® and the direction of α-amylase secretion needs to be further studied. In the native organ, α-amylase and fluid secretion must be directed into the lumen of the acinus so that it can subsequently travel unidirectionally through the ductal network until reaching the oral cavity. Additionally, HSG cells grown on this BM-like gel had decreased expression of vimentin, an intermediate filament expressed by undifferentiated salivary acinar cells in early development, and increased expression of cytokeratin, suggesting that Matrigel® drives the differentiation of salivary cells into a keratinocyte phenotype [66, 67]. This model may be useful for the study of differentiation from a progenitor-like cell into mature acinar-phenotype cells, as the HSG cells positively expressed progenitor/stem cell biomarkers CD44 and CD166. In summary, HSG cells or other human salivary gland-derived cells cultured in Matrigel® may serve as a 3D biological model to help elucidate the importance of BM components on the proper differentiation and organization of salivary cells, especially salivary acinar cells.

Examples from Other Tissue Systems in 3D

The mammary glands share many similarities with the salivary glands in terms of tissue architecture. Similar to the salivary gland, a highly branched ductal network connects the lobular secretory acini structures, while myoepithelial cells wrap around these acini lobules [68–70]. BM-rich 3D cultures of mammary gland cells have proven to be instrumental in their functional differentiation as noted by increases in production and secretion of milk proteins [70]. The importance of the mesenchyme also was revealed by tissue recombination experiments that led to cytodifferentiation and organization of the mammary epithelium [71].

The role of myoepithelial cells is poorly defined in the salivary gland literature. Studies involving the coculture of mammary acinar cells with myoepithelial cells have reported a differentiated and polarized acinus structure. Breast myoepithelial cells also secrete laminin, which can aid in the differentiation of acinar cells [72–75]. Clues from the mammary literature may help us better define the function of salivary myoepithelial cells and their possible involvement in establishing polarity in salivary acini, which is an essential requirement of secretory epithelia.

Researchers investigating epithelial organization into acini in 3D have been guided primarily by the efforts of the community of breast cancer investigators [76]. In one example, Ampuja and coworkers demonstrated acinus formation of the MCF-10A breast cell line in Matrigel®, with proper localization of integrin receptors at the apical surface of the structure [77]. In contrast, these same cells cultured in PEG-based hydrogels showed poor acinus formation and disorganized integrin expression. A recent comparison of three biomaterial models demonstrated the impact of elastic modulus on acinus formation

for human mammary gland cells [78]. Miroshnikova compared SAPs, assembled at both soft and stiff moduli, to similar Matrigel® matrices, and found that the stiffer SAPs could replicate the phenotype of a disorganized, invasive structure. The salivary community has benefited significantly from epithelium-mesenchyme recombination models also, which provide a 3D system for interrogating both soluble cell signals and physical interaction between these components during gland development.

Approaches for Tissue Engineering of an Artificial Salivary Gland

Glandular tissue engineering can be approached in two ways: The first is to isolate all necessary cell types and reengineer a model that will contain each of the distinct cues needed to make a gland, while the second approach is to regenerate the gland using glandular progenitor cells that can be transplanted into damaged glands or can be manipulated *in vitro* with the correct cues to reassemble into a functional, morphologically accurate glandular unit. Several groups in the past have worked with cell lines or primary cells in an attempt to seize the first approach. Neoplastic epithelial cell lines such as the HSY, HSG, SMIE, and RSMT-A5 have been used by a few groups for *in vitro* studies but remain questionable for use *in vivo* due to their tumorigenic background [79]. SMG C6 and SMG-C10 [80, 81], which are immortalized rat submandibular acinar cell lines capable of responding to muscarinic and β-adrenergic agonists, and Par-C10 and Par-C5 [82–85], which are immortalized rat parotid cell lines, capable of forming TJs, microvilli, and secretory granules but lack amylase expression [79, 86], are better models that display significant functionality. Work with primary human salivary gland cells has shown much promise for engineering artificial glands. Szlavik et al., Joraku et al., and Pradhan-Bhatt et al. have reported formation of spheroids in 3D, formation of tight junctions, and production of amylase [5, 6, 8, 87, 88]. Pradhan-Bhatt et al. have also reported response to neurotransmitter agonists and preservation and biomarker retention by

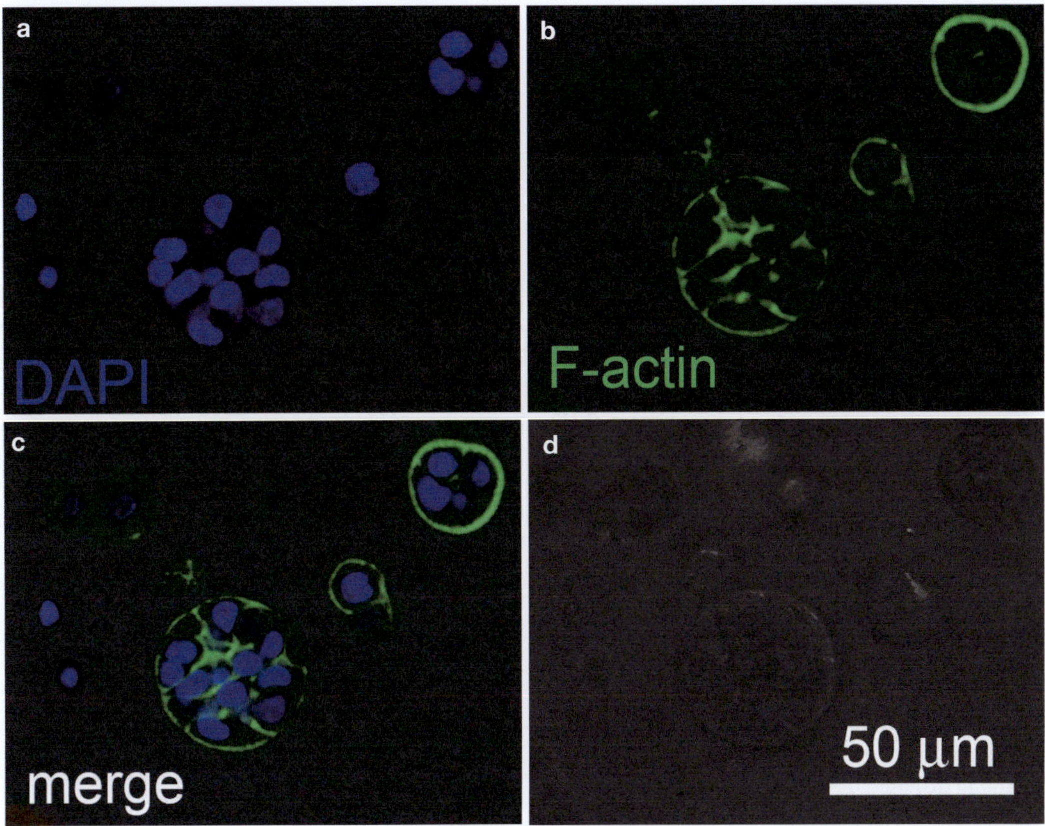

Fig. 8.1 Primary HSACs encapsulated in HA hydrogel. Single acinar cells are encapsulated and grown over 5 days to form multicellular spheroids indicated by (a) nuclear staining and delineated by (b) filamentous actin staining. (c) Confocal micrograph of merged image and (d) DIC image of the hydrogel

acini-like spheroids *in vivo* [7, 8]. One example from our team is shown in Fig. 8.1, a confocal microscopy image of primary HSACs, cultured in a 3D hyaluronic acid-based hydrogel (HyStem® from BioTime).

The use of progenitor cells poses as an attractive model for regenerating glandular tissue. Work by Knox et al., Nanduri et al., Kishi et al., and Lombaert et al. has shown much promise in this field [15, 89–92]. Transcription factors Ascl3 and Sox2, structural protein K5, and stem cell growth factor receptor c-kit have been used to identify progenitor and stem cell populations. Lombaert et al.'s report on the ability of a small population of c-kit-positive cells to rescue salivary gland morphology and function in irradiation glands has led the way to the possibility of successful stem cell therapy [90]. These studies can lead us to a combination approach where stem/progenitor marker-expressing cells are combined with just the correct bioactive scaffold that can be used to generate glands *in vitro*.

Efforts to Implement Vasculature and Innervation in a Tissue-Engineered Gland

One of the major challenges in tissue engineering is avoiding necrosis of implanted tissue. In order to ensure adequate nutrient flow to the engineered tissue, vascular supply is essential [93].

To overcome this problem, several strategies including overexpression of the angiogenic factor vascular endothelial growth factor (VEGF), incorporation of VEGF in engineered implants, or controlled release of VEGF from bioactive scaffolds have been sought [93–96]. Recent studies have suggested inclusion of mesenchymal stem cells to improve vascularization of tissues. Additionally, mesenchymal stem cells seeded in 3D environments form spheroid aggregates that have been found to secrete increased levels of VEGF and FGF-2 [93, 97].

Salivary fluid secretion is stimulated upon the binding of acetylcholine, a muscarinic agonist, which is released by parasympathetic nerves. Similarly, salivary protein secretion is dependent on the binding of β-adrenergic agonists, which are released by the sympathetic nerves [8, 13, 98]. Inclusion of the nerve growth factor (NGF), a neurotrophin, into implanted scaffolds has shown promise in nerve regeneration [99]. Complete functionality of salivary gland tissue cannot be achieved without adequate innervation of the engineered glands.

Modeling Salivary Gland Disorders

Studying disease-associated mechanisms is crucial for advancement toward generating new treatment, cures, and diagnostic tools for disease. Specifically, studying diseased tissues can yield new biomarkers for disease, or validate currently existing ones, and ultimately advance the establishment of accurate diagnostic tools. Salivary diagnostic tools would be a more feasible, economical, and accessible form of monitoring the patient's health. Diagnostic exams could be performed in the comfort of one's home due to how easy it is to collect saliva without the use of needles. However, in order to establish salivary diagnostic tools as the platform for monitoring health status, biomarkers must be adequately validated, and biomarker information must be easily accessible to all [100].

Biological models of diseased salivary gland tissue can be an available tool that can provide useful information on salivary gland diseases such as Sjögren's syndrome, radiation-affected glands, salivary gland cancers, and the like. An *in vitro* model of Sjögren's syndrome, an autoimmune disease in which your body's immune system attacks the lacrimal and salivary glands, could be accomplished by isolating healthy salivary acinar cells, growing them in an *in vitro* system, and comparing salivary secretions from before and after coculturing with lymphocytes or treatment with an immune system product in

question [101]. Such a model would be beneficial for studying the associated mechanisms because of the ability to control the added immune system products and more precisely measure an outcome. For example, this model could be used to further investigate the role of TGF-β (beta) in preventing autoimmune responses by suppressing proliferation and differentiation of lymphocytes [102]. Once an *in vitro* model is established, treatments could be tested *in vitro* before investing in *in vivo* animal models.

The effects of irradiation therapy on salivary glands can also be studied using an *in vitro* model. Approximately 40,000 head and neck cancer patients suffer from radiation-induced xerostomia every year [103]. Chemoradiation of head and neck cancers leads to a significant reduction in acinar cells, ductal metaplasia, and fibrosis [104]. The mechanism in which radiation therapy causes acinar cell loss needs to be further investigated. Furthermore, an *in vitro* salivary gland model could be used as a method to study radiation-induced effects on acinar cells and discover possible effective treatments.

Three-dimensional tissue culture systems also allow for the ex vivo growth of salivary gland tumor specimens and the study of the mechanisms associated with salivary gland cancers. The majority of tumors affecting the major salivary glands are benign and include pleomorphic adenomas and Warthin's tumor. Malignant tumors are rare in salivary glands and mostly affect people over the age of 60; these include mucoepidermoid carcinoma, adenocarcinoma, squamous cell carcinoma, malignant mixed tumors, adenoid cystic carcinoma, and acinic cystic carcinoma. Salivary gland tumor models would be extremely beneficial in discovering and characterizing new biomarkers for diagnostic use.

Modern Implementation of 3D Culture Systems

Salivary diagnostic platforms can be considered from multiple perspectives of the complete native gland system. Salivary secretions (i.e., saliva) may contain biomarkers that reflect an organism's health. *In vivo* interrogation of a living tissue (through live microscopy or other means) may yield information on tissue structure or permit the targeted collection of cells or biological materials. *In vitro* culture of salivary cell lines enables researchers to observe cell structure and behavior and assess cell response (e.g., protein/gene expression). Beyond all of these existing methods, 3D culture of salivary cells and tissues enables in situ access to the developing and functioning gland while promising a richer level of understanding of gland responses to environmental changes, e.g., drugs, altered extracellular matrix, or introduction of genes for targeted expression of necessary proteins.

The accuracy of salivary gland models relies on the replication of necessary minimal features of each element of the native gland. Cells can be cultured in 3D spheroids, but will require some surrogate of the ECM in order to receive and respond to the same mechanical and biological cues experienced by an intact gland. In the same way, an ECM system with high fidelity to native tissue requires a cell line (or primary cells) with accurate representation of *in vivo* phenotypes and likely also requires a mixture of multiple cell types, in proper ratio and geometry.

These same issues are fundamental to the broader field of tissue engineering and regenerative medicine, and advances in these fields can benefit similar efforts at advancing 3D salivary diagnostics models. The following sections will consider each element of the traditional tissue engineering model (ECM support and cell source), with a focus on their use *in vitro*.

Hydrogels Versus Microporous Scaffolds

Numerous reviews have documented the historical path of today's tissue engineering [105–109]. As researchers from the polymer and plastic communities intersected with colleagues in the clinical and biological disciplines, polymer engineers sought to mimic native ECM structures using existing polymeric materials. The key advances in this effort were the transitions from *biocompatible* to *bioinert* to *biodegradable* materials. Poly(α-esters), such as poly(glycolic acid) (PGA) and poly(lactic acid) (PLA) and their copolymers (PLGA), were primary entry points for nascent tissue engineers, since these offered physical properties similar to other common thermoplastics, but with degradation profiles that enabled the potential reentry of soluble hydrolysis products back into the cell cycle. The relative strength of these degradable plastics allowed them to be implemented in a manner similar to other thermoplastics; i.e., they could be extruded into fibers and woven into fabrics, as in Fig. 8.2, cast from organic solvent into complex structures or molded with sacrificial microparticles ("porogens") into microporous assemblies. These structures continue to find use in numerous tissue engineering applications, particularly in the regeneration of load-bearing musculoskeletal systems or in tissues with high native structural requirements.

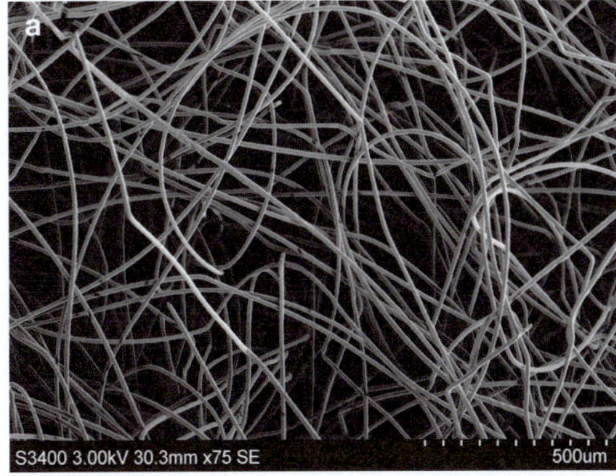
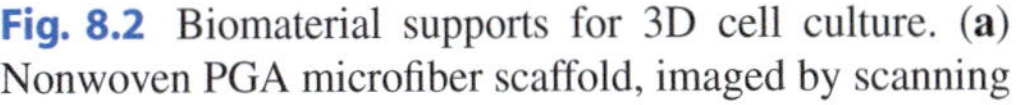

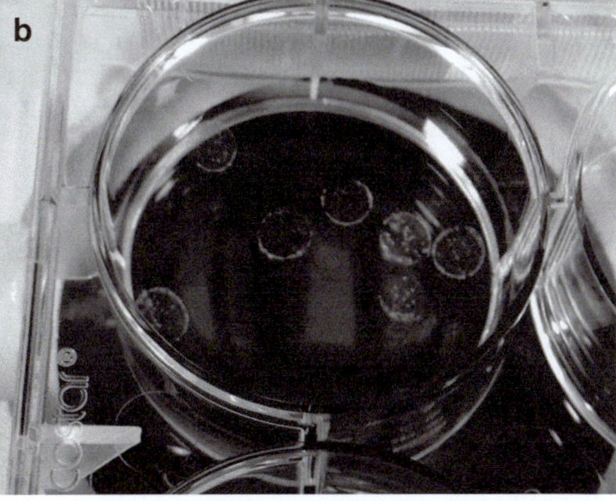

Fig. 8.2 Biomaterial supports for 3D cell culture. (**a**) Nonwoven PGA microfiber scaffold, imaged by scanning electron microscopy. (**b**) Hyaluronic acid polymer hydrogels, cast into discs 6 mm in diameter

However, a significant issue with these microporous scaffolds is that the polymer only mimics the *concept* of a 3D ECM, but not necessarily the mechanical, biological, or diffusive properties of the native 3D matrix. Polymer matrices such as PGA and PLA are orders of magnitude stiffer than the native ECM and prohibit the diffusion of important cell metabolites and signaling molecules—everything from oxygen to growth factors—across their boundary. Investigators soon discovered that *interconnected* pores were required for cell seeding and growth, since this would be the only path to allow cell-cell contact with other pores and (in the absence of vascularization) sufficient nutrient penetration into the core of a scaffold. While microporous scaffolds resemble 3D tissue structure, in many ways cells on these scaffolds experience a compact 2D structure, on an unnaturally stiff substrate. However, investigators continue to invent novel applications for these materials in modeling salivary structure and influencing salivary cell assembly, such as a recent description of micropatterned "craters" used to encourage acinar cell arrangement [110]. Electrospun solutions of PLGA in hexafluoroisopropanol (HFIP) yielded nanofibers in the range of 50–150 nm, which could be collected as a mat and molded to reproduce the pattern of microscale craters. These nanofibers, on the order of 100× smaller than conventional PGA microfibers, can better reproduce the native ECM and yield an improved application of this well-characterized biodegradable polymer.

In contrast, the modern hydrogel system employs an alternate 3D concept by using inherently hydrophilic molecules (either polymeric or small molecules) that can be triggered to surround and encapsulate cells fully, within a cross-linked network swollen with water. The triggers for gelation may be reversible (such as the use of Ca^{2+}, in the case of alginates and self-assembling peptides) or permanent covalent cross-links (through complementary reactive groups on adjacent polymer chains or through the use of a photocatalyst to initiate covalent cross-linking among chains). Microporous scaffolds employ pore sizes on the scale of 50–500 μm, to enable cell penetration during seeding; in contrast, hydrogel pore sizes are nearly three orders of magnitude lower in typical use—small enough that the diffusion of even some large proteins may be retarded.

For the replication of soft tissues, hydrogel scaffolds present a contrasting replication of two major elements of the native ECM:

Mechanical Properties

Numerous recent studies have demonstrated that a scaffold's mechanical properties are paramount to influencing the phenotype of the cells encapsulated within [111]. Cells sense and respond to their physical environment through multiple mechanisms, many of which are still being discovered. The assembly of integrin receptors into focal adhesions is a classic phenomenon of 2D culture on glass or tissue culture polystyrene substrates, and that behavior translates to cell attachment onto PLA/PGA microporous scaffolds. Such focal adhesions convey substrate stiffness through the cytoskeletal network, and additional intracellular signaling occurs through the proteins assembled at a focal adhesion structure. However, this behavior changes significantly when cells are fully encapsulated in a 3D hydrogel matrix [112] since moduli in the range of 100–1,000 Pa are most common for non-muscle soft tissues. The reduced stiffness of hydrogel matrices alters the size, frequency, and localization of focal adhesion plaques, as well as the arrangement of actin filaments, and these impact cell phenotype. Numerous reports have linked the abnormal expression of signaling proteins and cytoskeletal focal adhesions to a nonphysiological culture environment [113–115].

Swift et al. have recently examined a range of tissues, spanning nervous tissue to muscle to osteochondral tissues, and demonstrated a shift in the ratio of lamin isoforms (specifically lamin A to lamin B ratios) as a function of ECM modulus [116]. Lamins are present in the nuclear membrane of each cell, and the balance of isotypes influences nuclear membrane stiffness. As described by Swift, however, these proteins also affect transcription and enhance the lineage direction of cells. This example is only the most recent in a series of significant publications by Discher and coworkers, regarding the impact of substrate modulus on cell differentiation and its correlation to cytoskeletal components and nuclear mechanics [111, 117, 118].

Diffusion of Soluble Components

The diffusion of small molecules and growth factors through a tissue is regulated largely by the molecule's size, its molecular characteristics (e.g., hydrophilicity, charge), and its interaction with other ECM components. While such molecules do not pass through tissues unimpeded, their diffusion through fields of ECM components is possible due to the aqueous nature of body tissues. (Cartilage, a nearly avascular tissue, is an example of how nutrients and metabolites can be delivered via diffusion in aqueous networks.) Hydrogels and microporous scaffolds represent opposite extremes of this model: While microporous scaffolds with interconnected pores permit fluid flow across open interpore channels, cells may still remain isolated by largely impermeable walls that prevent contact between cells on opposite sides. Conversely, the open, swollen network structure of a hydrogel enables the diffusion of soluble molecules throughout the system, which then permits paracrine interaction among encapsulated cells. At low cell densities, this open network may reflect the opposite extreme, representing the lowest possible inhibition of nutrient diffusion. Under typical use, however, the hydrogel model best mimics the native ECM structure and function.

A third element of the native ECM has been implemented to varying degrees on hydrogel and macroporous scaffolds:

Biologically Relevant Native Epitopes

This group represents the set of minimal ECM features that have been identified as crucial to cell survival, migration, organization, or differentiation. Generally, these features are categorized as:

- *ECM Adhesion Sequences*: Minimal peptide sequences, particularly the RGDS sequence identified from fibronectin [119, 120], have been shown to promote integrin-based adhesion, which is crucial for many tissue-engineered model systems. Although intact adhesion-promoting proteins will quickly adsorb onto most scaffolds from fetal bovine serum in cell culture media, numerous applications require the deliberate integration of these sequences into or onto a scaffold.

- *Cell-Degradable Sequences*: Cell migration through the native ECM is mediated by the cell's toolbox of proteases and glycosidases. For *in vitro* applications using a non-proteinaceous scaffold material, investigators requiring cell migration must "build in" labile sites that are susceptible to the cell's inherent degradative enzymes. Matrix metalloproteinases (MMPs) have been well characterized, and numerous minimal substrate sequences have been identified (e.g., GPQG↓IAGQ, derived from collagen I) [121], which can be synthesized chemically and integrated into or onto a biomaterial. A classic example of synthetic PEG hydrogels, rendered susceptible to MMP degradation through the incorporation of an MMP substrate, was described by Lutolf et al. [122].

- *Polysaccharides*: This diverse class of macromolecules often influences cell behavior indirectly in the ECM, by either enabling or resisting the retention of proteins. Heparan sulfate oligomers, for example, may serve as depots for potent heparin-binding growth factors; conversely, heparin may be tethered to biomaterial surfaces to reduce clotting.

- *Cell Adhesion Molecule Mimics*: Many cells rely on cell-cell adhesion molecules (CAMs) for orientation and guidance, rather than cell-ECM interactions. Recombinant versions of these proteins or their fragments can be covalently incorporated into/onto 3D scaffolds to encourage the survival or phenotypic arrangement of such cells (e.g., ephA-ephrinA signaling in pancreatic β-cells [123] or ECM components such as perlecan fragments that may resemble CAMs and influence cell behavior in similar ways [6]).

The notable difference between the incorporation of biologically relevant epitopes in microporous scaffolds and hydrogels is a matter of "on" and "in." Such biomolecules can be covalently tethered onto the *surface* of microporous scaffolds through chemical modification of the scaffold surface and thus are typically present as a monolayer or a thin surface layer. Conversely, biorelevant peptides, proteins, and proteoglycans can be incorporated *throughout* a hydrogel, either through covalent attachment in the initial gelation step or simple diffusion into the established network.

A related consequence of these contrasting paradigms is their varying suitability for visual analysis by conventional techniques of confocal microscopy and histologic preparation. In general, hydrogels are sufficiently transparent that encapsulated cells can be observed via light microscopy (phase imaging or DIC), or fluorescence imaging of small molecules (live/dead stains, cell trackers, organelle tracers, etc.) and fluorescent proteins (e.g., GFP fusion proteins), or immunofluorescence, enabling real-time observation of cell response to culture conditions. Confocal microscopy methods enable the detailed reconstruction of cell features in 3D over several hundred microns. Conversely, these methods are difficult or impossible for most microporous scaffolds, since light cannot easily penetrate many common polymers or diffract so heavily that detailed imaging of cellular arrangement or phenotype beyond the exterior layer of a scaffold is obscured. Histologic methods are similarly affected by the scaffold composition; hydrogels with a high water content and low cell density or ECM density are not amenable to standard paraffin embedding, but can be adapted to cryoembedding, microtoming, and staining methods. Microporous polymer scaffolds can be more difficult to adapt to these methods, since standard paraffin embedding reagents may dissolve the most commonly used polymers, and cryomicrotome methods may be more difficult

with the higher stiffness of these scaffold materials. For our present interest in salivary diagnostic techniques, hydrogels are generally more amenable to assessment by conventional imaging methods (discussed in more detail later in this chapter).

Currently Available Biomaterials

Many synthetic materials may be modified with adhesive proteins to encourage cell attachment or promote a specific phenotype within a hydrogel. Collagen and laminin are common choices for this, and some commercial hydrogel kits (e.g., the HyStem series of hyaluronan-based hydrogels) include variations that incorporate proteins toward this purpose. It would be expected that such proteins would alter cell phenotype, given the presence of laminins and collagen IV within the basement membrane surrounding acinar structures. Conversely, other adhesive proteins contain binding sites that could promote a migratory phenotype, rather than a stabilized acinar structure. The details of the protein preparation are crucial, since covalent cross-linking of proteins or peptide fragments into another polymer network often requires chemical modification, and the degree of functionalization, nature of the cross-link chemistry, and steric accessibility will all influence the eventual consistency of the matrix structure. Similarly, specific processing details of these proteins can influence their biological function and their purity. One example of the influencing factors that may affect protein performance from biological perspective was described by Dhimolea et al. [124]. Collagen sourced from two different species (rat and bovine) performed differently in influencing mammary epithelial cell organization and phenotype. This could be attributed to differences in the species-specific sequence of the protein (which should be minimal, as many collagen structures are highly preserved), which could lead to changes in bundle formation, or differences in the protein processing steps, which could also lead to variation in collagen fibril isolation, and reassembly in the final hydrogel. Variations in collagen organization can lead to variations in matrix stiffness, which then influences cell behavior, as described previously.

The biomaterial literature describes numerous laboratories that synthesize traditional and/or custom matrices for the 3D *in vitro* culture of multiple cell types. Bulk biodegradable polymers, such as PGA, PLA, PLGA, poly(ε-caprolactone), and others, are also available commercially through chemical vendors (e.g., Sigma-Aldrich, Polysciences), and methods for creating porogen-leaching microporous scaffolds (most often manufactured using sodium chloride crystals, sieved to a selected size range, as a porogen) are well described in the literature. Similarly, multiple literature reviews describe methods for electrospinning these polymers from solutions in organic solvents into fibrous mats with fine micro- and nanoscale textures. Each of these methods for scaffold synthesis has matured over the past decade, along with complementary and necessary methods for characterization, sterilization, and seeding with cells, and all can be considered available and accessible to any laboratory.

While the majority of matrices used in tissue-engineered applications are polymeric, a unique class of biomaterial considered in this study is the self-assembling peptide (SAP) [125]. SAPs are small peptides that are preprogrammed to assemble into multimolecular hydrogel structures, with one or more levels of spatial organization, usually triggered by temperature, pH, or an ionic gradient. Self-assembled hydrogels often have weaker mechanical properties than polymeric gels, but are well within the desired range for cell encapsulation.

The commercial options for all of these are increasing and offer the benefits of quality control and specified parameters appropriate to each scaffold type (e.g., degradation rate, pore size distribution, cross-linking rate, endotoxin, sterility, etc.). A survey of current commercial options includes the following:

Commercial Microporous Scaffolds:

- *BIOFELT (Biomedical Structures)*—PLA, PGA, and PLGA woven (i.e., resembling a braided fabric) and nonwoven (i.e., random, resembling felt) scaffolds. The choice of polymer will dictate the degradation profile of the scaffold. One of the most common examples of these scaffolds is a nonwoven PGA matrix, with fibers 10–15 μm in diameter and pore sizes >100 μm in size.
- *Alvetex (reinnervate)*—polystyrene microporous scaffold. Although not biodegradable, these microporous scaffolds have an exceptionally open structure with high interpore communication.

Commercial Hydrogel Kits:

- *Matrigel (BD Biosciences)/Cultrex (Trevigen)*—One of the most widely used hydrogel matrices for modeling cell behavior in 3D culture, basement membrane extract (BME), is sold under the trade names of Matrigel and Cultrex as a solution of basement membrane proteins (largely comprising laminin, collagen IV, perlecan, and numerous potent growth factors) isolated from Engelbreth-Holm-Swarm (EHS) mouse sarcoma cells. Multiple formats and preparations of BME are available, including some with reduced growth factor content. While soluble at cold temperatures, BME proteins aggregate irreversibly to form a solid hydrogel structure at room temperature. Most cells adhere readily to BME-coated surfaces and gels.
- *Collagen I (multiple vendors)*—Most frequently derived from rat tail, collagen I gels have seen frequent use as matrices for cell culture, but their applicability to salivary gland models may be limited. Excess collagen I is often associated with specific tissue systems and/or a scar and repair phenotype in a wound response. These cues, along with the slow but persistent contraction of collagen gels, may induce an undesired phenotype in cells that prefer a more compliant tissue.
- *HyStem*—hyaluronic acid (HA)-derived hydrogels. HA from bacterial sources is thiolated at free carboxyl groups along the polymer and cross-linked with PEG-diacrylate. The thiol-acrylate "click"

chemistry proceeds quickly via a Michael addition mechanism, with no by-products and minimal reactivity with the surrounding biological components. Variations of HyStem include a thiolated gelatin component (HyStem-C) that can promote cell adhesion and a thiolated heparin component (HyStem-HP) that can retain heparin-binding growth factors for delayed release. The HyStem system's relevance is due to the pervasive presence of HA in the human body and the expression of HA receptors (RHAMM/CD168 and CD44) by many cells.

- *QGel MT 3D Matrix (QGel)*—PEG-based system, also based on a Michael addition for gelation within 10–20 min of gelation. PEG is an unnatural polymer that is biocompatible, but resists protein adsorption and is nondegradable by most native cell enzymes. QGel systems incorporate pendant RGD moieties, to enable cell adhesion, and integral MMP-degradable peptides, to allow for cell migration through the hydrogel.

- *AlgiMatrix (Life Technologies)*—alginate hydrogel derived from seaweed. Alginates can be purchased in this format, or in bulk, and gelled quickly in cationic solutions (e.g., $CaCl_2$). Encapsulated cells can be quickly released from the matrix (e.g., with EDTA). Alginates provide no sites for integrin-based adhesion by cells and are not easily degraded by cells. However, these systems have found great utility for 3D encapsulation and culture of many cell types (e.g., retention of chondrocyte phenotype, preservation of oocyte viability) and have been modified to include RGD sequences.

- *MAPtrix (Kollodis)*—ECM derived from recombinant mussel adhesive proteins (containing an 18 % lysine content), cross-linked with multiarm PEG-succinimide.

- *PuraMatrix (3D Matrix Medical Technology)*—unlike the other polymeric hydrogel matrices, PuraMatrix is an example of a self-assembling peptide system. The sequences of small peptides are engineered to enable their assembly upon trigger with ionic or pH gradients and form nanoscale structures that entangle to form a hydrogel structure.

The contrasting advantages and disadvantages of the aforementioned matrices—particularly the hydrogel systems—depend on the application. For researchers interested in cell encapsulation with an eventual application in regenerative medicine (i.e., implantation in humans), the animal-derived hydrogel systems (Matrigel/Cultrex, collagen I) are unsuitable, as these would not receive FDA approval for implantation. However, for salivary diagnostic models, particularly *in vitro* use, such protein-based systems may induce the optimal cell response. Researchers may consider some of the other listed materials to meet other criteria, such as cost, ease of use, or more granular control over hydrogel composition. In general, a wide range of biomaterial platforms are available, and only a small subset have been explored in the context of preserving, reconstituting, or analyzing salivary gland structure or function.

In Vitro and *In Vivo* Imaging

Advances in optical imaging hardware and software have increased the depth to which we can explore salivary gland physiology in situ and our ability to resolve objects, even down to the molecular scale. Improvements in fluorescent probe technology enable the detection of specific proteins, molecular processes, and cellular activation over extended length and timescales. Three-dimensional *in vitro* models in transparent hydrogels benefit from advances in both of these fields, particularly due to the longer working distances and multicellular assemblies that are characteristic of these cultures.

Imaging Techniques

Epifluorescence Microscopy

Epifluorescence microscopy uses a mercury or xenon arc lamp to illuminate the specimen or excite fluorophores within a specimen in the ultraviolet (UV) to visible light spectrum. The light is directed to and from the specimen by a series of mirrors and bandpass filters to allow photons of specific wavelengths to reach the eye port and/or camera for detection. Specific fluorophores targeting proteins of interest within a prepared specimen may be excited to emit photons that are detected by the epifluorescence microscope. The fluorescing areas will appear bright against the dark background and may be quantified using post-processing imaging software to determine protein expression and distribution within the specimen. Excited fluorophores undergo a "Stokes shift," in which the emitted light occurs at a longer wavelength (i.e., lower energy) than that of the incident light. Detection filters are therefore set to block the lower excitation wavelength and solely detect the longer emitted wavelength. Epifluorescence microscopy has been a powerful tool for determining protein distributions and live-2D visualization of the onset intercellular signaling using calcium indicators, voltage sensitive dyes, and small molecule fluorescent dye transfer *in vitro* and *in vivo* [126].

Confocal Microscopy

Confocal microscopy is an optical imaging technique that utilizes focused scanning beams of light across a specimen in the UV to visible light spectrum. Lasers are a more powerful light source and are used to excite molecular tracers or targeting fluorophores within a specimen. Emitted photons are collected and detected by sensitive photomultiplier tubes (PMTs) to generate an image. Light scatter within a specimen at these shorter wavelengths is proportionate to the thickness and translucence of the specimen, so it is important to consider these limitations when resolving anatomical or subcellular structures in hydrogel and tissue specimens. Compared to conventional epifluorescence microscopy, spatial resolution in confocal microscopy is considerably higher because of focused light and an adjustable pin hole to reduce photon scatter prior to detection. Sharp image slices may be captured through a specimen at intervals and reconstructed in 3D and are optimal for colocalization studies.

Confocal microscopy may be used to image 2D and 3D cell culture models as well as live animal models where lateral and axial resolution are determined by the excitation wavelength λ_{ex}, numerical aperture NA of the objective lens, and the refractive index n of the immersion medium [127] (see Eqs. 8.1 and 8.2). The refractive index n for air, water, and oil is 1.00, 1.33, and 1.52, respectively.

$$\text{Lateral resolution} = \frac{0.51\lambda_{ex}}{\text{NA}} \quad (8.1)$$

$$\text{Axial resolution} = \frac{0.88\lambda_{ex}}{\left(n - \sqrt{n^2 - NA^2}\right)} \quad (8.2)$$

Motion artifacts from animal respiration and heartbeat pose technical challenges in live imaging but may be overcome [128]. Also, phototoxicity and photobleaching may affect the integrity of the tissue as well as the intensity of fluorophores when imaging over time to create challenges when quantifying responses with respect to fluorescence intensity. Although presented with these challenges, confocal microscopy is still ideal where penetration depths are uniform to the surface to ensure optimal conditions and resolution of subcellular structures. Confocal microscopy has more recently been used to quantitatively determine the effectiveness of mouthwash on the oral flora [129].

Multiphoton Microscopy

This technology is based on nonlinear emissions and can image microstructures and intercellular processes beneath the skin. In this method, a fluorophore with a maximum excitation wavelength of λ_{ex} can be excited by the simultaneous "additive" absorption of two photons, each of a wavelength $2\lambda_{ex}$ (or corresponding energy $E/2$). For example, a fluorophore that normally excites maximally at λ_{ex} ~400 nm and has a maximum emission at λ_{em} ~550 nm can be excited by two coincident photons of λ ~800 nm each. (The excited fluor would still emit maximally at λ_{em} ~550 nm.) A much higher laser density is necessary in order to achieve this coordinated photon absorption, and specialized lasers ("pulsed" or "mode-locked") are required to obtain this high flux.

Although multiphoton microscopy offers no improvement in resolution over conventional confocal microscopy, the method does confer two other significant advantages. First, the use of $2\lambda_{ex}$ wavelengths in the IR range enhances laser penetration into the specimen of interest, since these longer wavelengths are less commonly absorbed by biological tissues. Secondly, the physical nature of multiphoton excitation relies not only on the exact *temporal* coincidence of the two low-energy photons but also a correspondingly high *spatial* focus. To understand the relevance of this idea, consider that, under conventional epifluorescence methods, an entire specimen is illuminated under the filtered light of a xenon/mercury lamp and the fluorescing moieties within a given depth of the focal plane are imaged. Because of this imaging configuration, the entire specimen may be gradually photobleached due to continual exposure to excitation wavelengths. Confocal microscopy offers the advantage of a scanning laser, with a reduced excitation cross section and dwell time, but it still exposes an entire specimen throughout its depth to extended excitation. In contrast to both of these methods, multiphoton excitation occurs solely at a precise point in space within the focal plane, where photon density is sufficiently high and coherent. All other laser light above and below the focal plane has insufficient coincidence to excite any fluorophores or induce any damage from photobleaching. These properties enable extended live imaging of thick *in vitro* samples or *in vivo* carriers with far less possibility of specimen damage.

Imaging intact tissue enables researchers to study biological processes in their native microenvironments and to extract physiologically relevant information. It has allowed researchers to image neuronal activity in brain tissue [130], macrophage motility during tumor cell invasion [131], secretory granule dynamics in salivary gland tissue [132], and Cl⁻ transport in salivary epithelium [133]. Two-photon excitation has been used to "uncage" bioactive compounds to visualize real-time intercellular communication in monolayers of cultured mouse skeletal muscle cells [134] and neuronal synaptic transmission in rat hippocampal slices [135]. Currently, two-photon microscopy is used to study various aspects of cell biology with cellular resolution in live mice under anesthesia [128] as well as in freely mobile rats [136].

Multiphoton microscopy allows for the observation of vascular and neuronal integration of seeded hydrogels implanted in the salivary bed. Longitudinal observations would be useful to track the progression of biological integration. Effects of pharmacological and mechanical perturbations on the system aimed to accelerate and encourage structural incorporation may also be observed with the native microenvironment.

Intensity-Based Imaging Techniques

A multitude of techniques take advantage of the consequential photobleaching of fluorophores in high-resolution, intensity-based imaging to study intercellular and subcellular molecular dynamics. Two well-established techniques are fluorescence recovery after photobleaching (FRAP) and fluorescence loss in photobleaching (FLIP). Focal regions within a specimen with fluorescently tagged molecules may be photobleached and imaged over time to determine molecular diffusion constants, protein synthesis and turnover rates, and subcellular connectivity.

Complementary techniques include fluorescence resonance energy transfer (FRET) and fluorescence correlation spectroscopy (FCS), which are used to observe interactions at the molecular scale. In FRET, if two fluorophores are within a very short distance of each other (usually <5 nm), some fraction of the excitation energy needed to excite the shorter wavelength fluorophore is transferred to excite the longer wavelength fluorophore through dipole-dipole coupling [137]. FRET donor-acceptor pairs are particularly sensitive to intermolecular distances, with FRET efficiency scaling on the order of R^6 (where R is the distance between fluors). A typical application of this technology is in the assessment of protein-protein interactions, either intramolecular (i.e., protein folding) or intermolecular. Individual proteins may be labeled with synthetic probes, or generated as fusion proteins, and assessed at the donor excitation wavelength. In theory, the proteins interact closely if the acceptor emission wavelength is observed and do not interact closely if the donor emission wavelength is observed. In practice, however, mixed populations of both wavelengths may be present, depending on the kinetics and stability of the system in question, and researchers must use population averaging and photobleaching controls to clearly delineate these effects. A FRET-based biosensor, Chameleon, uses the Ca^{2+} binding sites of calmodulin to link two fluorophores—yellow fluorescent protein (YFP) and cyan fluorescent protein (CFP)—so when Ca^{2+} binds to the construct, the binding domain folds to cause FRET. FRET has been used in live drosophila salivary gland to investigate caspase-mediated cell death during development [138]. FCS has been proposed as a less expensive and laborious method of detecting biomarkers in solution [139]. Another technique widely used to observe plasma membrane dynamics within 200 nm of the surface can be accomplished by total internal reflection fluorescence (TIRF) to observe cell adhesion [140] and receptor binding at the surface of the cell.

Small Animal Imaging

The great challenge of imaging physiological processes within small animals is overcoming the many biomolecular obstacles that absorb, distort, or scatter signals from the tissues, cells, or molecules of interest. This single challenge is additionally compounded for *living* animals under long-term observation. Noninvasive, nondestructive imaging can restrict the extent and quality of available information from a single animal, despite the investigator's goal of obtaining the greatest amount of data possible. High contrast therefore remains the ultimate goal for any imaging method. Luciferase-based (luminescent) reporter constructs continue to be popular for this reason, because, despite a comparably lower signal than many fluorescent probes, luminescent reporters are observed over a substantially lower background, yielding a greater signal-to-noise

ratio (S/N). The advent of high-resolution, low-noise, cooled CCD detectors has yielded significant improvements in signal detection and resolution. As an example, longitudinal evaluation of cell-seeded 3D scaffolds and hydrogel implants in the rodent salivary bed can be conducted using small animal imaging systems. Commercial examples include the multimodal IVIS® (Thermo Perkin-Elmer, formerly Caliper) and In-Vivo (Bruker, formerly Carestream/Kodak) imagers, which combine sensitive detectors for fluorescence, luminescence, and often X-ray imaging.

Selection of fluorescent and luminescent reporter probes (as described further in the next section) is critical and must provide appropriate image S/N ratio. In another example, optical-resolution photoacoustic microscopy (OR-PAM) has been employed in vascular imaging to provide structural information about vessel density and vascular permeability and integrity [141]. Available fluorescent vascular contrast agents fluoresce in the near-infrared and last for several minutes to hours. These contrast agents are injected in the tail vein and can be imaged beginning at 10–24 h after injection and depends on the experimental protocol. Alternatively, near-infrared (IR)-emitting quantum dots (QDs) can be noncovalently or covalently bound to various types of drug carriers to enable transport and tracking in living tissue [142]. Contrast agents or QDs may be introduced into the blood stream by traditional tail vein injection or directly into the salivary glands via major ducts in the oral cavity. It is therefore possible to image vascular changes and integration within implanted hydrogels in live animals at serial time intervals and in longitudinal studies without disturbing the salivary bed containing the implant. Real-time tissue distribution of luciferase transgene expression during targeted gene therapy in mice (imaged by IVIS) demonstrated that the treatment indeed remained localized to the parotid glands.

An overarching goal in the field of salivary tissue regeneration is to integrate the *in vitro* 3D model into the *in vivo* model to encourage salivation and restore tissue function, with clear applications in salivary diagnostics. Inspection of vascularization, innervation, structural integrity of the implant, as well as functional assessment of cellular structures may be performed in live animals by using animal imaging systems that quantitate luminescence and fluorescence in real time. A combination of imaging modalities and saliva collection would be used to determine the quality of integration and function of the *in vitro* implant within the salivary bed of small to larger animal models *in vivo*.

Advances in Fluorophores

The strong absorption of blue-green wavelengths by biological tissues (as described previously in the sections on *Multiphoton Microscopy* and *Small Animal Imaging*) has inspired investigators to engineer fluorescent proteins with excitation in the far-red. The ubiquity of 633 nm lasers, available in most confocal microscopes and flow cytometers, has facilitated this goal, along with an interest in replacing the fragile tandem probe pairs commonly used in flow cytometry. Key characteristics of a far-red fluorescent protein are a high quantum yield, extinction coefficient, photostability, low maturation time and cytotoxicity, and, of course, the longest possible excitation wavelengths. An additional preferred characteristic is that such proteins would be monomeric, as previous multimeric proteins have shown a propensity for intracellular precipitation with increased cytotoxicity and monomeric proteins are favored for their potential as fusion protein partners. However, bright and stable dimeric or multimeric proteins have clear utility in whole cell labeling and tracking applications, both *in vitro* and particularly *in vivo*, as recent animal imaging systems have been progressively updated with near-IR sources and detectors.

In the past decade, development of such probes has accelerated, as multiple laboratories have concurrently published several new far-red fluorescent proteins for all of the aforementioned applications. Most are derived from, or inspired by, the DsRed series of fluorescent proteins. Two of the earliest of the recent contributions, Katushka and its monomeric variant mKate

[143], have served as reference points for the rush of subsequent reports, including e2Crimson [144], mNeptune [145], eqFP650/eqFP670 [146], and Fusion Red [147]. Some of these are available commercially for cell labeling and as plasmids for fusion proteins. Vendors of small animal imagers have extended the far-red detection capabilities and sensitivities of their units and often offer far-red reagents (antibodies, small molecules, viral transfectants) that present the highest S/N compatibility with their systems. As researchers seek a broader range of *in vivo* probes for assessing salivary diagnostic applications, these far-red technologies represent lead options for improving signal quality.

In Vivo and *In Vitro* Platforms for Validation of Biomarkers

The predictive power of salivary diagnostics is dependent on the sensitivity and specificity of biomarkers in detecting a disorder or disease. Biomarkers in saliva associated with local, systemic, and infectious and neoplastic diseases may be detected in small volumetric amounts of saliva noninvasively collected from a patient. Early detection is critical when it comes to most disorders and diseases, particularly cancers that are difficult to detect with current imaging modalities. The noninvasive manner of this screening technique may appeal to more patients and identify at- or high-risk populations at earlier and treatable stages, decreasing the mortality rate of the disease or disorder. Promising methods that accurately screen for biomarkers for these diseases or disorders provide new tools for medical diagnosis of diseases and disorders.

Advancement in optical imaging has enabled researchers to visualize in real time the activation of molecular mechanisms, gene expression, anatomical and structural changes, effects of mechanical perturbation, and molecular transport on various length and timescales. Visualization of specific proteins and anatomical structures over time has aided in the identification of disease and the understanding of disease progression.

Currently it is unclear how particular biomarkers are transported to the oral cavity. Biomarkers may be fluorescently tagged and tracked to identify the mobilization of these targeted biomarkers and patterns as they travel through the localized regions or across biological systems. Tracking of currently identified salivary biomarkers will elucidate how biomarkers enter the oral cavity as well as serve as a platform for validation of the biomarkers associated with a particular disease or disorder. How the biomarker population differs in plasma versus saliva and the predictive power of the biomarker for a particular disease or disorder currently manifested may also be addressed. Selection of the imaging modality will depend on the task at hand and the information desired. Validation protocols using state-of-the-art imaging and fluorophore technologies *in vitro* and *in vivo* will greatly contribute to enhancing the predictive power of salivary biomarkers in the clinic.

Alternate Analyte Detection

Technological advances in the design of fluorescent probes allow for visual targeting of mRNA, RNA, genes, and proteins [148] *in vitro* and *in vivo*. Genetically encoded fluorescently tagged proteins enable the visualization and tracking of proteins of interest during development, organization, and disease progression. Fluorescent probes can also detect calcium responses [8, 149], intracellular pH, membrane potential, and electrical coupling [150]. Fluorescent probe technology is readily used in salivary diagnostics for the detection of particular biomarkers present in saliva.

In the past decade, numerous salivary biomarkers have been identified and quantified with respect to manifestations of local and systemic disorders as well as infectious diseases. Fluorescent probes are used to quantify mRNA, RNA, DNA, proteins, and various other molecules in a number of biological assays to investigate the predictive power of salivary biomarkers for cancer, periodontal disease, human immunodeficiency virus (HIV), hepatitis C, and a variety of other diseases and disorders. The enzyme-linked immunosorbent assay (ELISA), which is based on the binding of an analyte to a detection reagent that alters the transmitted light when measured by a spectrophotometer, is used to detect C-reactive protein associated with inflammatory diseases, such as periodontal and cardiovascular disease [151]. ELISAs are also routinely used to detect HIV-1 and HIV-2 analytes [152]. Other methods used based on fluorescence detection to quantify salivary biomarkers include mass spectrometry [153], human oral microbe identification microarrays (HOMIM) [154], and quantitative PCR (qPCR). The newly developed enzyme immunoassay (EIA) identifies hepatitis C virus antibodies in saliva with comparable results to serum immunoassays [155]. Technologies are increasingly improving in sensitivity and selectivity, and a handful of biomarkers are confidently used to detect certain diseases or disorders. Many researchers now look to *in vivo* or *in vitro* models as potential platforms to test and validate the sensitivity and specificity of these biomarkers [156–158].

Conclusion

The advances described throughout this chapter and their enabling technologies are almost universally found at the interface between multiple disciplines. The biomaterials employed in 3D tissue engineering scaffolds are born from the hybrid expertise of polymer chemists and clinical surgeons. In a similar way, advances in imaging technologies rely on contributions from protein engineers in the molecular design of fluorescent probes and from physical scientists in the improved detection limits of CCD cameras.

At a higher level, however, the creation of an *ex vivo* diagnostics platform is itself an intermediate, interdisciplinary effort. Researchers attempt to reduce the cost and labor involved in *in vivo* experimentation while expanding the complexity and accuracy of single-cell *in vitro* studies. The ongoing effort toward laboratory-scale 3D microtissues will change and improve our understanding of salivary gland structure/function relationships and yield more accurate assessments in applications of drug testing, health monitoring, and personalized medicine.

References

1. Lee YH, Wong DT. Saliva: an emerging biofluid for early detection of diseases. Am J Dent. 2009; 22(4):241–8 [Research Support, N.I.H., Extramural Research Support, Non-U.S. Gov't Review].
2. Greabu M, Battino M, Mohora M, Totan A, Didilescu A, Spinu T, et al. Saliva: a diagnostic window to the body, both in health and in disease. J Med Life. 2009;2(2): 124–32 [Review].
3. Blencowe T, Pehrsson A, Lillsunde P, Vimpari K, Houwing S, Smink B, et al. An analytical evaluation of eight on-site oral fluid drug screening devices using laboratory confirmation results from oral fluid. Forensic Sci Int. 2011;208(1–3):173–9 [Comparative Study Evaluation Studies Research Support, Non-U.S. Gov't].
4. Atkinson JC, Baum BJ. Salivary enhancement: current status and future therapies. J Dent Educ. 2001;65(10):1096–101.
5. Pradhan S, Liu C, Zhang C, Jia X, Farach-Carson MC, Witt RL. Lumen formation in three-dimensional cultures of salivary acinar cells. Otolaryngol Head Neck Surg. 2010;142(2):191–5.
6. Pradhan S, Zhang C, Jia X, Carson DD, Witt R, Farach-Carson MC. Perlecan domain iv peptide stimulates salivary gland cell assembly in vitro. Tissue Eng Part A. 2009;15(11):3309–20 [Research Support, N.I.H., Extramural].
7. Pradhan-Bhatt S, Harrington DA, Duncan RL, Farach-Carson MC, Jia X, Witt RL. A novel in vivo model for evaluating functional restoration of a tissue-engineered salivary gland. Laryngoscope. 2014; 124(2):456–61.
8. Pradhan-Bhatt S, Harrington DA, Duncan RL, Jia X, Witt RL, Farach-Carson MC. Implantable three-dimensional salivary spheroid assemblies demonstrate fluid and protein secretory responses to neurotransmitters. Tissue Eng Part A. 2013;19(13–14):1610–20 [Research Support, N.I.H., Extramural].
9. Feng J, van der Zwaag M, Stokman MA, van Os R, Coppes RP. Isolation and characterization of human salivary gland cells for stem cell transplantation to reduce radiation-induced hyposalivation. Radiother Oncol. 2009;92(3):466–71 [Comparative Study].
10. Tucker AS. Salivary gland development. Semin Cell Dev Biol. 2007;18(2):237–44 [Research Support, Non-U.S. Gov't Review].
11. Patel VN, Hoffman MP. Salivary gland development: a template for regeneration. Semin Cell Dev Biol. 2014;25–26:52–60.
12. Knosp WM, Knox SM, Hoffman MP. Salivary gland organogenesis. Wiley Interdiscip Rev Dev Biol. 2012; 1(1):69–82.
13. Ferreira JN, Hoffman MP. Interactions between developing nerves and salivary glands. Organogenesis. 2013;9(3):199–205 [Research Support, N.I.H., Intramural].
14. Witt RL. Salivary gland diseases: surgical and medical management. New York: Thieme; 2005.
15. Knox SM, Lombaert IMA, Reed X, Vitale-Cross L, Gutkind JS, Hoffman MP. Parasympathetic innervation maintains epithelial progenitor cells during salivary organogenesis. Science. 2010;329(5999): 1645–7.
16. Iden S, Collard JG. Crosstalk between small gtpases and polarity proteins in cell polarization. Nat Rev Mol Cell Biol. 2008;9(11):846–59.
17. LeBleu VS, MacDonald B, Kalluri R. Structure and function of basement membranes. Exp Biol Med. 2007;232(9):1121–9.
18. Kadoya Y, Yamashina S. Salivary gland morphogenesis and basement membranes. Anato Sci Int. 2005; 80(2):71–9.
19. O'Brien LE, Jou T-S, Pollack AL, Zhang Q, Hansen SH, Yurchenco P, et al. Rac1 orientates epithelial apical polarity through effects on basolateral laminin assembly. Nat Cell Biol. 2001;3(9):831–8.
20. Farach-Carson MC, Warren CR, Harrington DA, Carson DD. Border patrol: insights into the unique role of perlecan/heparan sulfate proteoglycan 2 at cell and tissue borders. Matrix Biol. 2014;34:64–79.
21. Hopf M, Göhring W, Kohfeldt E, Yamada Y, Timpl R. Recombinant domain iv of perlecan binds to nidogens, laminin–nidogen complex, fibronectin, fibulin-2 and heparin. Eur J Biochem. 1999;259(3):917–26.
22. Baker OJ. Tight junctions in salivary epithelium. J Biomed Biotechnol. 2010;2010:13.
23. Shin K, Fogg VC, Margolis B. Tight junctions and cell polarity. Annu Rev Cell Dev Biol. 2006;22(1): 207–35.
24. Melvin JE, Yule D, Shuttleworth T, Begenisich T. Regulation of fluid and electrolyte secretion in salivary gland acinar cells. Annu Rev Physiol. 2005; 67(1):445–69.
25. Yamada S, Nelson WJ. Localized zones of rho and rac activities drive initiation and expansion of epithelial cell–cell adhesion. J Cell Biol. 2007;178(3): 517–27.
26. Goldstein B, Macara IG. The par proteins: fundamental players in animal cell polarization. Dev Cell. 2007;13(5):609–22.
27. Yu W, Datta A, Leroy P, O'Brien LE, Mak G, Jou T-S, et al. B1-integrin orients epithelial polarity via rac1 and laminin. Mol Biol Cell. 2005;16(2):433–45.
28. Bornens M. Organelle positioning and cell polarity. Nat Rev Mol Cell Biol. 2008;9(11):874–86.
29. Masuda-Hirata M, Suzuki A, Amano Y, Yamashita K, Ide M, Yamanaka T, et al. Intracellular polarity protein par-1 regulates extracellular laminin assembly by

regulating the dystroglycan complex. Genes Cells. 2009;14(7):835–50.

30. Yamashita K, Suzuki A, Satoh Y, Ide M, Amano Y, Masuda-Hirata M, et al. The 8th and 9th tandem spectrin-like repeats of utrophin cooperatively form a functional unit to interact with polarity-regulating kinase par-1b. Biochem Biophys Res Commun. 2010;391(1):812–7.

31. Daley WP, Gervais EM, Centanni SW, Gulfo KM, Nelson DA, Larsen M. Rock1-directed basement membrane positioning coordinates epithelial tissue polarity. Development. 2012;139(2):411–22.

32. Wells CD, Fawcett JP, Traweger A, Yamanaka Y, Goudreault M, Elder K, et al. A rich1/amot complex regulates the cdc42 gtpase and apical-polarity proteins in epithelial cells. Cell. 2006;125(3):535–48.

33. Katsumata O, Sato Y-I, Sakai Y, Yamashina S. Intercalated duct cells in the rat parotid gland may behave as tissue stem cells. Anato Sci Int. 2009;84(3):148–54.

34. Kimoto M, Yura Y, Kishino M, Toyosawa S, Ogawa Y. Label-retaining cells in the rat submandibular gland. J Histochem Cytochem. 2008;56(1):15–24.

35. Cotroneo E, Proctor GB, Carpenter GH. Regeneration of acinar cells following ligation of rat submandibular gland retraces the embryonic-perinatal pathway of cytodifferentiation. Differentiation. 2010;79(2):120–30.

36. Lombaert IM, Hoffman MP. Epithelial stem/progenitor cells in the embryonic mouse submandibular gland. Front Oral Biol. 2010;14:90–106 [Review].

37. Patel VN, Rebustini IT, Hoffman MP. Salivary gland branching morphogenesis. Differentiation. 2006; 74(7):349–64.

38. Borghese E. The development in vitro of the submandibular and sublingual glands of *mus musculus*. J Anat. 1950;84(3):287–302, 283.

39. Borghese E. Explanation experiments on the influence of the connective tissue capsule on the development of the epithelial part of the submandibular gland of *mus musculus*. J Anat. 1950;84(3):303–18, 303.

40. Menko AS, Zhang L, Schiano F, Kreidberg JA, Kukuruzinska MA. Regulation of cadherin junctions during mouse submandibular gland development. Dev Dyn. 2002;224(3):321–33.

41. Proctor GB, Carpenter GH. Regulation of salivary gland function by autonomic nerves. Auton Neurosci. 2007;133(1):3–18.

42. Turner RJ, Sugiya H. Understanding salivary fluid and protein secretion. Oral Dis. 2002;8(1):3–11 [Research Support, Non-U.S. Gov't Review].

43. Rossi J, Luukko K, Poteryaev D, Laurikainen A, Sun YF, Laakso T, et al. Retarded growth and deficits in the enteric and parasympathetic nervous system in mice lacking gfrα2, a functional neurturin receptor. Neuron. 1999;22(2):243–52.

44. Heuckeroth RO, Enomoto H, Grider JR, Golden JP, Hanke JA, Jackman A, et al. Gene targeting reveals a critical role for neurturin in the development and maintenance of enteric, sensory, and parasympathetic neurons. Neuron. 1999;22(2):253–63.

45. Glebova NO, Ginty DD. Heterogeneous requirement of ngf for sympathetic target innervation in vivo. J Neurosci. 2004;24(3):743–51.

46. Garrett JR, Kidd A. The innervation of salivary glands as revealed by morphological methods. Microsc Res Tech. 1993;26(1):75–91.

47. Danielsson A, Hellstrom S, Henriksson R, Sundstrom S. Non-specific secretory supersensitivity in rat parotid gland following neonatal sympathetic denervation. Neurosci Lett. 1988;90(3):328–32.

48. Henriksson R, Carlsöö B, Danielsson A, Sundström S, Jönsson G. Developmental influences of the sympathetic nervous system on rat parotid gland. J Neurol Sci. 1985;71(2–3):183–91.

49. Proctor GB, Asking B. A comparison between changes in rat parotid protein composition 1 and 12 weeks following surgical sympathectomy. Exp Physiol. 1989;74(6):835–40.

50. Ekström J, Khosravani N, Castagnola M, Messana I. Saliva and the control of its secretion. In: Ekberg O, editor. Dysphagia. Berlin: Springer; 2012. p. 19–47.

51. Larrivée B, Freitas C, Suchting S, Brunet I, Eichmann A. Guidance of vascular development: lessons from the nervous system. Circ Res. 2009;104(4):428–41.

52. Gray H. Gray's anatomy: The unabridged running press edition of the american classic. In: Pick TP, Howden R, editors. Running Press, Philadelphia; 1974.

53. Modin A, Weitzberg E, Lundberg JM. Nitric oxide regulates peptide release from parasympathetic nerves and vascular reactivity to vasoactive intestinal polypeptide in vivo. Eur J Pharmacol. 1994;261(1–2):185–97.

54. Wang Y, Sudilovsky D, Cao M, Chen WG, Goetz L, Xue H, et al. Establishing efficient xenograft models of models of low-grade human prostate cancer. Eur Urol Suppl. 2003;2(6):30.

55. Parmar H, Melov S, Samper E, Ljung B-M, Cunha GR, Benz CC. Hyperplasia, reduced e-cadherin expression, and developmental arrest in mammary glands oxidatively stressed by loss of mitochondrial superoxide dismutase. Breast. 2005;14(4):256–63.

56. Wang Y, Xue H, Cutz J-C, Bayani J, Mawji NR, Chen WG, et al. An orthotopic metastatic prostate cancer model in scid mice via grafting of transplantable human prostate tumor line. Lab Invest. 2005;85(11):1392–404.

57. Cunha GR. Mesenchymal-epithelial interactions: past, present, and future. Differentiation. 2008;76(6):578–86 [Research Support, N.I.H., Extramural Review].

58. Grobstein C. Morphogenetic interaction between embryonic mouse tissues separated by a membrane filter. Nature. 1953;172(4384):869–70.

59. Grobstein C. Inductive epitheliomesenchymal interaction in cultured organ rudiments of the mouse. Science. 1953;118(3054):52–5.

60. Kratochwil K. Organ specificity in mesenchymal induction demonstrated in the embryonic development of the mammary gland of the mouse. Dev Biol. 1969;20(1):46–71.

61. Ekblom P, Lehtonen E, Saxen L, Timpl R. Shift in collagen type as an early response to induction of the metanephric mesenchyme. J Cell Biol. 1981;89(2):276–83.

62. Hoffman MP, Kidder BL, Steinberg ZL, Lakhani S, Ho S, Kleinman HK, et al. Gene expression profiles of mouse submandibular gland development: Fgfr1 regulates branching morphogenesis in vitro through bmp- and fgf-dependent mechanisms. Development. 2002; 129(24):5767–78 [Research Support, U.S. Gov't, Non-P.H.S. Research Support, U.S. Gov't, P.H.S.].

63. Larsen M, Hoffman MP, Sakai T, Neibaur JC, Mitchell JM, Yamada KM. Role of pi 3-kinase and pip3 in submandibular gland branching morphogenesis. Dev Biol. 2003;255(1):178–91 [Research Support, U.S. Gov't, P.H.S.].

64. Sakai T, Larsen M, Yamada KM. Fibronectin requirement in branching morphogenesis. Nature. 2003;423(6942):876–81 [Research Support, Non-U.S. Gov't Research Support, U.S. Gov't, P.H.S.].

65. Knox SM, Lombaert IMA, Haddox CL, Abrams SR, Cotrim A, Wilson AJ, et al. Parasympathetic stimulation improves epithelial organ regeneration. Nat Commun. 2013;4:1494. doi:10.1038/ncomms2493.

66. Maria OM, Maria O, Liu Y, Komarova SV, Tran SD. Matrigel improves functional properties of human submandibular salivary gland cell line. Int J Biochem Cell Biol. 2011;43(4):622–31 [Research Support, Non-U.S. Gov't].

67. Ogawa Y. Immunocytochemistry of myoepithelial cells in the salivary glands. Prog Histochem Cytochem. 2003;38(4):343–426 [Review].

68. Nelson CM, Bissell MJ. Modeling dynamic reciprocity: engineering three-dimensional culture models of breast architecture, function, and neoplastic transformation. Semin Cancer Biol. 2005;15:342–52.

69. Lee GY, Kenny PA, Lee EH, Bissell MJ. Three-dimensional culture models of normal and malignant breast epithelial cells. Nat Methods. 2007;4:359–65.

70. Barcellos-Hoff MH, Aggeler J, Ram TG, Bissell MJ. Functional differentiation and alveolar morphogenesis of primary mammary cultures on reconstituted basement membrane. Development. 1989;105: 223–35.

71. Sakakura T, Nishizuka Y, Dawe CJ. Mesenchyme-dependent morphogenesis and epithelium-specific cytodifferentiation in mouse mammary gland. Science. 1976;194(4272):1439–41.

72. Lakhani S, Bissell M. Introduction: the role of myoepithelial cells in integration of form and function in the mammary gland. J Mammary Gland Biol Neoplasia. 2005;10(3):197–8 [Editorial].

73. Gudjonsson T, Ronnov-Jessen L, Villadsen R, Rank F, Bissell MJ, Petersen OW. Normal and tumor-derived myoepithelial cells differ in their ability to interact with luminal breast epithelial cells for polarity and basement membrane deposition. J Cell Sci. 2002;115(Pt 1):39–50 [Comparative Study Research Support, Non-U.S. Gov't Research Support, U.S. Gov't, Non-P.H.S. Research Support, U.S. Gov't, P.H.S.].

74. Gudjonsson T, Adriance MC, Sternlicht MD, Petersen OW, Bissell MJ. Myoepithelial cells: their origin and function in breast morphogenesis and neoplasia. J Mammary Gland Biol Neoplasia. 2005;10(3):261–72 [Research Support, N.I.H., Extramural Research Support, U.S. Gov't, Non-P.H.S. Review].

75. Adriance MC, Inman JL, Petersen OW, Bissell MJ. Myoepithelial cells: good fences make good neighbors. Breast Cancer Res. 2005;7(5):190–7 [Research Support, N.I.H., Extramural Research Support, U.S. Gov't, Non-P.H.S. Research Support, U.S. Gov't, P.H.S.].

76. Vidi P-A, Bissell MJ, Lelièvre SA. Three-dimensional culture of human breast epithelial cells: the how and the why. Methods Mol Biol (Clifton, NJ). 2013;945:193–219.

77. Ampuja M, Jokimäki R, Juuti-Uusitalo K, Rodriguez-Martinez A, Alarmo E-L, Kallioniemi A. Bmp4 inhibits the proliferation of breast cancer cells and induces an mmp-dependent migratory phenotype in mda-mb-231 cells in 3d environment. BMC Cancer. 2013;13:429.

78. Miroshnikova YA, Jorgens DM, Spirio L, Auer M, Sarang-Sieminski AL, Weaver VM. Engineering strategies to recapitulate epithelial morphogenesis within synthetic three-dimensional extracellular matrix with tunable mechanical properties. Phys Biol. 2011;8(2):026013.

79. Nelson J, Manzella K, Baker OJ. Current cell models for bioengineering a salivary gland: a mini-review of emerging technologies. Oral Dis. 2013;19(3):236–44 [Research Support, N.I.H., Extramural].

80. Quissell DO, Barzen KA, Gruenert DC, Redman RS, Camden JM, Turner JT. Development and characterization of sv40 immortalized rat submandibular acinar cell lines. In Vitro Cell Dev Biol Anim. 1997;33(3):164–73 [Research Support, U.S. Gov't, Non-P.H.S. Research Support, U.S. Gov't, P.H.S.].

81. Liu XB, Sun X, Mork AC, Dodds MW, Martinez JR, Zhang GH. Characterization of the calcium signaling system in the submandibular cell line smg-c6. Proc Soc Exp Biol Med Soc Exp Biol Med. 2000;225(3):211–20 [Research Support, U.S. Gov't, P.H.S.].

82. Liu X, Mork AC, Sun X, Castro R, Martinez JR, Zhang GH. Regulation of ca(2+) signals in a parotid cell line par-c5. Arch Oral Biol. 2001;46(12):1141–9 [Research Support, U.S. Gov't, P.H.S.].

83. Quissell DO, Turner JT, Redman RS. Development and characterization of immortalized rat parotid and submandibular acinar cell lines. Eur J Morphol. 1998;36(Suppl):50–4.

84. Turner JT, Redman RS, Camden JM, Landon LA, Quissell DO. A rat parotid gland cell line, par-c10, exhibits neurotransmitter-regulated transepithelial anion secretion. Am J Physiol. 1998;275(2 Pt

1):C367–74 [Research Support, U.S. Gov't, Non--P.H.S. Research Support, U.S. Gov't, P.H.S.].

85. Quissell DO, Barzen KA, Redman RS, Camden JM, Turner JT. Development and characterization of sv40 immortalized rat parotid acinar cell lines. In Vitro Cell Dev Biol Anim. 1998;34(1):58–67 [Research Support, U.S. Gov't, Non-P.H.S. Research Support, U.S. Gov't, P.H.S.].

86. Baker OJ, Schulz DJ, Camden JM, Liao Z, Peterson TS, Seye CI, et al. Rat parotid gland cell differentiation in three-dimensional culture. Tissue Eng Part C Methods. 2010;16(5):1135–44 [Research Support, N.I.H., Extramural Research Support, Non-U.S. Gov't].

87. Szlávik V, Szabo B, Vicsek T, et al. Differentiation of primary submandibular gland cells cultured on basement membrane extract. Tissue Eng. 2008;14:1915–26.

88. Joraku A, Sullivan CA, Yoo J, Atala A. In-vitro reconstitution of three-dimensional human salivary gland tissue structures. Differentiation. 2007;75(4):318–24.

89. Lombaert IM, Knox SM, Hoffman MP. Salivary gland progenitor cell biology provides a rationale for therapeutic salivary gland regeneration. Oral Dis. 2011;17(5):445–9 [Review].

90. Lombaert IMA, Brunsting JF, Wierenga PK, Faber H, Stokman MA, Kok T, et al. Rescue of salivary gland function after stem cell transplantation in irradiated glands. PLoS ONE. 2008;3(4):e2063.

91. Nanduri LS, Maimets M, Pringle SA, van der Zwaag M, van Os RP, Coppes RP. Regeneration of irradiated salivary glands with stem cell marker expressing cells. Radiotherand Oncol. 2011;99(3):367–72 [Research Support, Non-U.S. Gov't].

92. Kishi T, Takao T, Fujita K, Taniguchi H. Clonal proliferation of multipotent stem/progenitor cells in the neonatal and adult salivary glands. Biochem Biophys Res Commun. 2006;340(2):544–52 [Comparative Study Research Support, Non-U.S. Gov't].

93. Melchiorri AJ, Nguyen BN, Fisher JP. Mesenchymal stem cells: roles and relationships in vascularization. Tissue Eng Part B Rev. 2014;20:218–28.

94. Koyama S, Sato E, Tsukadaira A, Haniuda M, Numanami H, Kurai M, et al. Vascular endothelial growth factor mrna and protein expression in airway epithelial cell lines in vitro. Eur Respir J. 2002; 20(6):1449–56.

95. Wernike E, Montjovent MO, Liu Y, Wismeijer D, Hunziker EB, Siebenrock KA, et al. Vegf incorporated into calcium phosphate ceramics promotes vascularisation and bone formation in vivo. Eur Cell Mater. 2010;19:30–40 [Research Support, Non-U.S. Gov't].

96. De la Riva B, Nowak C, Sanchez E, Hernandez A, Schulz-Siegmund M, Pec MK, et al. Vegf-controlled release within a bone defect from alginate/chitosan/pla-h scaffolds. Eur J Pharm Biopharm. 2009;73(1): 50–8 [Comparative Study Research Support, Non-U.S. Gov't].

97. Bhang SH, Cho SW, La WG, Lee TJ, Yang HS, Sun AY, et al. Angiogenesis in ischemic tissue produced by spheroid grafting of human adipose-derived stromal cells. Biomaterials. 2011;32(11):2734–47 [Research Support, Non-U.S. Gov't].

98. Lee MG, Ohana E, Park HW, Yang D, Muallem S. Molecular mechanism of pancreatic and salivary gland fluid and hco3 secretion. Physiol Rev. 2012;92(1):39–74 [Research Support, N.I.H., Extramural Research Support, N.I.H., Intramural Research Support, Non-U.S. Gov't Review].

99. He H, Yao Y, Wang Y, Wu Y, Yang Y, Gong P. A novel bionic design of dental implant for promoting its long-term success using nerve growth factor (ngf): utilizing nano-springs to construct a stress-cushioning structure inside the implant. Med Sci Monit. 2012;18(8):HY42–6.

100. Ai J-Y, Smith B, Wong DT. Bioinformatics advances in saliva diagnostics. In J Oral Sci. 2012;4(2):85–7.

101. Dawson LJ, Christmas SE, Smith PM. An investigation of interactions between the immune system and stimulus–secretion coupling in mouse submandibular acinar cells. A possible mechanism to account for reduced salivary flow rates associated with the onset of sjögren's syndrome. Rheumatology. 2000;39(11): 1226–33.

102. Mason GI, Hamburger J, Bowman S, Matthews JB. Salivary gland expression of transforming growth factor β isoforms in Sjogren's syndrome and benign lymphoepithelial lesions. Mol Pathol. 2003;56(1): 52–9.

103. Nagler RM, Baum BJ. Prophylactic treatment reduces the severity of xerostomia following radiation therapy for oral cavity cancer. Arch Otolaryngol–Head Neck Surg. 2003;129(2):247–50.

104. Sullivan CA, Haddad RI, Tishler RB, Mahadevan A, Krane JF. Chemoradiation-induced cell loss in human submandibular glands. Laryngoscope. 2005; 115(6):958–64.

105. Atala A, Kasper FK, Mikos AG. Engineering complex tissues. Sci Transl Med. 2012;4(160):160rv112 [Review].

106. Berthiaume F, Maguire TJ, Yarmush ML. Tissue engineering and regenerative medicine: history, progress, and challenges. Annu Rev Chem Biomol Eng. 2011;2:403–30 [Historical Article].

107. Griffith LG, Naughton G. Tissue engineering—current challenges and expanding opportunities. Science (New York, NY). 2002;295(5557):1009–14 [Review].

108. Langer R, Vacanti JP. Tissue engineering. Science (New York, NY). 1993;260(5110):920–6 [Review].

109. Vacanti CA. The history of tissue engineering. J Cell Mol Med. 2006;10(3):569–76 [Historical Article].

110. Soscia DA, Sequeira SJ, Schramm RA, Jayarathanam K, Cantara SI, Larsen M, et al. Salivary gland cell differentiation and organization on micropatterned plga nanofiber craters. Biomaterials. 2013;34(28):6773–84 [Research Support, N.I.H., Extramural Research Support, U.S. Gov't, Non-P.H.S.].

111. Engler AJ, Sen S, Sweeney HL, Discher DE. Matrix elasticity directs stem cell lineage specification. Cell. 2006;126(4):677–89.

112. Cukierman E, Pankov R, Stevens DR, Yamada KM. Taking cell-matrix adhesions to the third dimension. Science. 2001;294(5547):1708–12.

113. Paszek MJ, Zahir N, Johnson KR, Lakins JN, Rozenberg GI, Gefen A, et al. Tensional homeostasis and the malignant phenotype. Cancer Cell. 2005;8(3):241–54 [Research Support, N.I.H., Extramural Research Support, U.S. Gov't, Non-P.H.S. Research Support, U.S. Gov't, P.H.S.].

114. Hoffman BD, Grashoff C, Schwartz MA. Dynamic molecular processes mediate cellular mechanotransduction. Nature. 2011;475(7356):316–23 [Research Support, N.I.H., Extramural Research Support, Non-U.S. Gov't Review].

115. Plotnikov SV, Pasapera AM, Sabass B, Waterman CM. Force fluctuations within focal adhesions mediate ecm-rigidity sensing to guide directed cell migration. Cell. 2012;151(7):1513–27 [Research Support, N.I.H., Intramural].

116. Swift J, Ivanovska IL, Buxboim A, Harada T, Dingal PCDP, Pinter J, et al. Nuclear lamin-a scales with tissue stiffness and enhances matrix-directed differentiation. Science (New York, NY). 2013;341(6149):1240104.

117. Engler AJ, Carag-Krieger C, Johnson CP, Raab M, Tang H-Y, Speicher DW, et al. Embryonic cardiomyocytes beat best on a matrix with heart-like elasticity: scar-like rigidity inhibits beating. J Cell Sci. 2008;121(Pt 22):3794–802.

118. Pajerowski JD, Dahl KN, Zhong FL, Sammak PJ, Discher DE. Physical plasticity of the nucleus in stem cell differentiation. Proc Natl Acad Sci U S A. 2007;104(40):15619–24.

119. Pierschbacher MD, Ruoslahti E. Cell attachment activity of fibronectin can be duplicated by small synthetic fragments of the molecule. Nature. 1984;309(5963):30–3 [Research Support, U.S. Gov't, P.H.S.].

120. Ruoslahti E. Rgd and other recognition sequences for integrins. Annu Rev Cell Dev Biol. 1996;12:697–715 [Research Support, U.S. Gov't, P.H.S. Review].

121. Aimes RT, Quigley JP. Matrix metalloproteinase-2 is an interstitial collagenase. Inhibitor-free enzyme catalyzes the cleavage of collagen fibrils and soluble native type i collagen generating the specific 3/4- and 1/4-length fragments. J Biol Chem. 1995;270(11):5872–6 [Comparative Study].

122. Lutolf MP, Lauer-Fields JL, Schmoekel HG, Metters AT, Weber FE, Fields GB, et al. Synthetic matrix metalloproteinase-sensitive hydrogels for the conduction of tissue regeneration: engineering cell-invasion characteristics. Proc Natl Acad Sci U S A. 2003;100(9):5413–8.

123. Lin C-C, Anseth KS. Cell-cell communication mimicry with poly(ethylene glycol) hydrogels for enhancing beta-cell function. Proc Natl Acad Sci U S A. 2011;108(16):6380–5.

124. Dhimolea E, Soto AM, Sonnenschein C. Breast epithelial tissue morphology is affected in 3d cultures by species-specific collagen-based extracellular matrix. J Biomed Mater Res A. 2012;100(11):2905–12.

125. Boekhoven J, Stupp SI. 25th anniversary article: supramolecular materials for regenerative medicine. Adv Mater (Deerfield Beach, Fla). 2014;26:1642–59.

126. Timpson P, McGhee EJ, Anderson KI. Imaging molecular dynamics in vivo—from cell biology to animal models. J Cell Sci. 2011;124(17):2877–90.

127. Wilhelm S, Grobler B, Gulch M, Heinz H. Confocal laser scanning microscopy principles. Zeiss Jena [serial on the Internet]. 1997. Available from: http://zeiss-campus.magnet.fsu.edu/referencelibrary/pdfs/ZeissConfocalPrinciples.pdf.

128. Sramkova M, Porat-Shliom N, Masedunkas A, Wigand T, Amornphimoltham P, Weigert R. Salivary glands: a powerful experimental system to study cell biology in live animals by intravital microscopy. Curr Front Perspect Cell Biol. 2012;503–18. doi: 10.577/33524.

129. García-Caballero L, Quintas V, Prada-López I, Seoane J, Donos N, Tomás I. Chlorhexidine substantivity on salivary flora and plaque-like biofilm: an in situ model. PLoS ONE. 2013;8(12):e83522.

130. Pan F, Gan W-B. Two-photon imaging of dendritic spine development in the mouse cortex. Dev Neurobiol. 2008;68(6):771–8.

131. Narunsky L, Oren R, Bochner F, Neeman M. Imaging aspects of the tumor stroma with therapeutic implications. Pharmacol Ther. 2014;141(2):192–208.

132. Masedunskas A, Sramkova M, Parente L, Sales KU, Amornphimoltham P, Bugge TH, et al. Role for the actomyosin complex in regulated exocytosis revealed by intravital microscopy. Proc Natl Acad Sci. 2011;108(33):13552–7.

133. Hille C, Lahn M, Lohmannsroben H-G, Dosche C. Two-photon fluorescence lifetime imaging of intracellular chloride in cockroach salivary glands. Photochem Photobiol Sci. 2009;8(3):319–27. doi:10.1039/B813797H.

134. Denk W. Two-photon scanning photochemical microscopy: mapping ligand-gated ion channel distributions. Proc Natl Acad Sci. 1994;91(14):6629–33.

135. Pettit DL, Wang SSH, Gee KR, Augustine GJ. Chemical two-photon uncaging: a novel approach to mapping glutamate receptors. Neuron. 1997;19(3):465–71.

136. Helmchen F, Denk W, Kerr JND. Miniaturization of two-photon microscopy for imaging in freely moving animals. Cold Spring Harb Protoc. 2013;2013(10):904–13.

137. VanEngelenburg SB, Palmer AE. Fluorescent biosensors of protein function. Curr Opin Chem Biol. 2008;12(1):60–5.

138. Takemoto K, Kuranaga E, Tonoki A, Nagai T, Miyawaki A, Miura M. Local initiation of caspase activation in drosophila salivary gland programmed cell death in vivo. Proc Natl Acad Sci. 2007;104(33):13367–72.

139. Shahzad A, Knapp M, Lang I, Köhler G. The use of fluorescence correlation spectroscopy (fcs) as an alternative biomarker detection technique: a preliminary study. J Cell Mol Med. 2011;15(12):2706–11.

140. Axelrod D. Cell-substrate contacts illuminated by total internal reflection fluorescence. J Cell Biol. 1981;89(1):141–5.

141. Yang Z, Chen J, Yao J, Lin R, Meng J, Liu C, et al. Multi-parametric quantitative microvascular imaging with optical-resolution photoacoustic microscopy in vivo. Opt Express. 2014;22(2):1500–11.

142. Zintchenko A, Susha AS, Concia M, Feldmann J, Wagner E, Rogach AL, et al. Drug nanocarriers labeled with near-infrared-emitting quantum dots (quantoplexes): imaging fast dynamics of distribution in living animals. Mol Ther. 2009;17(11):1849–56.

143. Shcherbo D, Merzlyak EM, Chepurnykh TV, Fradkov AF, Ermakova GV, Solovieva EA, et al. Bright far-red fluorescent protein for whole-body imaging. Nat Methods. 2007;4(9):741–6 [Research Support, N.I.H., Extramural Research Support, Non-U.S. Gov't].

144. Strack RL, Hein B, Bhattacharyya D, Hell SW, Keenan RJ, Glick BS. A rapidly maturing far-red derivative of dsred-express2 for whole-cell labeling. Biochemistry. 2009;48(35):8279–81 [Research Support, N.I.H., Extramural Research Support, Non-U.S. Gov't].

145. Lin MZ, McKeown MR, Ng HL, Aguilera TA, Shaner NC, Campbell RE, et al. Autofluorescent proteins with excitation in the optical window for intravital imaging in mammals. Chem Biol. 2009;16(11):1169–79 [Research Support, N.I.H., Extramural Research Support, Non-U.S. Gov't].

146. Shcherbo D, Shemiakina II, Ryabova AV, Luker KE, Schmidt BT, Souslova EA, et al. Near-infrared fluorescent proteins. Nat Methods. 2010;7(10):827–9 [Research Support, N.I.H., Extramural Research Support, Non-U.S. Gov't].

147. Shemiakina II, Ermakova GV, Cranfill PJ, Baird MA, Evans RA, Souslova EA, et al. A monomeric red fluorescent protein with low cytotoxicity. Nat Commun. 2012;3:1204. doi:10.1038/ncomms2208.

148. Chalfie M, Tu G, Euskirchen G, Ward WW, Prasher DC. Green fluorescent protein as a marker for gene expression. Science. 1994;263(5148):802+ [Article].

149. Ryu S-Y, Peixoto PM, Won JH, Yule DI, Kinnally KW. Extracellular atp and p2y2 receptors mediate intercellular ca2+ waves induced by mechanical stimulation in submandibular gland cells: role of mitochondrial regulation of store operated ca2+ entry. Cell Calcium. 2010;47(1):65–76.

150. Wu D, Schaffler MB, Weinbaum S, Spray DC. Matrix-dependent adhesion mediates network responses to physiological stimulation of the osteocyte cell process. Proc Natl Acad Sci. 2013;110(29): 12096–101.

151. Christodoulides N, Mohanty S, Miller CS, Langub MC, Floriano PN, Dharshan P, et al. Application of microchip assay system for the measurement of c-reactive protein in human saliva. Lab Chip. 2005;5(3):261–9. doi:10.1039/B414194F.

152. Holmström P, Syrjänen S, Laine P, Valle SL, Suni J. Hiv antibodies in whole saliva detected by elisa and western blot assays. J Med Virol. 1990;30(4):245–8.

153. Xie H, Onsongo G, Popko J, de Jong EP, Cao J, Carlis JV, et al. Proteomics analysis of cells in whole saliva from oral cancer patients via value-added three-dimensional peptide fractionation and tandem mass spectrometry. Mol Cell Proteomics. 2008;7(3): 486–98.

154. Huyghe A, Francois P, Charbonnier Y, Tangomo-Bento M, Bonetti E-J, Paster BJ, et al. Novel microarray design strategy to study complex bacterial communities. Appl Environ Microbiol. 2008;74(6): 1876–85.

155. Cruz HM, Marques VA, Villela-Nogueira CA, do Ó KMR, Lewis-Ximenez LL, Lampe E, et al. An evaluation of different saliva collection methods for detection of antibodies against hepatitis C virus (anti-HCV). J Oral Pathol Med. 2012;41(10):793–800.

156. Elashoff D, Zhou H, Reiss J, Wang J, Xiao H, Henson B, et al. Prevalidation of salivary biomarkers for oral cancer detection. Cancer Epidemiol Biomarkers Prev. 2012;21(4):664–72.

157. Haeckel R, Hanecke P. Application of saliva for drug monitoring. An in vivo model for transmembrane transport. Eur J Clin Chem Clin Biochem. 1996;34(3):171–91.

158. Lau C, Kim Y, Chia D, Spielmann N, Eibl G, Elashoff D, et al. Role of pancreatic cancer-derived exosomes in salivary biomarker development. J Biol Chem. 2013;288(37):26888–97.

Using Saliva Secretions to Model Disease Progression

Charles F. Streckfus, Lenora Bigler,
Courtney Edwards, Cynthia Guajardo-Streckfus,
and Steven A. Bigler

Abstract

To date, because of the complexity and heterogeneity of cancer, no individual model recapitulates all aspects of this disease. The authors of this chapter developed a molecular model that utilizes one of the most easily obtained body fluids for tumor marker analysis. The in vivo model can fill in the current gaps in our understanding of cancer pathogenesis, signaling pathways, the efficacy of varying chemotherapeutics, identifying novel therapies, and, most importantly, shed new light on metastatic progression that is the principal cause of mortality. We propose that, secondary to cancer, the malignancy's rapid growth alters the proteomic content of the tissue microenvironment. These changes may manifest in up- or downregulation of salivary protein concentrations, which can be used as a sentinel for cancer modeling.

Introduction

Over the decades, biological modeling has been used to study disease progression in numerous types of carcinomas. To date, no one model can completely predict cancer progression. Consequently, there are a plethora of different types of models for numerous carcinomas. Additionally, cancer modeling lacks an in vivo system that reflects disease changes in a "real-time" approach.

Saliva is a complex and dynamic biological fluid, which over the years has been recognized for the numerous functions it performs in the oral cavity. However, modern technology has unveiled

C.F. Streckfus, DDS, MA, FAAOM, FAGD (✉)
Department of Diagnostic and Biomedical Sciences,
University of Texas School of Dentistry at Houston,
Houston, TX, USA

Department of Diagnostic and Biomedical Sciences,
Baylor College of Medicine, UT School of Nursing,
Houston, TX, USA
e-mail: charles.streckfus@uth.tmc.edu

L. Bigler, PhD
Department of Diagnostic and Biomedical Sciences,
University of Texas School of Dentistry at Houston,
Houston, TX, USA

C. Edwards, MD
Department of Surgery, Lehigh Valley Health
Network, Allentown, PA, USA

C. Guajardo-Streckfus, BS
Department of Pediatric Anesthesiology,
Baylor College of Medicine, Texas Children's
Hospital, Houston, TX, USA

S.A. Bigler, MD
Department of Pathology, Mississippi Baptist
Medical Center, Jackson, MS, USA

C.F. Streckfus (ed.), *Advances in Salivary Diagnostics,*
DOI 10.1007/978-3-662-45399-5_9, © Springer-Verlag Berlin Heidelberg 2015

a plethora of compounds never before detected in saliva such as drugs, pollutants, hormones, and, additionally, biomarkers of bacterial or viral infections and other systemic diseases. Interest in salivary biomarkers has led to improved methods of how saliva is collected, stored, and assayed, increasing its potential utility as a diagnostic medium in cancer research. This chapter will focus on the use of salivary protein alterations to study breast cancer progression. The authors of this chapter have studied the use of saliva in breast cancer progression for nearly two decades and our findings will be used to illustrate the hypothesis.

Current Models for Studying Breast Cancer Progression

Biological models, such as those for breast cancer, simulate the simultaneous operations and interactions of multiple processes and molecular networks, in an attempt to recreate and predict the appearance of complex phenomena such as breast cancer progression. A model that can reflect the presence and progression of malignancy among women would enhance our knowledge of breast cancer and serve as an enabling system for biomarker discovery and credentialing of candidate markers so that the biological causality of any analyte(s) can be assessed. With respect to the study of breast cancer, there are currently three major methods for creating models for studying breast cancer progression. The three modeling methods utilize either breast cancer tumor cell lines (BCTCL), xenografts of cell lines, and the third method uses animals—specifically genetically engineered mice [1]. All three models have generated useful insights into cancer progression; however, no individual model recapitulates all aspects of cancer progression.

For example, in the case of BCTCL research, the main question is: Are the cell lines representative of human breast cancer and how well do they capture breast cancer tumorigenesis in the context of the unique tumor–stroma microenvironment? This question is debatable, with strong evidence supporting both sides of the discussion. The fact is that no single cell line is representative of the

disease process. To date, there are 51 BCTCL used to detect genetic abnormalities associated with breast cancer. Moreover, the ability of ex vivo cell line experiments to recapitulate the tumor microenvironment is in question. Interactions between tumor cells, stromal cells, and extracellular matrix, involvement of the immune system, neovascularization, and the complex milieu of blood and tissue fluid all influence tumor cell biology and tumor progression in ways that cannot be completely recreated in ex vivo culture systems. Additionally, cell lines are prone to genotypic and phenotypic drift during their continual culture and there is always the problem of contamination [1–3]. One major concern is that multiple variants of the same cell line may exist and display distinct phenotypes, suggesting that subsequent to the establishment of the original cell line additional genetic changes have been acquired that might preclude comparison between different studies [1–3].

Xenograft models are also very useful in studying breast cancer and have certainly helped understand genetic pathways associated with breast cancers, but they are also problematic. Many of the problems that plague cell line studies also affect xenograft-driven modeling. One major problem is that xenografts must be established in immunocompromised mice [4–6]. The absence of an intact immune system may profoundly affect tumor development and progression as this microenvironment is entirely artificial. In fact, there is increasing evidence of roles for the immune system in both early stage breast cancer and metastasis [1, 4–6]. There are also differences in stromal cells and extracellular matrix between mouse and human breast tissues that must be taken into account. Xenograft models are different from breast cancer in patients in regard to the patterns of metastatic spread, preferentially colonizing the lungs in mice with decreased brain and liver metastasis. Nearly all xenograft models are hormone independent, whereas approximately half of human breast cancers are hormone dependent. There is a lack of histological concordance between tumors from genetically engineered mice and the common types of human breast cancers; most tumors from mice do not resemble the most common subtypes of breast cancer. Metastatic tumors in xenografts contain less fibrosis and inflammation than human tumors, due at least in part to the immunocompromised nature of the host.

Better model systems are needed for breast cancer tumorigenesis and prediction of response to treatment. This chapter provides evidence for use of salivary protein profiles as an adjunct model for studying breast cancer progression.

The Evidence for the Use of Salivary Protein Profiles as an Adjunct Model for Studying Breast Cancer Progression

Morphological Characteristics of Mammary and Salivary Gland Tissues

The mammary and salivary gland tissues are exocrine glands whose secretions pass into a system of ducts that lead ultimately to the exterior of the body. The inner surface of the glands and the ducts that drain them is topologically continuous with the exterior of the body and, when taken together, they produce a secretion that eventually exits into the *extracorporeal* milieu. The glands primarily consist of parenchyma and a supporting connective tissue framework or stroma [7].

The basic secretory units of the salivary glands are phenotypically similar to those of the mammary glands [7]. With the submandibular gland being the exception, they both have origins from the ectodermal germ layer. Both tissues are compound exocrine glands composed of specialized glandular epithelia. The tissues are characterized with two epithelial cell types, that is, ductal and acinar cells along with myoepithelial cells, which contract to move fluid from the acinar lumen to the ducts. The ductal epithelial cells (terminal ducts) adjacent to the acinar units are cuboidal [7, 8].

From an immunohistological perspective, there are a number of similarities between the mammary and salivary gland tissues. Both tissues have HER2/neu receptors on their ductal epithelial cells, which can be overexpressed in malignant transformation [9]. Additionally, epithelial cells of both tissues have estrogen, progesterone, and androgen receptors that can be overexpressed [10]. The p53 tumor suppressor gene is often mutated with overexpression of ineffective, mutated protein in carcinomas of the breast or the salivary glands. More interesting is that these proteins can be found in mammary ductal fluids and saliva [11, 12].

Besides the obvious fact that the mammary glands produce milk and the salivary glands produce saliva, there are numerous differences between the exocrine glands. For example, the mode of secretion for the mammary glands is primarily apocrine. Materials such as lipids accumulate at the apical portion of the cell and, when ample, the apex of the cell "pinches off" into the lumen. In contrast, the salivary glands are merocrine glands and secrete by exocytosis, depositing their products into the lumen as they are produced through specific secretory vesicles using well-developed transport mechanisms [8, 13]. It is also worth noting that of all the exocrine glands, only the salivary glands have striated ducts, which reabsorb sodium producing a solution that is hypotonic to serum. This mechanism does not occur in the intercalated ducts of the mammary glands; and, therefore, the resultant milk product is isotonic to serum. The epithelium of the mammary ducts principally functions as a conduit for the transport of milk to the nipple.

Another striking difference between the two tissues is that mammary glands do not function through the course of the individual's life span. The mammary tissues prominently develop during puberty due to the influence of increased levels of ovarian steroids. Generally speaking, estrogen promotes ductal development while progesterone facilitates lobular or acinar growth. During pregnancy, the placenta produces a lactogen factor that initiates further, rapid growth of the tissue. Postpartum, prolactin becomes the most important hormone maintaining breast function as it initiates and maintains milk production. Active lactation is achieved via a neuroendocrine reflex in which oxytocin is produced, resulting in the contraction of myoepithelial cells that force milk to the nipple. Once the infant is weaned and nursing activities cease, the lobules decrease in size and the tissues return to their prepregnancy state. After menopause, a portion of the mammary lobules and ducts is obliterated and replaced with connective tissue. No other exocrine gland demonstrates this degree of dependence on hormonal and aging factors. Considering that the mammary gland tissues are minimally functional during most of a woman's life may be an advantage in detecting carcinoma, as the initiation of a new biological process and metabolic activity within the tissues may become molecularly evident when compared to the tissues' quiescent state of lower molecular activity. Indeed, this is largely the rationale for breast cancer detection by magnetic resonance imaging (MRI).

Salivary Protein Alterations Secondary to Carcinoma of the Breast

Various analytical methods have been used to determine the salivary proteome. These include mass spectrometry, Western blot, and enzyme-linked immunosorbent assay (ELISA). Additionally, unstimulated whole saliva and stimulated whole saliva (SWS) have been biochemically analyzed for protein alterations secondary to carcinoma of the breast. Considering that there is a paucity of information on the topic of salivary breast cancer biomarkers and that the majority of the 15 manuscripts in the PubMed.gov database are from the author of this chapter, the ensuing discussion will focus on the findings from the biochemical analysis of SWS [14–19]. Table 9.1 represents a list of proteins found in the saliva from patients with ductal carcinoma of the breast cancer. The subjects contributing to the list were from various cancer stages and differing receptor status. In total, there are 87 proteins in Table 9.1, of which all but four have at least one reference indicating activity associated with carcinoma of the breast.

The overall salivary protein profile in Table 9.1 is a reflection of the proteomic analysis of breast cancer tissue and cell lines [20–48]. For example, 15 % of the proteins are associated with the cytoskeleton, 8 % with apoptotic inhibition, 7 % with molecular

chaperones, and 6 % with nucleosome activity (histones). The list also exhibits numerous proteins associated with immune–response/anti-inflammatory activity (14 %) and with cell growth and proliferation regulation (7 %). The remaining 43 % are related to calcium binding, detoxification/redox function, and extracellular activity. Despite the heterogeneity of carcinoma of the breast, the panel of core proteins appears to be consistent with those found in breast cancer tissues and individual human cell lines [20–49]. Additionally, the panel of salivary proteins is also consistent with healthy mammary gland tissue [50].

Possible Molecular Mechanisms of Action That Are in Relation to Salivary Modeling for Breast Cancer Development and Progression

What is the mechanism linking saliva protein expression with breast cancer? As previously suggested, one should examine the similarities that salivary tissue and fluid have to breast tissue and fluid. Pia-Foshini et al. describe how breast glands and salivary glands are both tubuloacinar exocrine glands sharing similar morphological features [51]; consequently, it is reasonable to expect similarities in pathological processes, particularly oncogenesis and tumor progression between these two types of glandular tissue [52]. Indeed, similarities can be identified despite the fact that primary carcinomas of the breast and salivary glands differ in incidence and clinical behavior.

Many of the proteins of interest expressed in saliva are large, and there are several hypothetical mechanisms, which may explain their presence in saliva. One might postulate that the proteins in saliva originate from the gingival crevicular fluid (GCF). This is a possibility as GCF is a serum exudate and is considered a portion of the total whole saliva; however, the authors have found elevated salivary proteins such as HER2/neu concentrations among edentulous patients where no GCF is present and in saliva collections sampled directly from the parotid and submandibular glands [53]. With this in mind, the concept that

Table 9.1 Constitutes salivary proteins that have been discovered to be differentially expressed secondary to carcinoma of the breast

Accession number	Gene ID	Protein name	References
P31947	1433S	14-3-3 protein sigma	[20, 21]
P63104	1433Z	14-3-3 protein zeta/delta	[22, 23]
P11021	GRP78	78 kDa glucose regulated	[21, 24]
P63261	ACTG	Actin, cytoplasmic 2	[25]
Q15848	ADIPO	Adiponectin	[26]
P02763	A1AG1	Alpha-1 acid glycoprotein 1 precursor	[27]
P06733	ENOA	Alpha-enolase	[21–23, 28]
P04083	ANXA1	Annexin A1	[22, 23]
P12429	ANXA3	Annexin A3	[23]
P46193	ANXA1	Annexin I	[23]
P07355	ANXA2	Annexin II	[21–23]
P02647	APOA1	Apolipoprotein A-I	[23, 27]
P02649	ApoE	Apolipoprotein -E	[25]
O14727	Apaf-1	Apoptotic protease activity factor-1	[29]
P61769	B2MG	Beta-2 microglobulin precursor	[22, 27]
Q8WZ76	Bcrp	Breast cancer resistance protein	[30, 31]
P12830	CDH1	Cadherin-1	[32]
P05109	S10A8	S100-A8	[33, 34]
P14211	CRP55	Calreticulin	[22, 23, 33]
P15941	CA 15-3	Cancer antigen 15-3, MUC-1	[27, 35]
P00915	CAH1	Carbonic anhydrase 1	[23, 36]
P07339	CATD	Cathepsin D	[23, 24, 27, 28]
P38936	p21	Cyclin-dependent kinase	[23]
P01034	CYTC	Cystatin C	[22, 27]
P20813	CYP2B6	Cytochrome p450	[29, 37]
P04264	K2C1	Cytokeratin 1	[23, 28, 33]
P13645	KRT10	Cytokeratin 10	[[24]]
P19012	KRT15	Cytokeratin-15	[23]
Q04695	KRT17	Cytokeratin-17	[38]
P08727	KRT19	Cytokeratin-19	[27, 35]
P13647	K2C5	Cytokeratin-5	[38, 39]
Q96SD1	K2C6A	Cytokeratin-6A	[24]
P08729	KRT7	Cytokeratin-7	[24, 35]
P35527	K1C9	Cytokeratin-9	[22, 39]
Q02487	DSC2	Desmocollin-2 precursor	–
P20585	MSH3	DNA mismatch repair	[40]
P98170	XIAP	E3 ubiquitin-protein ligase	[41]
P01133	EGF	Epidermal growth factor	[27, 35]
P00533	EGFR	Epidermal growth factor receptor	[27, 35]
P04626	HER2/neu	Epidermal growth factor receptor	[27, 35]
Q01469	FABPE	Fatty acid-binding protein	[21, 22]
P02675	FIBB	Fibrinogen beta chain	[25]
Q15151	JUP	g-Catenin	–
P06396	GELS	Gelsolin	[24, 25, 36]
P09211	GSTP1	Glutathione S-transferase P	[[22, 23]]

(continued)

Table 9.1 (continued)

Accession number	Gene ID	Protein name	References
P29354	GRB2	Growth factor receptor-bound protein 2	[20, 23]
P00738	HPT	Haptoglobin precursor	[24, 27]
P11142	HSP10	Heat shock 10 protein	–
Q12988	HSP27	Heat shock 27 protein	[20–23, 28, 33]
P08107	HSP70	Heat shock 70 protein	[22, 28]
P25685	HSP40	Heat shock protein 40	–
P16403	H12	Histone H1.2	[42]
Q8IUE6	H2A2B	Histone H2A	[42]
P16104	H2AX	Histone H2A.x (H2a/x)	[39, 42]
Q71DI3	H32	Histone H3.2	[43]
P62805	H4	Histone H4	[43]
P22301	IL-10	Interleukin—10	[27]
P18510	IL1RA	IL-1ra	[27]
Q14764	LRP	Lung-resistance protein	[[31]]
P61626	LYSC	Lysozyme C precursor	[44]
Q9HC84	MUC5B	Mucin-5B precursor	[[32]]
Q8TAX7	MUC7	Mucin-7	[35]
O15438	MDRP	Multidrug resistance protein	[30, 31]
P29474	NOS Type 3	Nitric oxide synthase	[45]
P49024	Paxillin	Paxillin	[46]
P62937	PPIA	Peptidyl-prolyl cis-trans	[22, 23, 33]
Q06830	PRDX1	Peroxiredoxin-1	[21–24]
P01833	PIGR	Poly-IG receptor protein	[[21]]
P07737	PROF1	Profilin-1	[21–23]
P12273	PIP	Prolactin-inducible protein precursor	[27, 35, 47]
P04637	p53	Protein 53	[27]
P07237	PDIA1	Protein disulfide-isomerase	[22, 28, 36]
Q92730	Rho	Rho-related GTP	[33, 34]
P31949	S10AB	S100-A11	[21, 34]
P26447	S10A4	S100-A4	[22, 34]
P06703	S10A6	S100-A6	[34]
P31151	S100P	S100-A7	[21, 33, 34]
P29508	SPB3	Serpin B3	[44]
P42224	Stat1	Signal transducers and activators of transcription 1	[24]
P10599	THIO	Thioredoxin	[22, 33]
P02787	TRFE	Transferrin	[24, 27]
P01135	TGFα	Transforming growth factor alpha	[33]
P60174	TPIS	Triosephosphate isomerase	[23]
P62988	UBIQ	Ubiquitin	[21, 22]
P15692	VEGF	Vascular endothelial growth factor	[27]
P08670	VIME	Vimentin	[22, 23, 33]
P25311	ZA2G	Zinc-alpha-2-glycoprotein	[25, 47]

The proteins were analyzed by mass spectrometry, Western blot, and ELISA in stimulated whole saliva. They are listed by accession number, genomic identifier, protein name, and by references that have shown the proteins to be changed in other media such as serum, nipple aspirate fluid, cell culture lysates, or by breast tissue analysis

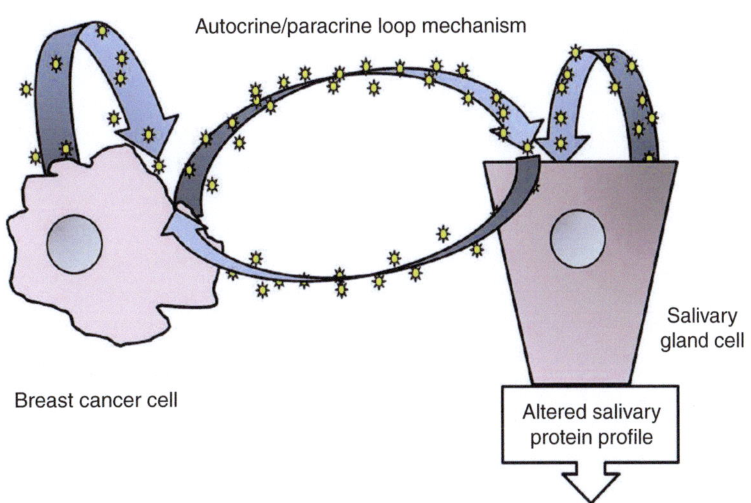

Fig. 9.1 Representation of an autocrine/paracrine "loop" mechanism, which may explain how membrane-bound proteins such as EGFR, HER2/*neu*, CA 15-3, and VEGF, for example, influence secretions from one exocrine gland to another

GCF is a major contributor of the protein alterations currently cannot be substantiated.

It is conceivable that the presence of biomarkers in saliva is due to "leakage" from the extracellular fluid into the secretory system of the salivary glands resulting from hydrostatic pressure, which widens the space between the tight junctions of the acinar epithelium allowing the molecules to enter the saliva. This may be possible, but a study in rats using a sustained HER2/neu delivery system implanted in the peritoneum exhibited classic "dose–response" curves when HER2/neu was assayed in saliva over time, suggesting that the concentration of Her2/neu was the key factor and not the leakiness or tightness of the junctions. This evidence taken with the predictable clinical presence of this protein in saliva suggests that the mechanism by which a biomarker enters the saliva is probably not by leakage [54].

An alternative hypothesis is active transport of the proteins into saliva by the salivary glandular epithelium. This could also account for the presence of membrane-bound proteins such as CA 15-3. Protein markers may be secreted into saliva as a consequence of localized regulatory function in the oral cavity via signal transduction [12]. In health, these intracellular and extracellular feedback loop mechanisms are in equilibrium, with each pathway promoting normal phenotypic processes of growth, proliferation, cell death, and differentiation. We postulate that, in the presence of carcinoma of the breast, there is an overabundance of various bioactive proteins associated with the rapid, abnormal growth of the neoplasm, which in turn produces a response in the salivary glands (Fig. 9.1). This response results in elevated salivary biomarkers. Similar phenomena have been reported in breast fluid [12], where elevated levels of HER2/neu were detected in nipple aspirates from breasts diagnosed with ductal carcinoma, and interestingly, concentrations of HER2/neu in nipple aspirates from the opposite healthy breast were also correspondingly elevated. This independent study suggests from a different perspective that there may be signaling between carcinoma of the breast and distant exocrine glandular tissues [12].

One more theory, related to the hypothesis, is that cellular communication may occur via extracellular vesicles (EVs). It is known that cells secrete numerous EVs into the extracellular space [55, 56]. These nanostructures range in size from 30 to 100 nm (exosome-like vesicles) to 0.2 μ(mu) m (larger microvesicles) and are antigenically diverse depending upon their function and cellular origin. The vesicles have numerous names, but in this discussion they will be collectively referred to as EVs. Figure 9.2 illustrates the appearance of these entities as observed by electron microscopy [58]. They are found in most body fluids, but more importantly in this context they are present in saliva, breast milk, and serum [56].

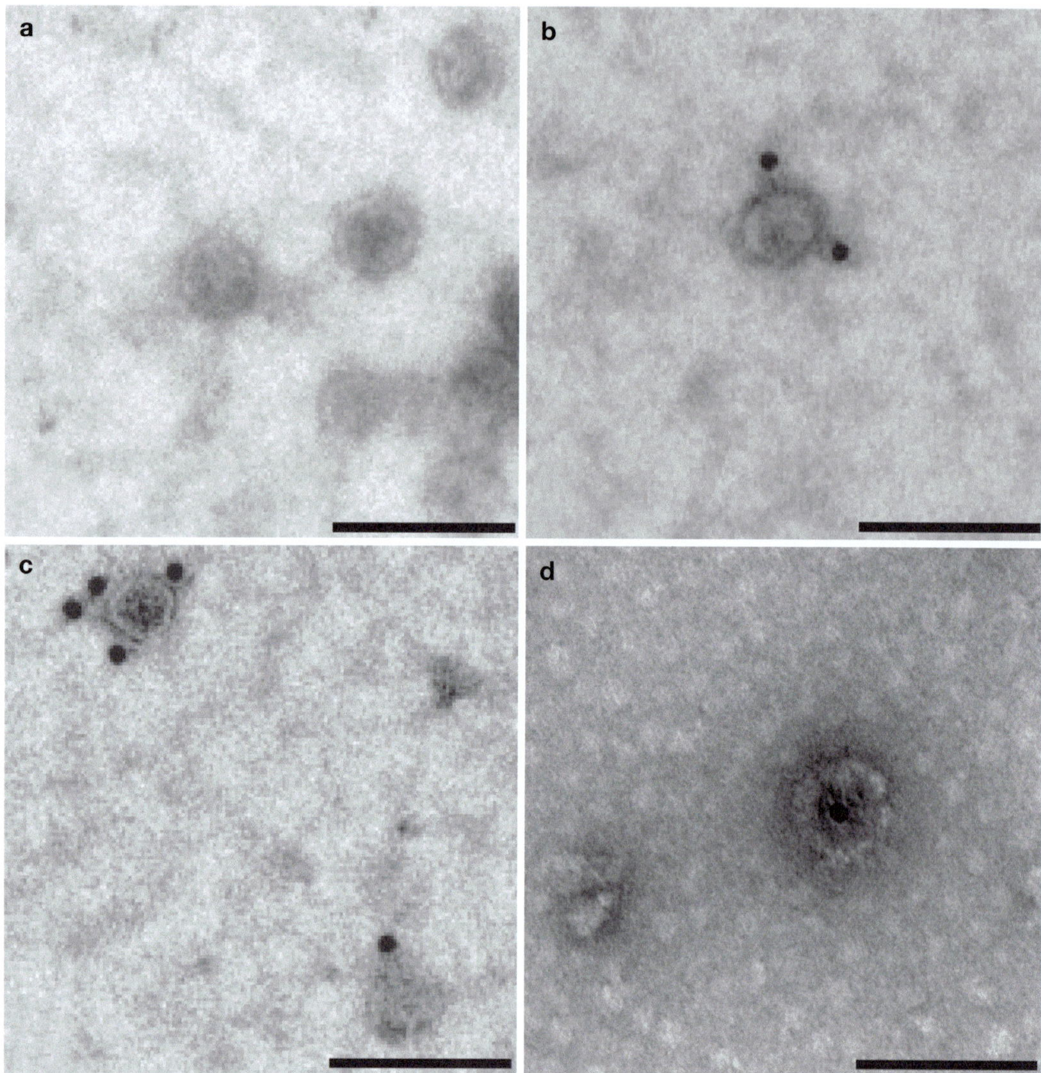

Fig. 9.2 Illustration of exosomes from saliva, plasma, and breast milk detected with electron microscopy. Exosomes from human saliva (**a**, **b**), plasma (**c**), and breast milk (**d**) were examined in the electron microscope. No isotype control antibody (**a**), but anti-CD63 antibody (**b**, **d**), was detected by 10 nm gold-labeled secondary antibody. The scale bars represent 100 nm (Reprinted from Lässer et al. [57]. http://www.translational-medicine.com/content/9/1/9. Used under the terms of the Creative Commons Attribution License)

EVs are packaged in the cell of origin, merge with the cell membrane, and are released into the extracellular space. They are then dispersed throughout the body by macrophages (Fig. 9.3). Consequently, they can play a role in intercellular signaling. Once released and disseminated throughout the body, they can merge with and release their contents into cells that are distant from their cell of origin. This, in turn, may influence processes in the recipient cell.

We suggest that EVs from breast cancer cells are shed and are transported to salivary gland parenchyma. There they bind to the glandular epithelial membrane and change the normal salivary protein profile in the presence of carcinoma of the breast [55–62].

In a study conducted by Palazzolo et al. in 2012, they performed an "in-depth" proteomic analysis of EVs from breast cancer cells. The results of the study revealed 179 proteins, 32 pro-

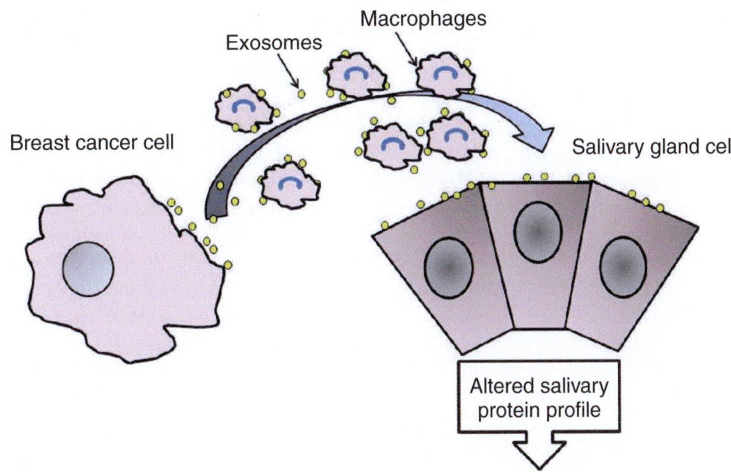

Fig. 9.3 Illustration of exosomes emanating from the breast, influencing salivary protein secretion. The nanoparticles are released into the extracellular environment and may be shuttled to their destination via microphages

tein isoforms corresponding to 22 genes [62]. Among those proteins listed in that manuscript [62]: annexin A1, apolipoprotein A-1, beta-2-microglobulin, carbonic anhydrase-1, calreticulin, alpha-enolase, fatty acid-binding protein, peptidyl-prolyl cis-trans isomerase, gelsolin, glutathione S-transferase, heat shock protein 70 kDa, cytokeratin-9, peroxiredoxin-2, profilin-1, S100-A6, S100-A11, thioredoxin, triosephosphate isomerase, and ubiquitin—all of which can be found in Table 9.1. These proteins also have been found in salivary EVs [61]. Currently, relatively little is known about the signals and mechanisms that initiate cellular secretion of EVs carrying these proteins. Until these and other questions are answered, we can only postulate as to how and why these large proteins are regulated and secreted into the oral cavity in patients with carcinoma of the breast [55–62].

Conclusion

Based on the evidence provided in this chapter, using breast cancer as our example, the investigators feel that salivary secretions may have great potential for studying systemic disease development and progression—especially for cancer. We have seen evidence of this phenomenon in other malignant neoplasms, including lymphoma and head and neck carcinoma [63, 64]. Considering the logistical advantages of saliva collection and its noninvasive acquisition, it would be extremely useful to continue to explore the possibility of using saliva as an in vivo medium to study oncogenesis and tumor progression. Further studies using new technologies are clearly warranted based on these promising preliminary developments.

Acknowledgments The research presented in this chapter was supported by the Avon Breast Cancer Foundation (#07-2007-071), Komen Foundation (KG080928), Gillson-Longenbaugh Foundation, and the Texas Ignition Fund. The authors would also like to thank Applied Biomics Inc. for the 2D-Gel analyses.

References

1. Eccles SA, Aboagye EO, Ali S, Anderson A, et al. Clinical research gaps and translational priorities for the successful prevention and treatment of breast cancer. Breast Cancer Res. 2013;R92. http://breast-cancer-research.com/content/15/5/R92.
2. Kulkarni YM, Suarez V, Klinke DJ. Inferring predominant pathways in cellular models of breast cancer using limited sample proteomic profiling. BMC Cancer. 2010;10:291–303.
3. Vargo-Gogola T, Rosen JM. Modelling breast cancer: one size does not fit all. Nat Rev Cancer. 2007;7:659–72.
4. Tordai A, Wang J, Andre F, Liedtke C, Yan K, Sotiriou C, Hortobagy G, Symmans WF, Pusztai L. Evaluation of biological pathways involved in chemotherapy response in breast cancer. Breast Cancer Res. 2008;10:R37.
5. Hennighausen L. Mouse models for breast cancer. Breast Cancer Res. 2000;2(1):2–7.
6. Francia G, Cruz-Manos W, Man S, Xu P, Kerbel RS. Mouse models of advanced spontaneous metastasis

for experimental therapeutics. Nat Rev Cancer. 2011;11:135–41.

7. Gartner LP & Hiatt JL. Female reproductive system. In: Gartner LP, Hiatt JL, editors. Color atlas and text of histology. 6th ed. Baltimore: Lippincott Williams and Wilkins; 2009. p. 430–31.

8. McManaman JL, Reyland ME, Thrower EC. Secretion and fluid transport mechanisms in the mammary gland: comparisons with the exocrine pancreas and the salivary gland. J Mammary Gland Biol Neoplasia. 2006;11:249–68.

9. DeRoche TC, Hoschar AP, Hunt JL. Immunohistochemical evaluation of androgen receptor, HER-2/*neu*, and p53 in benign pleomorphic adenomas. Arch Pathol Lab Med. 2008;132(12):1907–11.

10. Nasser SM, Faquin WC, Dayal Y. Expression of androgen, estrogen, and progesterone receptors in salivary gland tumors: frequent expression of androgen receptor in a subset of malignant salivary gland tumors. Am J Clin Pathol. 2003;119:801–6.

11. Streckfus CF, Bigler L, Tucci M, Thigpen JT. The presence of CA 15-3, c-*erb*B-2, EGFR, Cathepsin-D, and p53 in saliva among women with breast carcinoma. Can Invest. 2000;18(2):101–9.

12. Kuerer HM, Thompson PA, Krishnamurthy S, Fritsche HA, Marcy SM, Babiera GV, Singletary SE, Cristofanilli M, Sneige N, Hunt KK. High and differential expression of Her2/neu extracellular domain in bilateral ductal fluids from women with unilateral invasive breast cancer. Clin Cancer Res. 2003;9:601–6.

13. Turner R, Sugiya H. Understanding salivary fluid and protein secretion. Oral Dis. 2002;8:3–11.

14. Streckfus CF, Arreola D, Edwards C, Bigler L. A comparison of salivary protein profiles between her2/neu receptor positive and negative breast cancer patients: support for using salivary protein profiles for modeling breast cancer progression. J Oncol. 2012; Article ID 413256, 9 pages. doi:10.1155/2012/413256.

15. Streckfus CF, Bigler L, Storthz K, Dubinsky WP. A comparison of the oncoproteomic profiles in pooled saliva specimens from individuals diagnosed with stage IIa and stage IIb ductal carcinoma of the breast and healthy controls. J Oncol. 2009;1–12. Article ID 737619.

16. Streckfus CF, Mayorga-Wark O, Daniel Arreola D, Edwards C, Bigler L, Dubinsky WP. Breast cancer related proteins are present in saliva and are modulated secondary to ductal carcinoma *in situ* of the breast. Can Invest. 2008;26(2):159–67.

17. Streckfus CF, Bigler L. The use of soluble, salivary c-*erb*B-2 for the detection and post-operative follow-up of breast cancer in women: the results of a five year translational study. J Adv Dent Res. 2005;18:17–22.

18. Bigler LG, Streckfus CF. A unique protein screening analysis of stimulated whole saliva from normal and breast cancer patients. Preclinica. 2004;2(1):52–6.

19. Streckfus CF, Bigler L, Dellinger TD, Dai X, Kingman A, Thigpen JT. The presence of c-erbB-2, and CA 15-3 in saliva and serum among women with breast carcinoma: a preliminary study. Clin Cancer Res. 2000;6(6):2363–70.

20. Hudelist G, Singer CF, Pischinger KI, et al. Proteomic analysis in human breast cancer: identification of a characteristic protein expression profile of malignant breast epithelium. Proteomics. 2006;6:1989–2002.

21. Wulfkuhle JD, Sgroi DC, Krutzsch H, et al. Proteomics of human breast carcinoma *in situ*. Cancer Res. 2002;62:6740–9.

22. Minafra IP, Cancemi P, Fontana S, et al. Expanding the protein catalogue in the proteome reference map of human breast cancer cells. Proteomics. 2006;6:2609–25.

23. Lai TC, Chou HC, Chen YW, Lee TR, Chan HT, Shen HH, Lee WT, Lin ST, Lu YC, Wu CL, Chan HL. Secretomic and proteomic analysis of potential breast cancer markers by two-dimensional differential gel electrophoresis. J Proteome Res. 2010;9(3):1302–22.

24. Alldridge L, Metodieva G, Greenwood C, Al-Janabi K, Thwaites L, Sauven P, Metodiev M. Proteome profiling of breast tumors by gel electrophoresis and nanoscale electrospray ionization mass spectrometry. J Proteome Res. 2008;7(4):1458–69.

25. Varnum SM, Covington CC, Woodbury RL, et al. Proteomic characterization of nipple aspirate fluid: identification of potential biomarkers of breast cancer. Breast Cancer Res Treat. 2003;80(1):87–97.

26. Kaklamani VG, Wisinski KB, Sadim M, Gulden C, et al. Variants of the adiponectin (ADIPOQ) and adiponectin receptor 1 (ADIPOR1) genes and colorectal cancer risk. JAMA. 2008;300(13):1523–31.

27. Polanski M, Anderson NL. A list of candidate cancer biomarkers for targeted proteomics. Biomark Insights. 2006;2:1–48.

28. Chamberry A, Farina A, Di Maro A, et al. Proteomic analysis of MCF-7 cell lines expressing the zinc finger or proline-rich domain of retinoblastoma-in reacting-zinc-finger protein. J Proteome Res. 2006;5:1176–85.

29. Reed JC. Dysregulation of apoptosis in cancer. J Clin Oncol. 1999;17(9):2941–53.

30. Kawabata S, Oka M, Soda H, Shiozawa K, Nakatomi K, et al. Expression and functional analyses of breast cancer resistance protein in lung cancer. Clin Cancer Res. 2003;9(8):3052–7.

31. Li XQ, Li J, Shi SB, Chen P, Yu LC, Bao QL. Expression of MRP1, BCRP, LRP and ERCC1 as prognostic factors in non-small cell lung cancer patients receiving postoperative cisplatin-based chemotherapy. Int J Biol Markers. 2009;24(4):230–7.

32. Valque H, Gouyer V, Gottrand F, Desseyn JL. MUC5B leads to aggressive behavior of breast cancer MCF7 cells. PLoS One. 2012;7(10):e46699. doi:10.1371/journal.pone.0046699. Epub 2012 Oct 2.

33. Nagaraja GM, Othman M, Fox BP, Alsaber R, Pellegrino CM, Zeng Y, Khanna R, Tamburini P, Swaroop A, Kandpal RP. Gene expression signatures and biomarkers of noninvasive and invasive breast cancer cells: comprehensive profiles by representational difference analysis, microarrays and proteomics. Oncogene. 2006;25(16):2328–38.

34. Cancemi P, Di Cara G, Albanese NN, Costantini F, et al. Large-scale proteomic identification of S100 proteins in breast cancer tissues. BMC Cancer. 2010;10:476.

35. Lacroix M. Significance, detection and markers of disseminated breast cancer cells. Endocr Relat Cancer. 2006;13(4):1033–67.

36. Somiari RI, Sullivan A, Russell S, et al. High – throughput proteomic analysis of infiltrating ductal carcinoma of the breast. Proteomics. 2003;3:1863–73.

37. Murray GI, Taylor MC, McFadyen MCE, et al. Tumor-specific expression of cytochrome P450 CYP1B1. Cancer Res. 1997;57:3026–31.

38. Alshareeda AT, Soria D, Garibaldi JM, Rakha E, Nolan C, Ellis IO, Green AR. Characteristics of basal cytokeratin expression in breast cancer. Breast Cancer Res Treat. 2013;139(1):23–37.

39. Wu SL, Hancock WS, Goodrich GG, Kunitake ST. A approach to the proteomic analysis of a breast cancer cell line (SKBR3). Proteomics. 2003;3:1037–46.

40. Benachenhou N, Guiral S, Gorska-Flipot I, et al. Frequent loss of heterozygosity at the DNA mismatch-repair loci hMLH1 and hMSH3 in sporadic breast cancer. Br J Cancer. 1999;79:1012–7.

41. Zhi X, Zhao D, Wang Z, Zhou Z, Wang C, Chen W, Liu R, Chen C. E3 ubiquitin ligase RNF126 promotes cancer cell proliferation by targeting the tumor suppressor p21 for ubiquitin-mediated degradation. Cancer Res. 2013;73:385–94.

42. Hadnagy A, Beaulieu R, Balicki D. Histone tail modifications and noncanonical functions of histones: perspectives in cancer epigenetics. Mol Cancer Ther. 2008;7(4):740–8.

43. Chervona Y, Costa M. Histone modifications and cancer: biomarkers of prognosis? Am J Cancer Res. 2012;2(5):589–97.

44. Collie-Duguid ES, Sweeney K, Stewart KN, Miller ID, Smyth E, Heys SD. SerpinB3, a new prognostic tool in breast cancer patients treated with neoadjuvant chemotherapy. Breast Cancer Res Treat. 2012;132(3):807–18.

45. Thomsen LL, Miles DW, Happerfield L, Bobrow LG, Knowles RG, Moncada S. Nitric oxide synthase activity in human breast cancer. Br J Cancer. 1995;72(1):41–4.

46. Short SM, Yoder BJ, Tarr SM, Prescott NL, et al. The expression of the cytoskeletal focal adhesion protein paxillin in breast cancer correlates with HER2 overexpression and May help predict response to chemotherapy: a retrospective immunohistochemical study. Breast J. 2007;13(2):130–9.

47. Alexander H, Stegner AL, Wagner-Mann C, Du Bois GC, Alexander S, Sauter ER. Proteomic analysis to identify breast cancer biomarkers in nipple aspirate fluid. Clin Cancer Res. 2004;10(22):7500–10.

48. Kao J, Salari K, Bocanegra M, et al. Molecular profiling of breast cancer cell lines defines relevant tumor models and provides a resource for gene discovery. PLoS ONE. 2009;4(7):e6146.

49. Pitteri SJ, Kelly-Spratt KS, Gurley KE, et al. Tumor microenvironment–derived proteins dominate the plasma proteome response during breast cancer induction and progression. Cancer Res. 2011;71(15):5090–100.

50. Costa GG, Kaviski R, Souza LE, Urban CA, Lima RS, Cavalli IJ, Ribeiro EM. Proteomic analysis of non-tumoral breast tissue. Genet Mol Res. 2011;10(4):2430–42.

51. Pia-Foschini M, Reis-Filho JS, Eusebi V, et al. Salivary gland-like tumours of the breast: surgical and molecular pathology. J Clin Pathol. 2003;56:497–506.

52. Wick MR, Ockner DM, Mills SE, Ritter JH, Swanson PE. Homologous carcinomas of the breasts, skin, and salivary glands: a histologic and immunohistochemical comparison of ductal mammary carcinoma, ductal sweat gland carcinoma and salivary duct carcinoma. Am J Clin Pathol. 1988;109:75–84.

53. Streckfus C, Bigler L, Dellinger T, Kuhn M, Chouinard N, Dai X. The expression of the c-*erb*B-2 receptor protein in glandular salivary secretions. J Oral Pathol Med. 2004;33:595–600.

54. Brinkley J, Copeland L, Streckfus C, Tucci M, Benguzzi H. Sustained delivery of *HER-2/NEU* antibody by TCPL delivery device using adult male rats as a model. Biomed Sci Instrum. 2003;39:324–8.

55. Vlassov AV, Magdaleno S, Setterquist R, Conrad R. Exosomes: current knowledge of their composition, biological functions, and diagnostic and therapeutic potentials. Biochim Biophys Acta. 2012;1820(7):940–8.

56. Hendrix A, Hume AN. Exosome signaling in mammary gland development and cancer. Int J Dev Biol. 2011;55:879–87.

57. Lau CS, Wong DTW. Breast cancer exosome-like microvesicles and salivary gland cells interplay alters salivary gland cell-derived exosome-like microvesicles in vitro. PLoS One. 2012;7(3):e33037. doi:10.1371/journal.pone.0033037. Epub 2012 Mar 20.

58. Lässer C, Alikhani VS, Ekström K, et al. Human saliva, plasma and breast milk exosomes contain RNA: uptake by macrophages. J Translat Med. 2011;9:9. http://www.translational-medicine.com/content/9/1/9. Accessed 17 Jan 2014.

59. Luga V, Zhang L, Viloria-Petit AM, Ogunjimi AA, et al. Exosomes mediate stromal mobilization of autocrine Wnt-PCP signaling in breast cancer cell migration. Cell. 2012;151(7):1542–56.

60. Ma XJ, Dahiya S, Richardson E, Erlander M, Sgroi DC. Gene expression profiling of the tumor microenvironment during breast cancer progression. Breast Cancer Res. 2009;11(1):R7.
61. Ogawa Y, Miura Y, Harazono A, Kani-Azuma M, et al. Proteomic analysis of two types of exosomes in human whole saliva. Biol Pharm Bull. 2011;34(1):13–23.
62. Palazzolo G, Albanese NN, DI Cara G, Gygax D, Vittorelli ML, Pucci-Minafra I. Proteomic analysis of exosome-like vesicles derived from breast cancer cells. Anticancer Res. 2012;32(3):847–60.
63. Streckfus CF, Romaguera J, Streckfus CE. The use of salivary protein secretions as an in vivo model to study mantel cell lymphoma progression and treatment. Cancer Invest. 2013;31(7):494–9.
64. Ohshiro K, Rosenthal DI, Koomen JM, Streckfus CF, Chambers M, Kobayashi R, El-Naggar AK. Preanalytic saliva processing affect proteomic results and biomarker screening of head and neck squamous carcinoma. Int J Oncol. 2007;30:743–9.

Index

C.F. Streckfus (ed.), *Advances in Salivary Diagnostics,*
DOI 10.1007/978-3-662-45399-5, © Springer-Verlag Berlin Heidelberg 2015

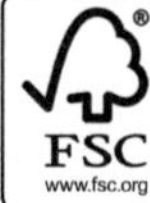